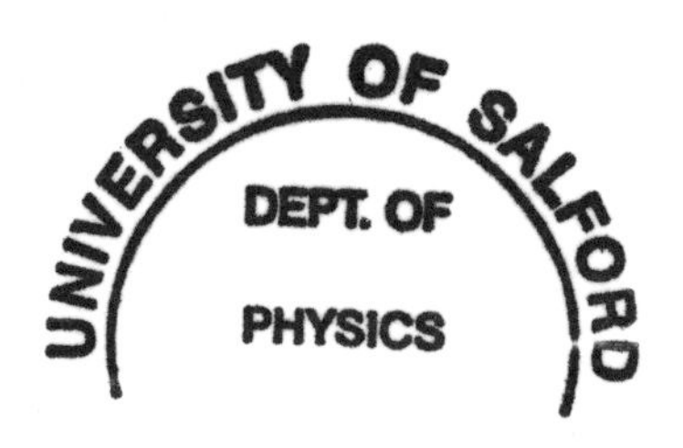

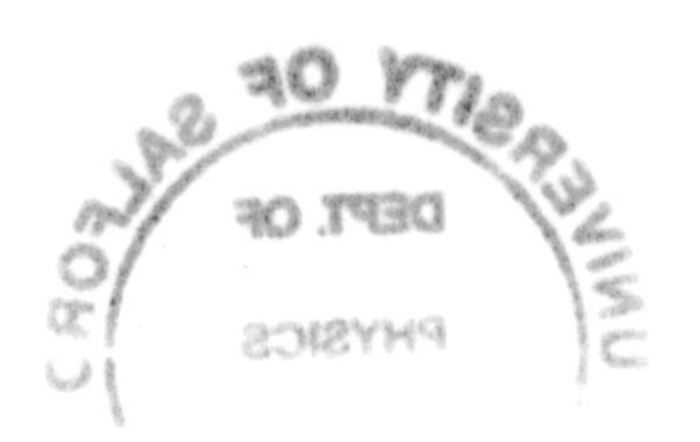

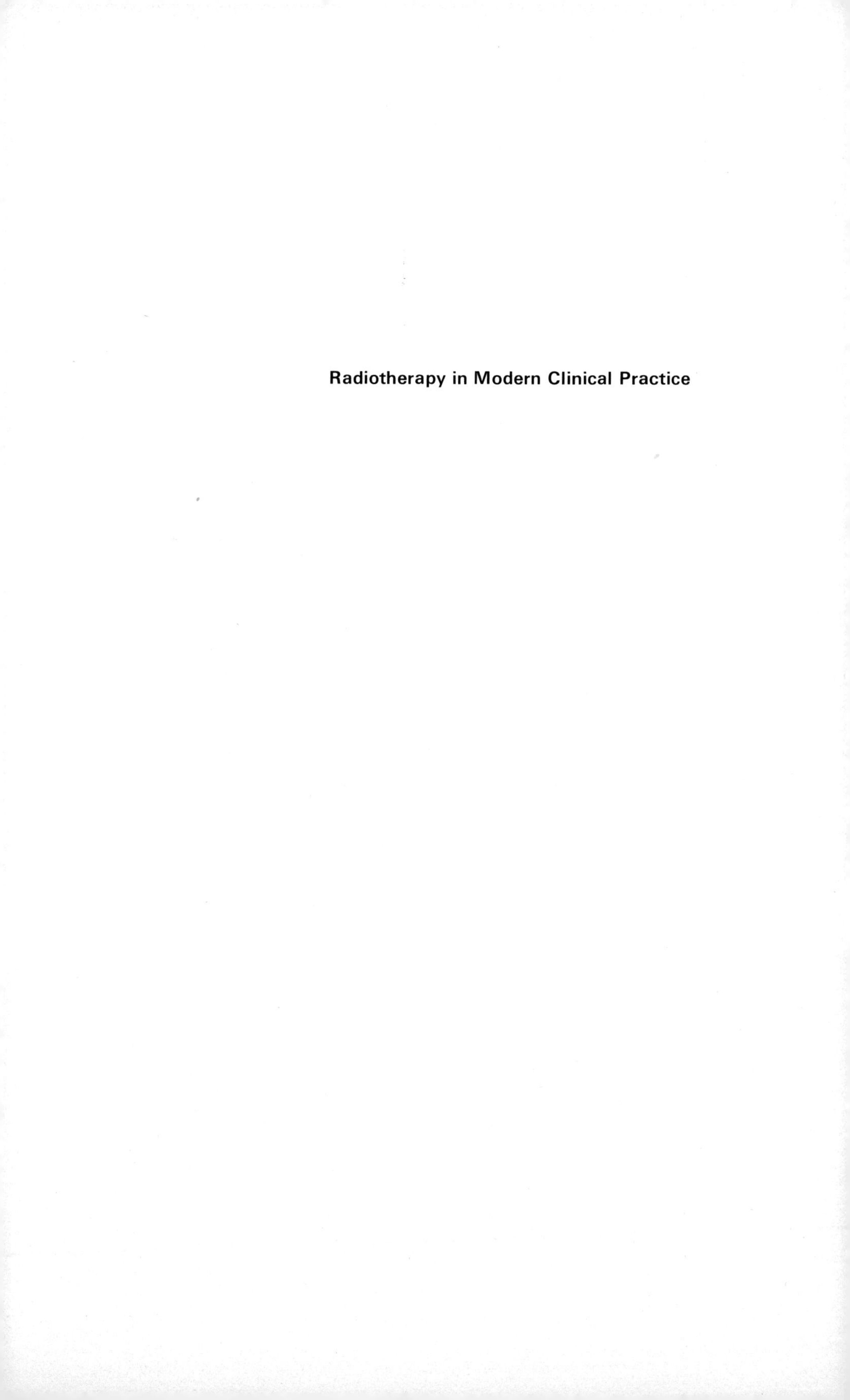

Radiotherapy in Modern Clinical Practice

Radiotherapy in Modern Clinical Practice

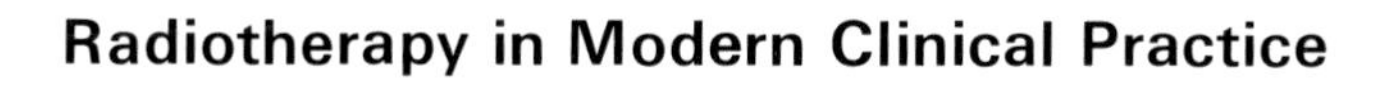

EDITED BY H. F. HOPE-STONE

Crosby Lockwood Staples London

Granada Publishing Limited
First published in Great Britain 1976 by Crosby Lockwood Staples
Frogmore St Albans Herts and 3 Upper James Street London W1R 4BP

ISBN 0 258 96978 4

Filmset in Photon Times 12 on 13 pt by
Richard Clay (The Chaucer Press) Ltd, Bungay, Suffolk
and printed in Great Britain by
Fletcher & Son Ltd, Norwich

Preface

The aim of this book is to highlight some of the advances that have been made in the past decade in the treatment of malignant disease by irradiation.

Oncology is a subject of growing importance in the practice of medicine today, and it will continue to be so in the future, as with an ageing population there is a 2–3 per cent annual increased incidence of malignant disease. Irradiation is only one of the many methods used in the management of neoplastic disease. This book stresses the importance of a multi-disciplinary approach so that all clinicians associated with different aspects of the disease will closely correlate their ideas and aims in order that the best forms of treatment can be formulated.

Clinical and radiobiological research is an active and continuous process with which radiotherapists are closely associated. Let it be realised, however, that the chances of any dramatic improvement in the management of malignant disease is unlikely to occur; nevertheless we must try, if not to cure our patients, at least to mitigate their sufferings both with technical skill and with compassion.

In editing this book I would like to thank and to acknowledge the help of all the contributors and in particular of Dr B. S. Mantell, who from the start has provided very helpful criticism and advice. Finally I would like to thank my secretary, Miss Sandra Gibby, without whose help this book would never have been written.

H.F.H-S.

September, 1975

List of Contributors

Mary Catterall, MB, BS, FRCR, DMRT
Consultant in Charge of the Fast Neutron Clinic,
Hammersmith Hospital, London

M. Cohen, BSc, PhD, ARCS, FInstP
Director of the Department of Medical Physics,
The London Hospital
Honorary Senior Lecturer in Medical Physics,
The London Hospital Medical College

J. M. Henk, MA, MB, BChir, FRCR, DMRT
Consultant Radiotherapist,
South Glamorgan Area Health Authority (Teaching)
Clinical Teacher,
Welsh National School of Medicine

H. F. Hope-Stone, MB, BS, LRCP, MRCS, FRCR, DMRT
Consultant Radiotherapist,
The London Hospital
Honorary Consultant Radiotherapist,
Whipps Cross Hospital, London and

Harold Wood Hospital, Romford, Essex
Teacher of Radiotherapy,
University of London

N. Howard, MA, DM(Oxon), FRCR, DMRT
Consultant in Radiotherapy and Oncology,
Charing Cross Hospital, London
Honorary Consultant Radiotherapist,
Wembley Hospital, Middlesex

G. W. H. Jardine, MB, ChB, FRCR, DMRT
Consultant Radiotherapist,
Newcastle and Cumbrian Area Health Authorities
Clinical Lecturer in Radiotherapy,
University of Newcastle-upon-Tyne

B. S. Mantell, MB, BS(London), MRCP, FRCR, DMRT
Consultant Radiotherapist,
The London Hospital and the London Chest Hospital

G. Newsholme, MD, FRCP, DMRT
Consultant Radiotherapist,
The General Hospital, Birmingham

D. O'Connell, KM, KSG, BA, MD, FFR(Ire)
Physician in Charge of the Departments of Radiotherapy and Oncology,
Charing Cross Hospital, London

C. R. H. Penn, MA, MB, BChir, FRCR, DMRT
Consultant Radiotherapist,
Royal Devon and Exeter Hospital, Exeter

George Wiernik, MD, BS(London), FRCR, DMRT
Physician in Administrative Charge,
Department of Radiotherapy and Oncology,
Oxfordshire Area Health Authority (Teaching)
Radcliffe Infirmary and Churchill Hospital, Oxford
and Horton General Hospital, Banbury, Oxfordshire
Clinical Lecturer in Radiotherapy,
University of Oxford

Contents

CHAPTER ONE

The Technical Aspects of Radiotherapy

B. S. Mantell

Historical Background

Radiotherapy began during the closing years of the nineteenth century, when the discovery of X-rays by Röntgen in 1895 and of radium by Pierre and Marie Curie, in 1898, placed two sources of ionising radiation at the disposal of medicine. The realisation that these rays were biologically active led to the trial of their use in many different conditions. Superficial cancers had been cured by radiotherapy before the turn of the century, but a blissful ignorance of the risks of radiation together with an almost magical belief in its 'stimulating' properties also led to much indiscriminate overexposure for diagnostic, therapeutic and cosmetic purposes for many years.

The early X-ray apparatus was simple and crude. Induction coils were used to power the X-ray tubes which were often completely unprotected, emitting rays in all directions. Development of the transformer and introduction of the Coolidge tube in 1913 resulted in improved performance, and enclosure of X-ray tubes in adequately screened casings became mandatory. By 1920 X-ray apparatus working at 200 kV was available and the era of deep X-ray therapy had begun.

The Curies obtained only 100 mg of radium from a ton of pitchblende, and it was many years before radium became available in reasonably large quantities. However, the first few years of the twentieth century saw radium used for the treatment of carcinoma of the cervix and implanted in tubes into malignant tumours, while the radioactive gas, radon, which emanates from radium was collected in brass tubes for therapy. The permanently implanted gold seed containing radon was introduced by Failla in 1924, and has only recently been totally replaced by the solid radioactive gold grain.

A turning point in radiotherapy was reached in 1928, when a unit of radiation dose, precisely defined in terms of ionisation in air, was accepted by the Second International Congress of Radiology and named the roentgen. It is only in recent years that this has become superseded by the unit of radiation absorption, the rad. In 1934 Paterson and Parker described a system for arranging radium sources to produce homogeneous dosage when implanted interstitially into tumours or arranged on surface moulds. Thus by the time of the Second World War radiotherapy was an established specialty with well-tried techniques of superficial, deep and radium therapy, and steadily improving results in terms of palliation and cure.

The Megavoltage Era

It had been known for many years that 'hard' X-rays of higher energy were more penetrating and therefore more useful for deep therapy, while 'soft' or low-energy X-rays were absorbed heavily in the skin and superficial tissues where they produced severe reactions. Metal filters were constructed to absorb these soft rays, and so 'harden' the beams, and techniques using multiple fields with beams 'crossfiring' deep-seated tumours were developed. Even then 'radiation burns' were often produced; the scattering of the radiation within the patient produced damage outside the tumour area, and patients complained of discomforts such as malaise and nausea. Furthermore, even the 'hard' X-rays were heavily absorbed by bone, and necrosis of ribs, pelvis, mandible and other bones often followed irradiation of adjacent tumours. These considerable side-effects, which frequently made curative irradiation or even palliation impossible, were less marked when higher voltages were used to excite still harder X-rays. But it was found difficult to apply much more than about 250 kV across an ordinary X-ray tube. In this the electrons generated by a heated cathode are accelerated by the voltage difference towards the anode, where they are stopped and where they give up their energy in the form of X-rays and heat. Insulation becomes difficult to achieve above about 250 kV under these circumstances.

Attempts to solve this problem led to two different lines of development. On the one hand, workers sought to construct devices for accelerating electrons which would overcome the above difficulty – true 'megavoltage' apparatus. On the other hand, X-rays were abandoned, and 'bombs' of radioactive material emitting beams of high energy gamma rays for 'telecurie' therapy were built. Strictly speaking, 'megavoltage' means a voltage of one million or more. In modern radiotherapeutic idiom it is taken to refer to X-rays generated by the arrest of electrons whose energy is at least two million volts. The term is also loosely extended to include telecurie apparatus producing gamma rays of similar quality to these X-rays. Two million volts is chosen because only at this energy are the skin- and bone-sparing maximal, and scatter of the radiation minimal.

As early as 1931 a multisection X-ray tube, 25 ft long, was in use at the California Institute of Technology, producing X-rays at 700 kV; by the end of the decade, one-million-volt tubes had been constructed. At the same time enough radium had been collected to form the first telecurie units, each containing several grams. Advances in technology during the Second World War provided the basis for development of the megavoltage and telecurie apparatus which today has largely replaced the deep X-ray or 'orthovoltage' equipment of a few years ago, and which enables high doses of radiation to be administered to deeply sited tumours with no skin reaction or bone damage, and a minimum of discomfort to the patient.

The principal machines now in use for producing megavoltage X-rays are the Van de Graaff generator, the linear accelerator and the betatron.

The Van de Graaff Generator (Fig. 1.1)

Introduced in 1931, this apparatus has been developed and improved over the years and is still used in many radiotherapy centres. A metal

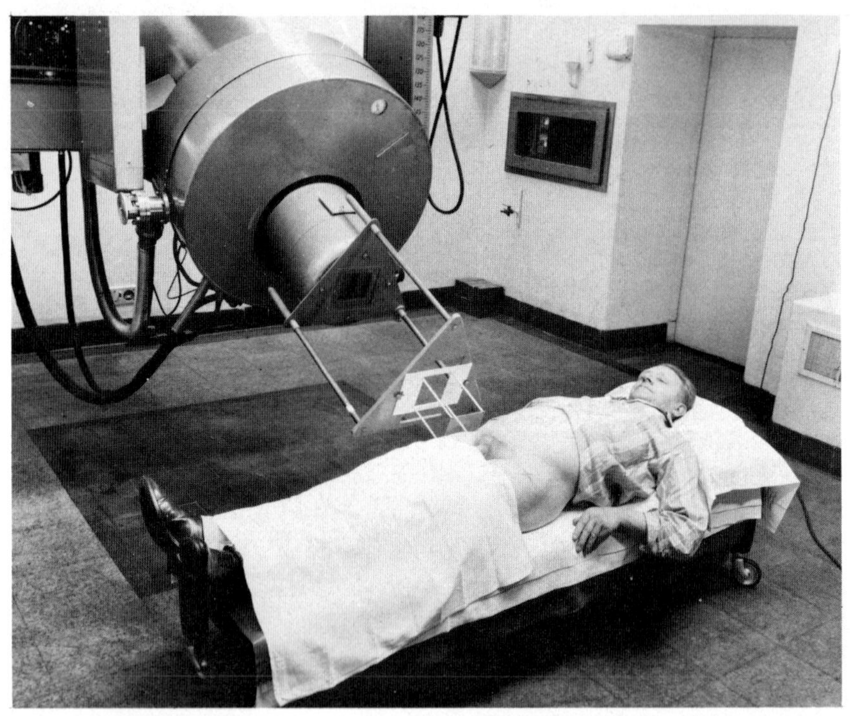

Fig. 1.1. Treatment of bladder cancer with the Van de Graaff generator (courtesy Dr K. A. Newton, Westminster Hospital).

dome is housed within a cylindrical tank filled with an insulating gas under very high pressure, and is supported by insulating pillars. Electrons from a brush of needle points maintained at a negative potential flow onto a rapidly moving non-conducting belt which passes over a pulley inside the dome. Here another set of needle points collects the electrons which pass to the outside of the dome, where a large electrostatic charge soon accumulates. In the modern Van de Graaff unit the dome reaches a negative voltage of two million. The dome is constantly discharged to earth through a high resistance. An evacuated accelerating tube with an electron source and a series of intermediate electrodes is connected to the high resistance so that succeeding intermediate electrodes are maintained at progressively diminishing negative voltage. A constant stream of electrons is thus accelerated down the evacuated tube to strike a gold target at its lower end. This target is connected to earth, and is cooled by water. A beam of X-rays with a maximum energy of two million volts is produced. As the focal point where the electron beam strikes the target is only about 3 or 4 mm in diameter, the beam has very sharp, clearly-defined edges; it is produced continually as long as the machine is energised.

The usefulness of the Van de Graaff generator is somewhat limited by its bulkiness; it cannot be used on an isocentric mounting (see below).

The Linear Accelerator (Fig. 1.2)

This apparatus developed as a result of the research on microwave (radar) beams during the Second World War. Like the Van de Graaff

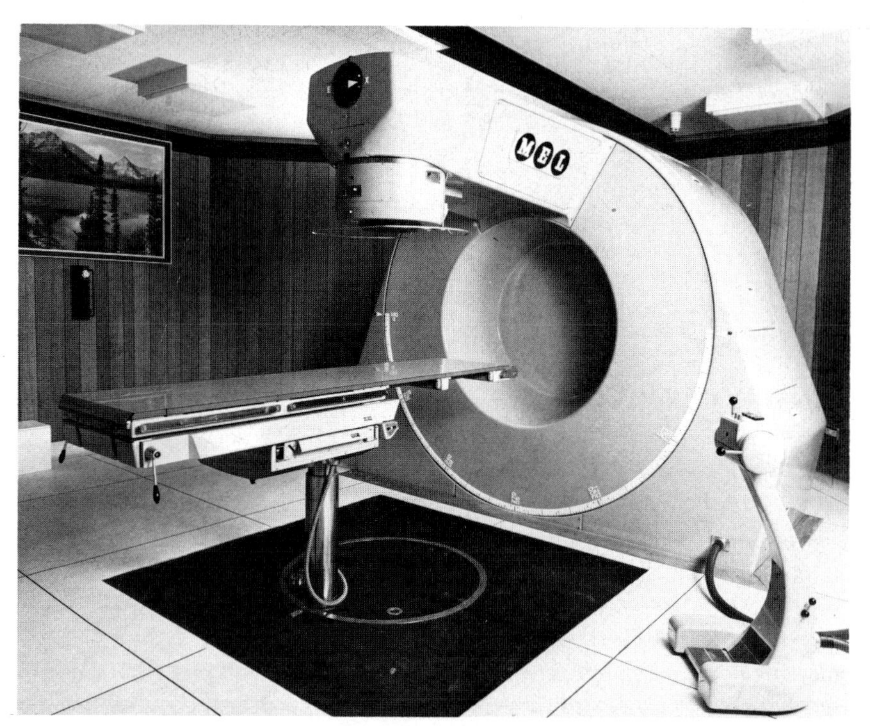

Fig. 1.2. 10 MV linear accelerator with isocentric mounting (courtesy MEL Ltd).

generator, it too has an evacuated accelerating tube with a source of electrons at one end and a target at the other. The tube is known as a wave guide, since it is designed specially to conduct along its length a microwave or radar beam, introduced at the same end as the electron source. The microwave beam consists of alternate peaks of positive and negative potential, and moves down the tube with the speed of light. The electrons injected into the tube are attracted towards the positive peaks and repelled by the negative, and are thus built up into a series of bunches, accelerating down the tube to strike the target to produce X-rays. The electron source or 'gun' and the microwave generator or 'magnetron' are energised simultaneously many times each second by a timing device or 'modulator'. The frequency with which the bunches of electrons strike the target depends upon the frequency of the modulator, which is controllable. Thus the X-rays are produced as a rapid series of bursts rather than a steady stream, but the dose rate is readily adjustable. The energy of the X-rays depends upon the power of the microwave beam and the length of the accelerating tube. Energies equivalent to 4, 6 or 8 million volts are commonest, but energies up to 40 million volts have been obtained. In many linear accelerators the target is removable so that the electron beam itself is available for use in therapy, although the changeover may be inconveniently time-consuming in a busy department.

The Betatron (Fig. 1.3)

Invented in 1941, the betatron is a cyclic accelerator in which electrons are accelerated around a circular path to very high energies. The accelerating tube or 'doughnut' is circular and is maintained at a high vacuum. It is placed between the poles of a large electromagnet energised by a rapidly alternating current. Electrons are injected into the doughnut by an electron gun, and move in a circle around the doughnut as the power of the electromagnet increases with the phase of the alternating current. The electrons become established in an orbit at very high speeds. Then, as the alternating current declines, the strength of the electromagnet diminishes and it no longer holds the electrons in their orbit. They therefore spiral out and are extracted from the doughnut

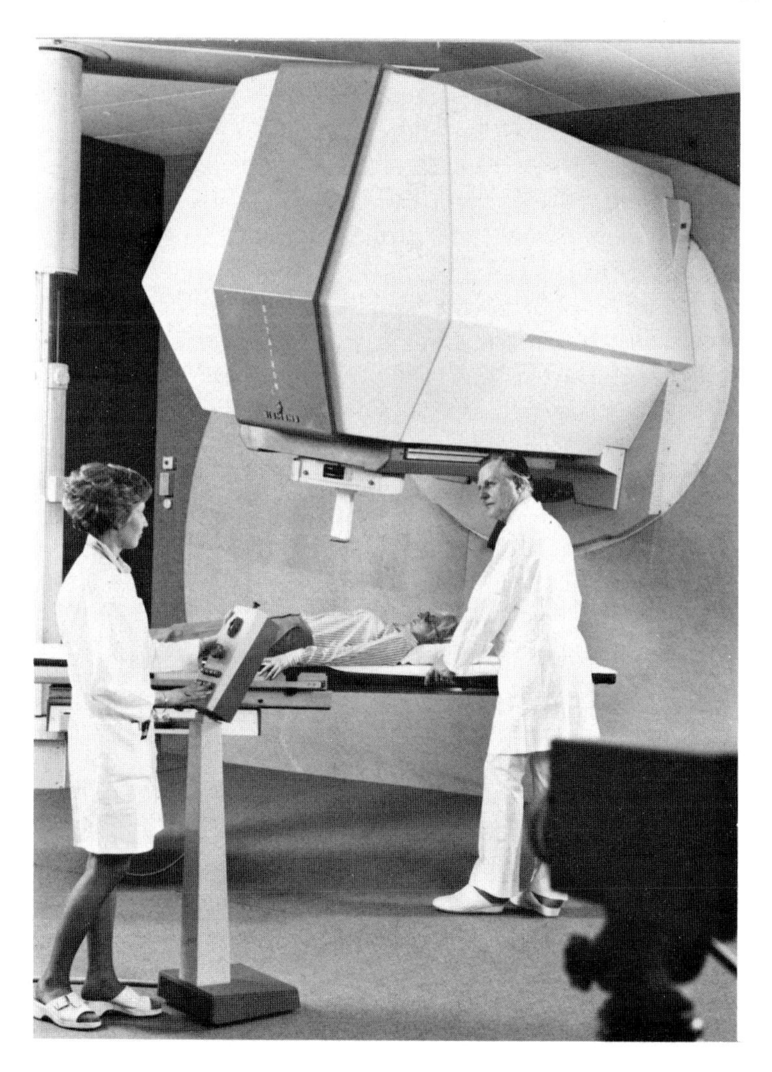

Fig. 1.3 42 MV betatron (courtesy Siemens AG).

as a beam. This electron beam may be directed on to a target to produce X-rays, or may be used directly for electron beam therapy. The energy of the radiation produced is readily controllable. X-ray and electron beams equivalent to 40 million volts or more are obtainable by present day betatrons.

Telecurie Beam Units

As early as 1917 fairly deep-seated tumours were being treated by 'radium packs' applied to the skin. When larger quantities of radium became available it was found possible to move the source several centimetres from the skin; the advantage of this was that, although the dose-rate was diminished at the surface in accordance with the inverse square law, the relative dose-rate at depth was increased. For example, 4 grams of radium placed 9 cm from the skin gave a dose-rate of about five roentgens per minute at the skin, while at 14 cm it gave only about two. However, for every 100 roentgens at the skin only 20 reached a depth of 10 cm in the first case, while more than 30 roentgens reached 10 cm in the second. Still larger quantities of radium could be used to increase the dose-rate, allowing shorter treatment times. Alternatively, they could be used to increase the source–skin distance, thus further improving the depth dose for the same treatment time, and allowing more deeply-seated lesions to be treated without giving excessive skin doses.

Such large quantities of radium required special provision for shielding so that radiation escaped only in a controlled beam and only when required. Ingenious devices were constructed for moving the radium by remote control from a safe to the treatment head and back again. However, radium was of limited value as a telecurie source. It was never possible to obtain more than a few grams for a source, and the gamma ray output was never high enough to construct units with a source–skin distance of the 60 cm or so required to give good depth doses, without impossibly long treatment times. Radium gives off the radioactive gas radon which would represent a major hazard should leakage of a source occur. Also, the gamma rays of radium are equivalent only to X-rays generated at about 1·5 million volts, barely within the megavoltage range. The full development of the telecurie beam unit had therefore to await the arrival in the 1950s of radioactive cobalt – ^{60}Co.

Cobalt Units (Fig. 1.4)

^{60}Co is manufactured in the atomic pile. It is a very powerful emitter of gamma rays which are equivalent to X-rays generated at about 2·5

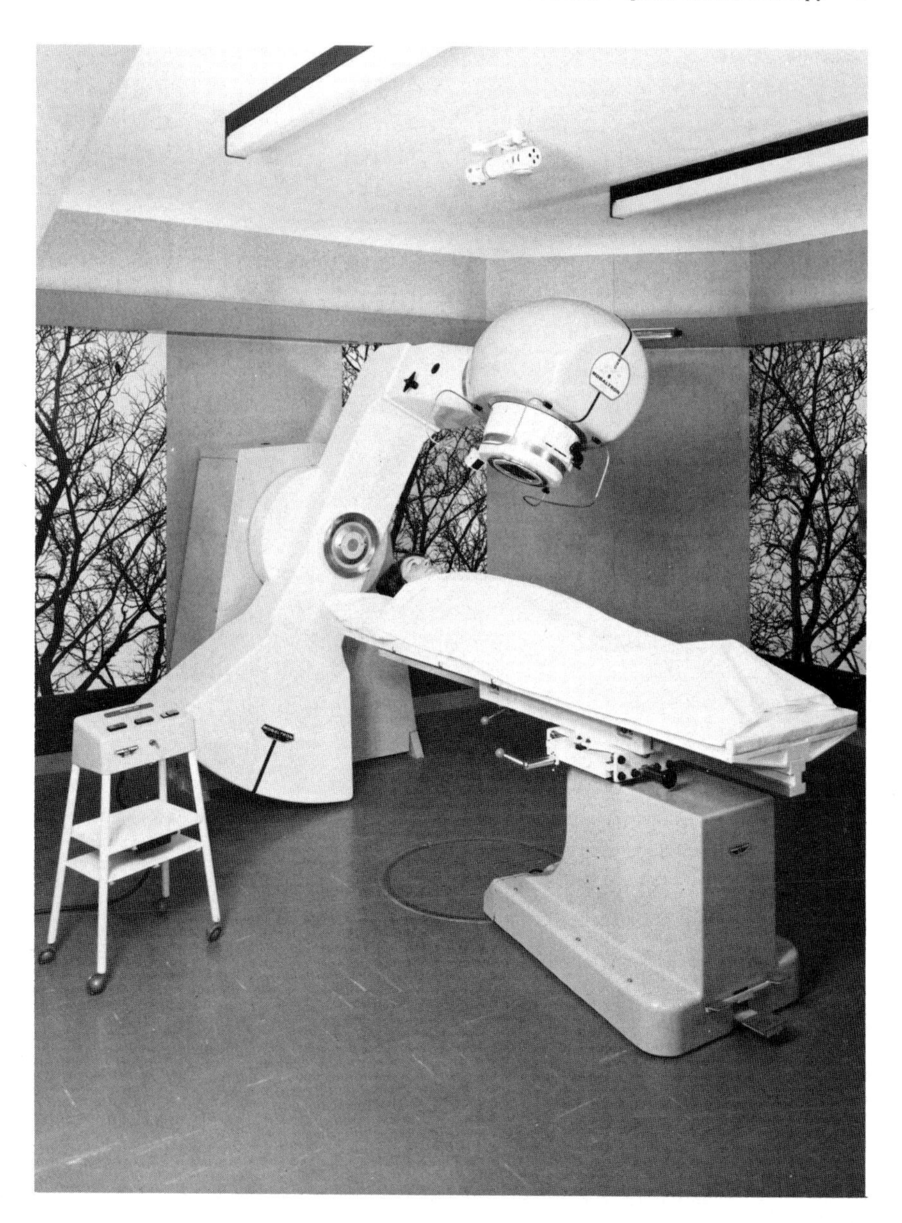

Fig. 1.4. Cobalt unit with isocentric mounting (courtesy TEM Ltd).

million volts. It is possible to produce samples each gram of which emits as much radiation per unit time as 200 grams of radium. A cobalt source may be used at a distance of 80 or 100 cm from the patient's skin to produce depth doses and treatment times within the range of the megavoltage X-ray machines already described. Its disadvantage is its short half-life – only 5·3 years compared with the 1600 years of radium. This means that after 5·3 years any treatment will take twice as long to give, so sources must be renewed every three years or so to keep treatment times within reasonable limits.

Massive shielding is required to protect staff and patients from the radiation streaming from a cobalt source. The treatment head of a cobalt unit is essentially a block of lead, uranium or other heavy metal. Within it is housed the source with a mechanical device for bringing it to an aperture in the head when required. Various forms of wheel, slide or shutter are used for this purpose in different units. The beam of radiation passes through a collimator, consisting of jaws of heavy metal which limit the beam to the dimensions required.

Units have been constructed using caesium-137 instead of ^{60}Co. Such units are of limited value, in spite of the fact that ^{137}Cs has a relatively long half-life of 30 years. The energy of its gamma rays is not sufficient to bring it into the megavoltage range, and its output per gram is so low that sources of ^{137}Cs need to be physically large: for example, 4 cm diameter compared with 2 cm for ^{60}Co. This produces a large penumbra at the edge of the beam, which thus lacks sharpness. The source must be fairly close to the patient's skin if the low gamma-ray output is not to result in very long treatment times, and so poor depth doses result.

The Housing and Mounting of Megavoltage and Telecurie Units

Equipment producing X-rays or gamma rays in the megavoltage range must be housed in a room specially constructed to prevent the highly-penetrating radiation from reaching the outside. Such rooms are normally sited on the lowermost floor of the building. Any part of the walls or ceiling which may receive the main beam is described as a 'primary barrier'. It is usually constructed of concrete several feet thick, and may contain several inches' thickness of steel. Other parts of the walls or ceiling receive only scattered radiation, and are less thick 'secondary barriers'. Such rooms are not entered directly, but through a protected passageway or 'maze'. Electrical interlocks are provided, operated by opening of the door to the room or breaking of the light beam on a photocell, which causes the apparatus to be switched off automatically should any person enter the room while it is operating. The patient is observed by means of a radiation-absorbing window sited in a 'secondary barrier', or by closed-circuit television or periscope.

The equipment may be mounted on a gantry which enables it to be raised or lowered and the beam directed within certain confines. Many cobalt units and linear accelerators are mounted on a rotating gantry which allows the beam to pass through the patient as the source is rotated around him in a vertical plane. This may be combined with a treatment couch which rotates in a horizontal plane; the axes of rotation of beam and couch coincide at a point known as the 'isocentre'. Treatments are planned so that the patient's tumour lies on the isocentre. By this 'isocentric' method the beam always passes through the tumour, however the couch and treatment head are disposed (Figures 1.2 and 1.4).

An interesting development is the tracking technique described by Green (1959), where movement of the couch under automatic control, combined with rotation of the beam, allows a zone of high dosage to be produced which follows any tortuous anatomical site, for example the oesophagus. The movement of the couch is governed by a template constructed from radiological studies.

Electron Therapy

Unlike X-rays and gamma rays which are absorbed exponentially, electrons have a finite range in tissue. Instead of the progressive attenuation of an X-ray beam, an electron beam produces a plateau of high dose extending in from the skin surface. The depth of this plateau depends upon the energy of the electrons, but beyond it the dose falls off very rapidly to zero. This property may be exploited for radiotherapy. The electrons may be generated by a linear accelerator or a betatron. Alternatively, beta particles, the electrons emitted by certain radioactive isotopes such as ^{90}Sr, may be utilised. The electron beam is of use for irradiating superficial structures while sparing deeper tissues.

Indications for Electron Therapy

Extensive Skin Malignancy

Trump *et al.* (1953) described the use of an electron beam from a Van de Graaff machine for the treatment of widespread superficial malignancies. Such a beam, generated at 2 million volts, produces its maximum dose about 4 mm below the surface, with a maximum range in tissue of about 7 mm. Extensive areas or even the whole body can be irradiated by moving the patient through the beam, while producing none of the haematological or systemic effects of similar treatment using X-rays. Szur *et al.* (1962) used the electron beam from a linear accelerator to irradiate the whole body surface, anteriorly then posteriorly, particularly for the control of mycosis fungoides. Bratherton (1972) reports the experience at Cambridge using specially constructed strontium-90 beta-particle units. Such units are relatively simple, but can deliver 200 rad to the whole of the anterior or posterior aspect of the body in about ten minutes. (See Chapter 7.)

Localised Superficial Malignancy

Very superficial basal cell carcinomas or carcinoma-in-situ (Bowen's disease) may be treated by application of a beta-particle-emitting plaque, usually of strontium-90. Mantell and Morgan (1969) described the construction and use of an exactly-fitting mould impregnated with yttrium-90 for the beta-particle irradiation of Queyrat's erythroplasia, carcinoma-in-situ of the penis.

Infiltrating Skin Tumours

Most skin tumours are readily treatable by superficial X-rays generated at 50 to 140 kV. The thicker growths may require deep X-rays (200–300 kV) or even a specially planned megavoltage technique. An electron beam from a linear accelerator or betatron is an alternative. The depth of the plateau of high dosage may be selected by adjusting the energy of the machine, or by placing an absorber of wax or perspex on the skin surface. A 10 MV electron beam enables the first 3 cm of tissue to be irradiated to more than 90 per cent of the incident dose, while less than 10 per cent reaches 5 cm (Jackson, 1970).

Other Accessible Tumours

The limited penetration of the electron beam may be used to advantage in a variety of sites such as the lip, parotid gland, and lymph nodes (Zuppinger, 1967). Electrons from a 24 MV betatron have been used in the treatment of breast carcinoma (Chu *et al.*, 1963). Jackson and Gibb (1972) have used an 8 MV single-field electron beam from a linear accelerator for the irradiation of the chest wall after mastectomy.

The Eye

Irradiation of the cornea or conjunctiva may be required, often for a benign lesion such as pterygium, or to prevent vascularisation of a corneal graft. Specially constructed ophthalmic applicators containing ^{90}Sr may be used. The beta particles emitted allow the surface of the cornea to be treated while almost no radiation reaches the posterior pole of the lens, thus avoiding the risk of cataract. Such applicators may be used also for treatment of malignant melanoma of the conjunctiva (Lederman, 1961).

Brachytherapy

This term is used to include interstitial therapy, which involves the implantation of radioactive sources into the tissues; intracavitary treatment, i.e. the insertion of sources into body cavities such as the uterus; and the application of radioactive moulds to the skin surface. For many years radium was the only isotope available for brachytherapy. It was enclosed in needles for implantation, and techniques were developed for irradiating planes of tissues such as the edge of the tongue bearing a carcinoma, or cylindrical volumes for bulkier tumours. The quantity of radium required and its arrangement was obtained by a series of rules and tables which also governed the arrangement of radium sources on felt plaques for the treatment of surface tumours. The radioactive gas, radon, emanating from radium was collected into gold 'seeds' for implantation. Having a half-life of only 3·8 days these seeds could be left permanently in the tissues, which was of great advantage in sites such as the bladder where removal of an implant would be difficult.

Radium proved of great value in the treatment of carcinoma of the cervix. Various techniques were perfected in centres such as Paris,

Stockholm and Manchester, but all essentially consisted of the insertion of a tube containing radium into the uterine cavity, with the addition of further radium in suitable containers in the vagina.

Radium has a half-life of approximately 1600 years, so the activity of any radium tube or needle remains for all practical purposes constant. It has certain disadvantages, however: its gamma rays are very penetrating and require several centimetres of lead to absorb them. Also it produces radon gas which could represent a health hazard should it escape due to damage to a radium needle or tube. The manufacture of radon seeds has recently ceased because of the risk of escape of the gas. They have been replaced by 'grains' of radioactive gold for permanent implants; these have a half-life of 2·7 days.

In recent years radium needles and tubes have been largely replaced by those containing isotopes which do not emit radioactive gas. ^{60}Co is of limited value, as its half-life is only 5·3 years and its gamma rays require even more shielding than do those of radium. ^{137}Cs, however, has a half-life of more than 30 years, and its gamma rays, having less energy than the mean of those of radium, are more readily absorbed by shielding material.

Afterloading Methods

The techniques mentioned above involve the handling of radioactive sources in the operating theatre, with the associated (minimal) irradiation of staff. In afterloading, only the source containers are inserted in the first instance. These can be manipulated and adjusted as required with no radiation hazard. Only when their position has been verified as optimal are they loaded with the radioactive sources, a simple and quick manoeuvre carried out on the ward from behind protecting lead screens.

Iridium-192 is available as wire and is very suitable for afterloaded implants (Fig. 1.5). It is highly flexible and its gamma rays are readily absorbed by a few millimetres of lead, making protection much easier than with radium; its half-life is 74 days. Thin nylon tubing is first implanted into the tissues and loaded with non-active wire for verification by radiography. The inert wires are easily and quickly replaced by active iridium wires when the position of the implant has been approved and the loading and time calculated. Such an implant is flexible

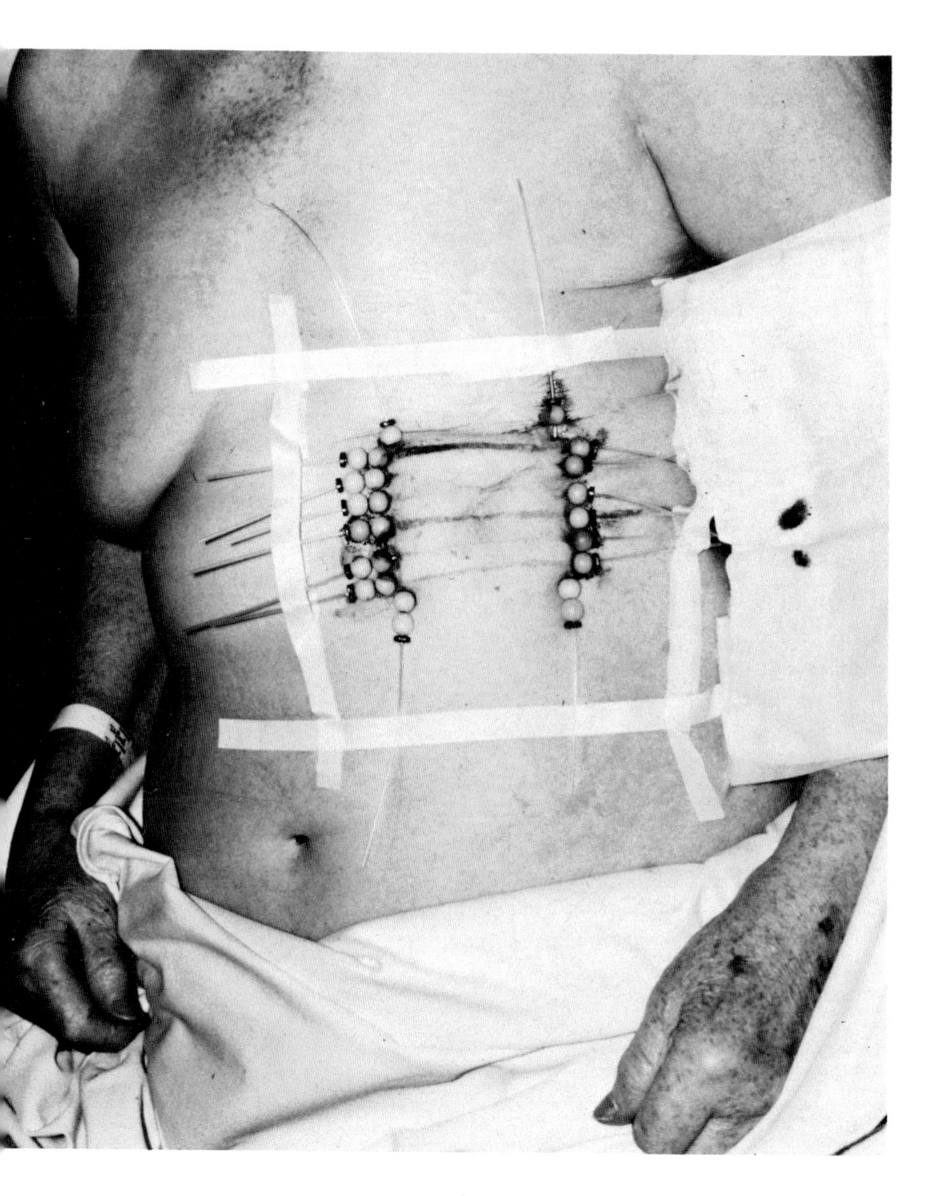

Fig. 1.5. Iridium wire implant of the chest wall in a case of breast carcinoma.

and readily adapted to tissue contours, unlike the conventional rigid needles (Paine, 1972). For this reason, as well as the simpler protection requirements, ^{192}Ir is also very suitable for the construction of radioactive surface moulds.

Similar hand-afterloading techniques have also been used in intracavitary therapy. Suit *et al.* (1963) described such a method for treatment of carcinoma of the cervix, using radium sources afterloaded with special inserters into applicators already placed accurately in the uterus and vagina. The quantities of radioactive material used in intracavitary therapy, however, are usually considerably greater than in interstitial, with a correspondingly increased risk of exposure of staff. Attention has been directed therefore to the development of mechnical methods of afterloading with remote control.

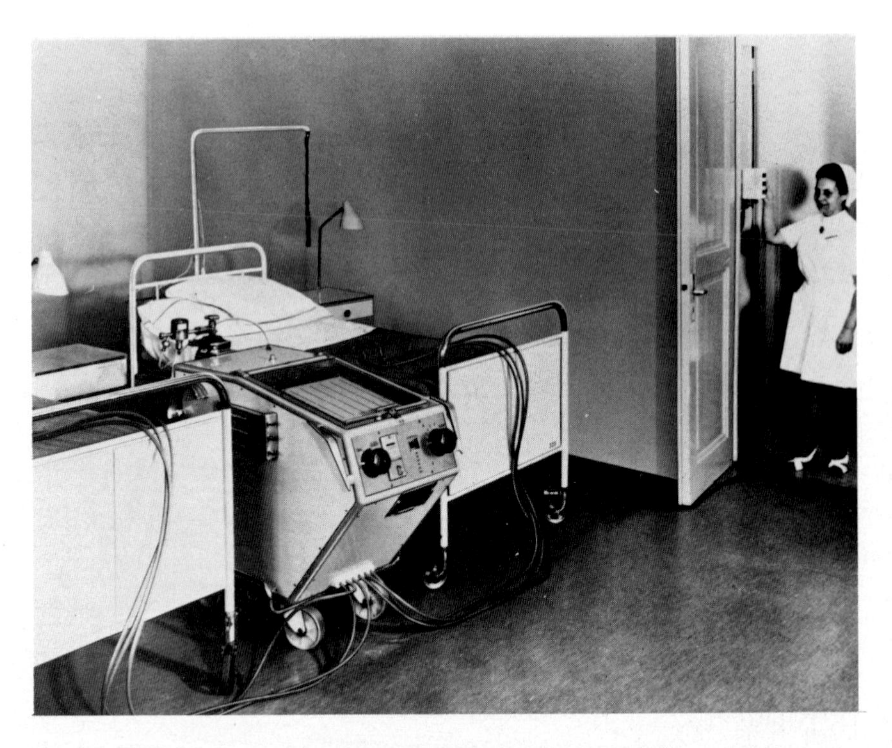

Fig. 1.6. The Cervitron II apparatus for gynaecological malignancy. Note the flexible tubes for conveying the sources to the catheters inserted into the patient (courtesy Old Delft Ltd).

All such methods involve a shielded safe in which the radiation sources are stored. The sources are driven by a suitable mechanism out of the safe and through long flexible catheters which are connected to applicators already in position in the patient. Some method of selection of sources is provided to allow flexibility of treatment. Two types of equipment for mechanical afterloading are available, one giving a low dose-rate and the other a high.

The low dose-rate method resembles the older radium insertion techniques in that treatment times are of the order of 40 to 60 hours per insertion, and thus the dosage of radiation given may be expected to be similar biologically to the older régimes. Because the dose-rate is low, protection requirements are relatively simple. The Cervitron-II (Nuclear Engineering and Equipment, Geneva) is one such system (Fig. 1.6). Capable of treating two patients at the same time, the apparatus is housed in a lightly protected room. The sources are prepared by manipulation of controls on the equipment. There is a choice of 36 beads of ^{137}Cs, and 12 inert spacer beads, giving great variability. The sources are propelled down the connecting catheters to the applicators, already inserted in the patient, by compressed air. A timing device controls the total duration of treatment, and the apparatus is connected to a switch outside the treatment room. When staff wish to enter for nursing or other purposes, operation of the switch causes the sources to return to the safe and stops the timer. Further operation of the switch on leaving the room brings the sources back to the patient and re-starts the timer. The Curietron is a similar but less sophisticated device.

The Cathetron (O'Connell *et al.*, 1967) is a high dose-rate system. The sources here are composed of capsules of high-activity ^{60}Co, together with inert spacers, and are propelled down the connecting catheters by drive-cables. Treatment times are very short, of the order of minutes, and the dose is usually given as a series of fractions. Thus the treatment might be expected to resemble biologically a course of external irradiation rather than the slow prolonged exposure given by radium. This new concept of high dose-rate, fractionated intracavitary treatment is not yet widely accepted.

The high dose-rate means that heavy protection is required. The Cathetron is in fact housed in a room similar to that used for megavoltage or telecurie apparatus (Fig. 1.7). (See Chapter 10.)

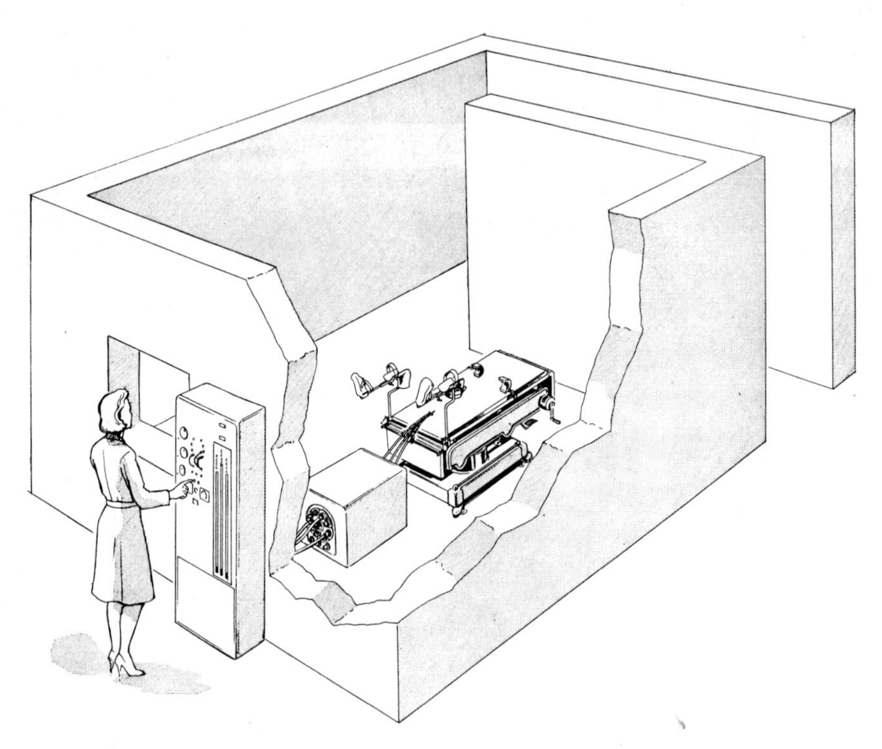

Fig. 1.7. The Cathetron high-dose-rate intracavitary system (courtesy TEM Ltd).

Particle Beam Therapy

The subatomic particles which are of particular interest to the radiotherapist are electrons, neutrons, alpha particles, protons and negative pi-mesons. The production and properties of electron beams in radiotherapy have been described earlier in this chapter.

The characteristic of proton and alpha particle beams is that a 'peak' of energy deposition occurs at the limit of the beam's penetration into tissue. A 'plateau' of relatively low dose extends in from the skin surface until the 'peak' in the region in which the particles are coming to rest, where they give up the greater portion of their energy; the depth of the peak depends upon the energy imparted to the particles in the generating device. Thus it is possible to deliver a high dose of radiation to a deeply-seated organ while giving a relatively small dose to the overlying tissues. By adjusting the diameter of the beam and choosing the correct energy, the size and position of the high dose-volume can be controlled with great accuracy. Such a technique may be used, for example, to produce stereotactic lesions in the brain for the treatment of Parkinsonism. Possibly the most important application is in the treatment of pituitary disease, where part or all of the pituitary gland can be irradiated as required, for acromegaly, Cushing's disease or to produce pituitary ablation in breast carcinoma or diabetic retinopathy (Kjellberg and Kliman, 1974). Direction and control of the beam must be extremely exact as a few millimetres' inaccuracy may be disastrous.

The peak effect is even more marked with the negative pi-meson beam, which causes disintegration of the nuclei of the elements in tissue at the limit of its penetration. The densely ionising fragments produced cause intense localised radiation effects.

Accelerators for Particle Beams

The linear accelerator and betatron for producing electron beams have already been described. The other machines which will be considered are the synchrotron, the proton synchrotron, the cyclotron and the synchrocyclotron.

Synchrotron

Electrons are accelerated in an evacuated ceramic 'doughnut' under the influence of an increasing magnetic field, as in the betatron. Further energy is imparted to the electrons by a radio-frequency field applied at the appropriate instant to coincide with the time an electron takes to pass once around the doughnut. The electrons thus acquire great energy, as a result of which a relativistic increase in their mass takes place as their speed approaches that of light (see synchrocyclotron, below).

Proton Synchrotron

This is a development of the synchrotron for accelerating heavy positively-charged protons instead of light negative electrons. The core of the electromagnet of a proton synchrotron may weigh several thousand tons. The proton beam may be used to bombard a carbon target to produce pi-mesons.

Cyclotron

This device was first constructed in 1931 by Lawrence and Livingston. It consists of two 'Ds', semicircular hollow metal boxes resembling the letter D. The straight sides of the Ds are open and face each other as the Ds lie between the poles of a large and powerful magnet, enclosed in an evacuated chamber. A very high frequency alternating current is applied to the Ds so that one is positive and the other negative, alternately.

The ions to be accelerated are introduced at the centre of the cyclotron between the Ds. These ions may be alpha particles which are helium nuclei, protons which are hydrogen nuclei, or deuterons which are the nuclei of heavy hydrogen, deuterium; all are positively charged. They are formed by introducing a small amount of the appropriate gas and ionising it by a heated filament. The ions move from the interior of one D to that of the other under the influence of the electrical field between the Ds. As they move, the magnetic field in which the Ds lie causes the ions to adopt a curved path; the rapidly alternating polarity of the Ds forces the ions to oscillate between them, and the combined effect is that the ions follow a spiral track outward as they gain energy. With each turn of the spiral the ions travel a greater distance in the same time, and they eventually leave the cyclotron with a very high energy, for example 15 million volts.

The principal use of the cyclotron in radiotherapy is to bombard a beryllium target with a beam of deuterons. This causes the target to emit an intense beam of fast neutrons which may be used for treatment (Chapter 3). Cyclotrons are not suitable for accelerating electrons.

Synchrocyclotron

The increase in mass experienced by particles whose speed approaches that of light was referred to in the description of the synchrotron and its electron beam. A particle being accelerated in a cyclotron takes longer to complete a revolution between the Ds when its mass increases. It therefore ceases to move in phase with the alternating current which is applied to the Ds, and is no longer in the correct position to be accelerated further as the polarity of the Ds changes. This phenomenon limits the amount of energy that a cyclotron can impart to the particles.

In the synchrocyclotron the frequency of the alternating current is progressively decreased as the ions spiral out from the centre of the Ds to their outer edge. This allows the ions to remain in phase with the alternating current as their mass increases, and thus they acquire enormous energies of the order of hundreds of millions of volts. They emerge from the synchrocyclotron as a series of pulses instead of the constant stream emitted by the conventional cyclotron.

Use of Particle Beam Accelerators

The betatron is a relatively compact machine, and many are installed in radiotherapy departments. The other machines which have been described are very large, and extremely expensive to build and to operate.

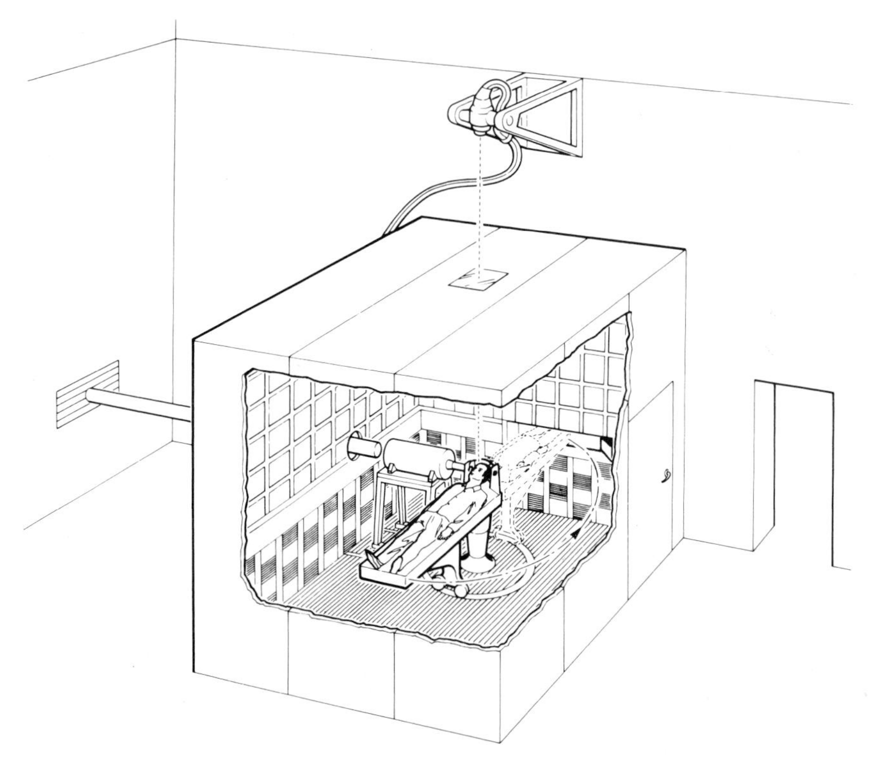

Fig. 1.8. Proposed treatment room for proton beam therapy using the Harwell synchrocyclotron (courtesy Dr C. Whitehead, AERE Harwell, and the Editor, *Proceedings of the Royal Society of Medicine*).

The Harwell synchrocyclotron has a magnet weighing 700 tons, and a proton synchrotron installed in California uses one weighing 10 000 tons. Such machines are far beyond the resources of an ordinary hospital; but as they provide many facilities for physical, chemical and biological research and the production of radioisotopes they may be installed in a university complex and time allowed for a radiotherapy programme, as in the case of the Medical Research Council's cyclotron sited at the Hammersmith Hospital, London. It is proposed to use the proton beam of the Harwell synchrocyclotron (Fig. 1.8) for radiotherapy (Whitehead, 1974). The recently built TRIUMF cyclotron in British Columbia represents a joint project financed by the Canadian Atomic Energy Control Board and four Canadian universities, producing simultaneous proton, pi-meson and neutron beams for multiple research projects and radiotherapy which may all continue at the same time.

References

BRATHERTON, D. G. (1972) in *Modern Trends in Radiotherapy – 2*, ed. Deeley, T. Butterworth, London, 176–187.

CHU, F. C. H., NISCE, L. and LAUGHLIN, J. S. (1963) *Radiology*, **81**, 871–879.

GREEN, A. (1959) *Proceedings of the Royal Society of Medicine*, **52,** 344–346.

JACKSON, S. M. (1970) *British Journal of Radiology*, **43**, 431–440.

JACKSON, S. M. and GIBB, R. (1972) *British Journal of Radiology*, **45**, 745–747.

KJELLBERG, R. N. and KLIMAN, B. (1974) *Proceedings of the Royal Society of Medicine*, **67**, 32–33.

LEDERMAN, M. (1961) *British Journal of Radiology*, **34**, 21–42.

MANTELL, B. S. and MORGAN, W. Y. (1969) *British Journal of Radiology*, **42**, 855–857.

O'CONNELL, D., JOSLIN, C. A., HOWARD, N., RAMSEY, N. W. and LIVERSAGE, W. E. (1967) *British Journal of Radiology*, **40**, 882–887.

PAINE, C. H. (1972) *Clinical Radiology*, **23**, 263–272.

SUIT, H. D., MOORE, E. B., FLETCHER, G. H. and WORSNOP, R. (1963) *Radiology*, **81**, 126–131.

SZUR, L., SILVESTER, J. A. and BENTLEY, D. K. (1962) *Lancet*, **1**, 1373–1377.

TRUMP, J. G., WRIGHT, K. A., EVANS, W. W., ANSON, J. H., HARE, H. F., FROMER, J. L., JAQUE, C. I. and HOME, K. W. (1953) *American Journal of Roentgenology*, **69**, 623.

WHITEHEAD, C. (1974) *Proceedings of the Royal Society of Medicine*, **67**, 29–31.

ZUPPINGER, A. (1967) in *Modern Trends in Radiotherapy – 1*, ed. Deeley, T. Butterworth, London.

CHAPTER TWO

Radiobiological Studies of Clinical Problems in Radiotherapy

George Wiernik

Evolution of the Radiobiology of Clinical Problems

Cancer research at the present time is undergoing a radical reappraisal. When cancer research on a systematic basis became widespread in the latter part of the nineteenth century the research workers had the problems of human cancer as their immediate task. The ethical difficulties which presented themselves channelled the work progressively into methodologies which involved laboratory techniques and laboratory animals. The first generation of research workers gradually became replaced by a younger group who entered the laboratories directly and had had little exposure to the clinical problems posed by the cancerous process. The lines of enquiry naturally followed the most exciting scientific leads which resulted from their research efforts and, not infrequently, experimental methods and objectives were chosen because they would provide results more easily and more quickly than the tackling of similar problems in the clinical cancer field.

The diagnosis of any of the ubiquitous manifestations of the cancerous process raises today, in the same way as it has done for centuries untold, a tremendous emotive force that finds expression in the generous donation of very large sums of money for cancer research.

Money has always been hard to come by, and hence research workers in many fields of fundamental scientific enquiry have linked their work nominally to cancer research so as to obtain access to such funds. This mixture of the gradual evolutionary move by the laboratory cancer research workers away from the clinical cancer problem, and the entry into the field of workers in the general biological sciences, has tended to reduce the immediate value of cancer research for the patients actually suffering from the disease; this in turn has led to the recent general move towards a reappraisal of the current situation.

There is another side to this as to any other coin, and this relates to the clinicians who are face to face with the day-to-day problems posed by their patients who are suffering from cancer. The majority of these clinicians have received the hospital training considered appropriate to their specialty which, in the main, is anecdotal and based on their own and their teachers' personal experiences. Currently there is a wide gulf between the precise methodology that is possible in the experimental laboratory and the rather imprecise clinical assessment which is frequently recorded. With some laboratory training in their formative years and the influence of laboratory scientists on their education, the younger generation of clinicians now performs much more assessable research work, but the time available to the clinician for research purposes remains at a premium so that the quantity of such high quality work is still, unfortunately, very small.

It was against this background that the Churchill Hospital Research Institute was founded to try to re-establish a centre where geographical proximity, which is of prime importance, allowed a group of clinicians from widely diverse clinical specialties to work with laboratory scientists on those problems which are directly related to the radiotherapeutic treatment of patients suffering from cancer. To be effective, such a group must of necessity be small enough to allow personal interaction and, consequently, their work is concentrated on a very small sector. No attempt has been made in this chapter to provide a wide-ranging review of the excellent radiobiological research work currently being performed throughout the world, whether this relates directly to the requirements of clinical practice or to the work being done by our group, as it is considered that the literature is too extensive to make this a worthwhile exercise; the reader wishing to enter this field would find a good starting-point in the 'Biological Basis of Radiotherapy' (Wiernik, 1973).

The contents of this chapter are confined to only a part of the work being performed at the Churchill Hospital Research Institute; that part which will lead to a better understanding of the effects of irradiation on those normal human tissues which limit the radiotherapist's efforts to eradicate a tumour in a patient. Many of the experimental methods were designed to evaluate radiation damage to the vascular system, in various organs, and to test whether damage to blood vessels is responsible for late radiation changes. Quantitative histological techniques have been applied to test whether such late radiation damage can be correlated with direct injury to the epithelial or mesenchymal tissues. The effects of irradiation have been studied by variations in the fractionation régimes and by the effects of radiosensitisers such as hyperbaric oxygen.

Effects of Irradiation on the Skin

Improvement in clinical radiation techniques may be regarded from both the social aspects as well as from the point of view of the cure rate compared with the degree of radiation damage caused by any given régime. Currently, the majority of patients undergoing irradiation treatment receive this on a daily basis. For those attending as outpatients this frequently necessitates very long and wearing road journeys; for many, admission to hospital is required because this burden is too great, especially as a large number of patients are old and often suffer from additional debilitating diseases. If, therefore, the number of attendances for treatment can be diminished without detriment to the effectiveness of the treatment, much will have been achieved for individual patients, especially during these times of financial stringency when staff and equipment shortage threaten the service that can be offered to them.

With this in view, a national clinical trial to test a very limited sector of this field (BIR, 1963; 1972) has been undertaken, and preliminary results suggest that treatment given on alternate days is equally effective to that given daily. To enable the individual radiotherapist to predict the changes in the dose–time relationship necessitated by such changes in fractionation, a number of theoretical systems have been proposed (Fowler and Stern, 1963; Cohen, 1968; Ellis, 1971; Liversage, 1971). Comparison of these simple models with experimental results has demonstrated the paucity of adequate, clinically applicable data, and the disaster which might ensue from their uncritical application in clinical practice (Fowler, 1971). We therefore set out to obtain the necessary experimental data in animals and then to test these results in clinical practice.

Animal Studies

Radiation Skin Reactions

The pig has been chosen as a suitable experimental animal because of the similarity of its skin and subcutaneous tissue to that of humans, and because the distribution and volume of the internal organs in the pig is very close to that in man. Previous irradiation studies involving the skin of pigs (Bewley *et al.*, 1963; Fowler *et al.*, 1963) had shown that quantitative evaluation of different radiation régimes was possible, but we felt that the numerical system of these authors had certain limitations and so we devised a modification of their system in which the

Oxford scoring system

Erythema		*Pigmentation*		*Desquamation*		*Numerical score*
Minimal	A	Minimal	K	—		1·0
						1·5
Moderate	B	Light brown	L	—		2·0
						2·5
Bright red	C	Dark brown	M	Dry	R	3·0
Dusky red	D	—		—		3·5
—	—			Moist, less than half field area	S	4·0
—		—		Moist, more than half field area	T	5·0
—		—		Slough	U	6·0
Fading	E	Localised	N	Healing	V	No numerical score
		confluent	0			

observers recorded separately, by alphabetical symbols, the presence and degree, or absence, of erythema, pigmentation and desquamation, and also changes that had occurred since the same animal was last scored.

These observations were then converted to numerical scores which, during the development of the reaction, corresponded closely with the score which would have been recorded under the Hammersmith system. The initial objective scoring without numbers, however, preserves the raw data so that suitable numerical weighting factors can be allocated subsequently and the value of any one component can be reassessed at a later stage.

Fields on the flanks of domestic pigs, that were anaesthetised with halothane for all procedures, were irradiated with 250 kVp X-rays in courses of one, six or thirty fractions. The doses chosen allowed us to test whether the Nominal Standard Dose hypothesis (Ellis, 1971) was valid and, in order to obtain a spread of values, 15 per cent incremental variations above and below the NSD value were also used. According to the NSD hypothesis the doses which we used should have represented normal tissue tolerance, but we have found that there was very poor correlation between the doses predicted by the NSD system and the experimental observations on acute skin reactions (Berry, Wiernik and Patterson, 1972; 1974). An approximately 30 per cent higher equivalent dose was required when administered in six fractions over 18 days to produce either dry or moist desquamation than was required when given in thirty fractions over 39 days.

In this lies the great danger of employing a simple, theoretical model such as the NSD hypothesis, because most radiotherapists have been trained in clinical practice to judge their dose-level by the acute radiation damage which they observe and, in the majority of instances, clinicians will find themselves in the position of wishing to reduce their customary régime of daily fractionation over 6 weeks to a new system involving fewer fractions over a shorter period. A dose which will give rise to similar late radiation damage will cause quite different levels of acute radiation damage. We found that the equivalent doses predicted by the NSD system for the three fractionation schemes tested gave rise to similar degrees of late radiation damage.

When taking, as late radiation damage, the dose which marginally did not cause skin necrosis and comparing it with clinically observed skin-tolerance levels for comparable field-sizes irradiated with 250 kVp X-rays, we were able to show that our experimental system gave results which ran exactly parallel with the data from clinical practice (Fig. 2.1). It will be seen that the absolute tolerance of pig skin is approximately 30 per cent above that of human skin.

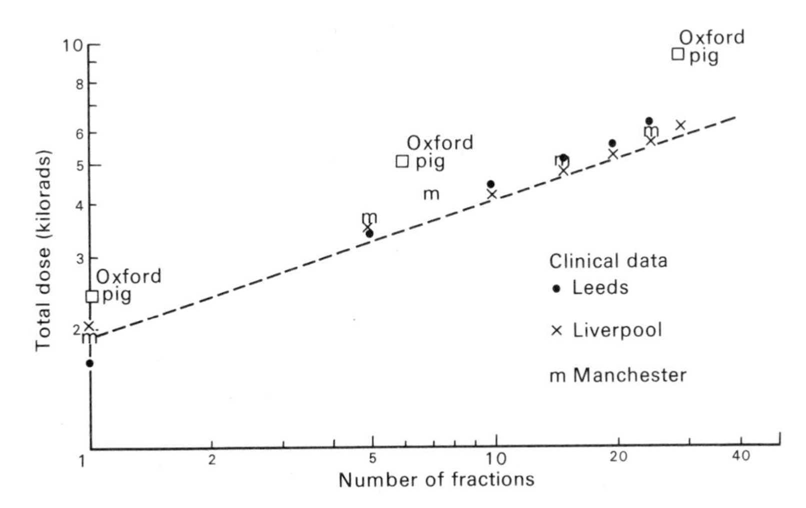

Fig. 2.1. Comparison of variation in tolerance to 250 kVp X-rays with dose fractionation in human and pig skin. Clinically derived dose limits for a 64 cm^2 field are shown for three large radiotherapy centres. The dotted line represents the variation in tolerance dose with number of fractions predicted by the NSD formula. The pig skin data represent the highest dose used which failed to produce any necrotic skin-fields at one year after the end of irradiation. (*British Journal of Radiology* 1974, **47**, 188. Reproduced by permission of the Editors.)

Subcutaneous Fibrosis

The method of assessing late radiation damage which we used in our experimental animals, by exceeding normal tissue tolerance and causing a radiation necrosis, then extrapolating backwards to arrive at the dose which will not cause a necrosis, is not applicable in clinical practice. We therefore looked for another parameter which we could measure and which could later be assessed in patients. Subcutaneous fibrosis, which has become the limiting factor as far as the skin is concerned since the introduction of megavoltage therapy, appeared to provide the necessary criteria.

The same Large White pigs as those used for the study of early and late skin tolerance were used for this study. As well as the 16 × 4 cm field on the left flank which was irradiated, these pigs had a similar field delimited by Indian ink tattoo on the right flank. The area of these fields was traced on to translucent paper so that a permanent record could be retained. Three measurements were taken from each field, along both outside edges and up the middle, and a mean length was calculated.

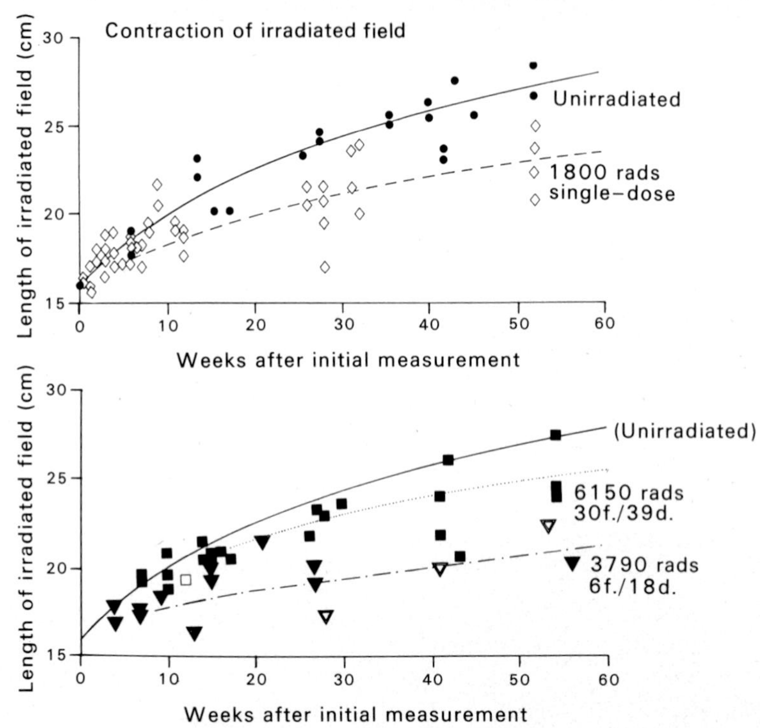

Fig. 2.2. Length of skin-fields on the flank of the pig at various times after initial tattooing of a 16 × 4 cm area. Each symbol represents one field on one animal. The upper panel shows data for unirradiated fields (●) and for those irradiated with a single dose of 1800 rad (◇). The lower panel duplicates the mean line drawn through the measurements on unirradiated skin fields, and shows the data for fields irradiated in courses of 6 f/18 d (▼ ▽) and 30 f/39 d (■ □). The open symbols represent measurements made on the two slow-growing 'runt' animals, corrected for the increase in size of the unirradiated fields on the normally-growing animals. (*British Journal of Radiology* 1974, *47*, 278. Reproduced by permission of the Editors.)

The irradiated pigs were approximately 18 weeks old at the time of treatment and so the length of the unirradiated field increased from the original 16 cm to about 27 cm at one year, due to growth of the animals. Two pigs proved to be slow-growing 'runts' and the data for these had to have a correction factor applied to make all the data comparable. The data from the irradiated fields were then compared with those from the unirradiated fields, as shown graphically in Fig. 2.2.

The upper panel shows that no difference in length can be discerned until about the twelfth week after irradiation, when comparing the unirradiated with the single-treatment fields, after which there is a relative diminution in the length of the irradiated fields. Similar features can be seen in the lower panel, though there is a wider spread in the data for the 30 f/39 d fractionation régime.

These data on subcutaneous fibrosis reveal a poor correlation with the data referred to above for skin reactions when, according to the NSD hypothesis, they should have been similar. For instance, in the 6 f/18 d régime the dose of irradiation which gave rise to only a minor degree of skin reaction is associated with a severe degree of late subcutaneous fibrosis so that, had the clinician raised the dose initially by 30 per cent in order to achieve a skin reaction approaching normal tissue tolerance, he would have caused grossly excessive, i.e. necrotic, late radiation damage. These results are in agreement with one report in the literature (Hayashi and Suit, 1972) but differ materially from the only other similar work which has been reported (Field, 1969).

The onset of fibrosis can be identified in Fig. 2.2 approximately six weeks after the start of fractionated irradiation. This finding correlates well with our data from skin flaps, discussed later in the chapter. From six months onwards there does not appear to be a material increase in the relative amount of fibrosis.

When our data for subcutaneous fibrosis are plotted as an iso-effect curve, the slope of our experimental line between 6 f/18 d and 30 f/39 d has a value of 0·46 as compared with the NSD prediction, for the combined fractionation and time factors, of 0·35 (Berry, Wiernik, Patterson and Hopewell, 1974).

Vascular System Damage

The thread that runs through the whole of this part of our research work is the hypothesis that the effects of irradiation of human tissue can be correlated directly with the effect on the vascular system. In order to validate this hypothesis it must be shown that the various end-points which are amenable to scientific measurement can be shown to give results consistent with each other, and that variations in the component parts of a fractionated course of irradiation affect these end-points in a manner which is predictable on the basis of damage to the vascular system. Hopewell (Hopewell and Wright, 1970) has proposed the 'sausage' segment theory to explain the effects of irradiation on blood vessels, which suggests that blood flow is interrupted or slowed by obstruction to the vessels caused by clones of proliferating endothelial cells. Some histological evidence, in rat brain, to support the hypothesis has been reported (Hopewell, 1974).

Skin Flaps

Another way of testing our general hypothesis is to assess the functional capacity of irradiated blood vessels by measuring the quantity of tissue which these vessels can maintain in a viable condition. A combination of surgery and radiotherapy is frequently used in the treatment of malignant disease. In the treatment of recurrent disease or of late radiation damage it is always difficult to assess how far the blood supply in the area has been damaged, as this dictates the design of local skin flaps and whether grafts will 'take' or wounds will heal. We have, therefore, evolved an experimental system, which can also be applied in clinical practice (Patterson, 1968), with which we can measure the degree of radiation damage to the blood vessels by assessing the length of a rectangular skin flap that can be maintained by the damaged vessels (Patterson *et al.*, 1972; Wiernik, Berry and Patterson, 1974; Wiernik, Patterson and Berry, 1974). The skin of young pigs is relatively non-hairy, it is not completely freely mobile on the deep fascia, and, on the flank, it has a segmental pattern of blood supply which is much more like that of man than that of any other standard laboratory mammal. Three areas 16 cm long by 4 cm wide were marked out on the flank of the pig with intervening areas of 4 cm between each; these outlines were lightly scored with Indian ink and received courses of fractionated irradiation as previously described.

At varying intervals from one day to 28 weeks after the last dose of irradiation, randomly allocated treated areas were raised as conventional single pedicle skin flaps by incising round three sides and dissecting back until they were attached only by a 4 cm wide ventral pedicle. The flaps were then laid back in their beds and sutured into place. The length of the flap was designed so that even unirradiated skin flaps were too long to survive throughout their full length and the terminal part became necrotic. The 'surviving length' of flap is proportional to the blood supply through the pedicle and is dependent on the state of the inherent blood supply within the flap. The 'surviving length' could be accurately forecast immediately by the intravenous injection of a vital dye, Disulphine Blue, and the actual 'surviving length' measured at one week by determining the length between the base of the flap and the line of demarcation.

Maximum survival was seen in those flaps which were raised at short times after irradiation, but between six weeks and six months after the start of irradiation the survival of these flaps was poor, approximately 40 per cent of the control length, and varied little with time (Fig. 2.3).

From our observations it appears that pre-operative courses of irradiation should be relatively short so that the operation can be performed as soon as the acute radiation reaction has passed (Patterson *et al.*, 1974). These experimental findings in the pig correlate well with clinical practice in the treatment of carcinoma of the cervix uteri (Stallworthy, 1971).

Skin Blood-flow Measurements

Blood flow in irradiated vessels in the skin may also be quantitatively evaluated by external counting following the intradermal injection of $^{99}Tc^{m}$ using sodium iodide crystal detectors. This technique has been elaborated in our laboratory by Hopewell following reports in the literature of preliminary studies by Keyeux *et al.* (1971). The effect of the volume of injected isotope, the site of injection and the repeatability of the technique have been investigated. The curves obtained are a double exponential function from which two modes of isotope clearance can be derived (Moustafa and Hopewell, 1974).

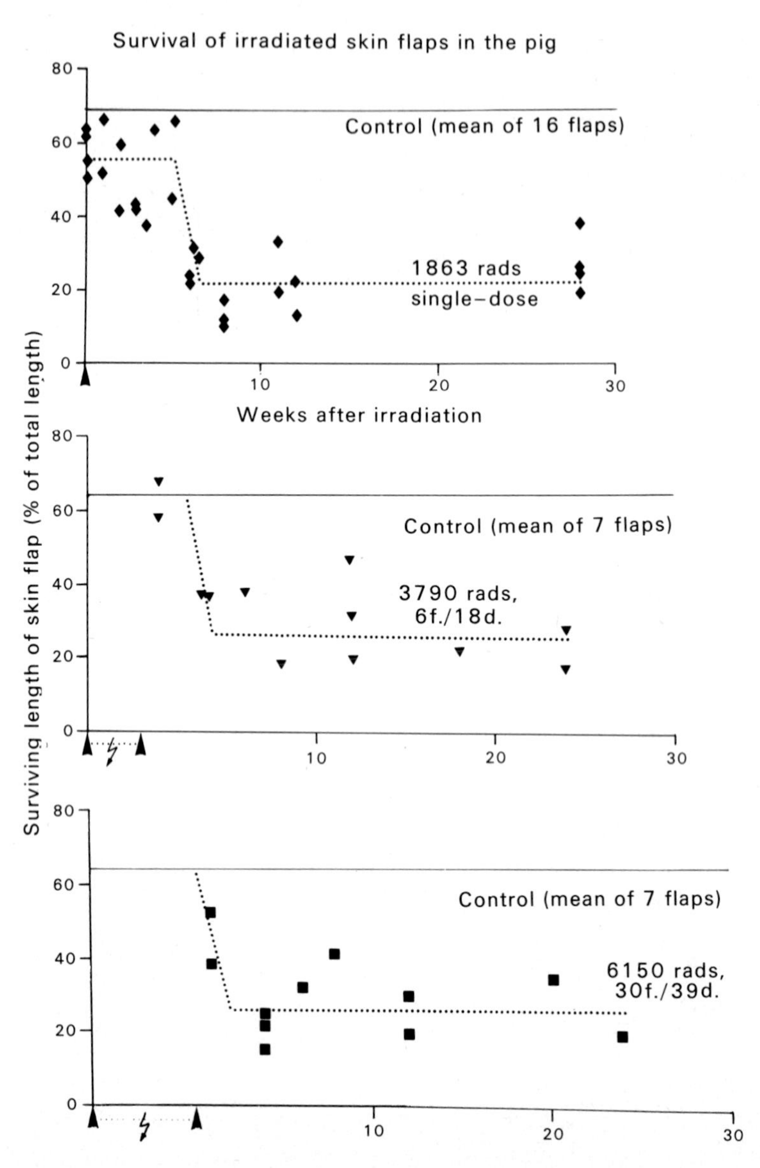

Fig. 2.3. Survival of irradiated skin flaps in the pig. Note that the time on the abscissa is given in weeks after the last irradiation but the intersection with the ordinate is at the first irradiation. The surviving length of skin flap was assessed one week after operation. (*British Journal of Radiology* 1974, **47**, 344. Reproduced by permission of the Editors.)

This method of assessment to investigate the effects of single and fractionated courses of irradiation on the blood vessels in the skin is being performed at the present time and will be correlated with the other end-points such as skin reactions, subcutaneous fibrosis, wound healing and the survival of skin flaps.

Clinical Studies

We have applied the Oxford skin scoring system to test the predictive value of the NSD system over a small range of variation in the treatment of patients with skin cancers by scoring the skin reaction in the margin of normal skin included in the irradiation field. The percentage cure rate in this form of cancer is so high that these variations did not influence the effective eradication of the tumours and so this study could not assess the predictive value of the NSD formula on tumour cure rate.

Three régimes were tested which involved three, seven or ten fractions given in the same overall time of 14 days, and our results showed that over this very limited range of variation the NSD formula was applicable, a result, which was consistent with our animal studies (Brennan, *et al.*, 1973; 1975).

Effects of Irradiation on the Kidney

Functional Studies in Pig Kidneys

Renal radiation tolerance is well below that of other tissues in the body and, because of this, restricts the radiotherapist's ability to give tumourocidal doses of irradiation to many intra-abdominal neoplasms. Whether this is due to the effect of radiation on the renal blood vessels being materially different to that on blood vessels in other organs remains to be resolved. In the first instance we have had to make the assumption that, by testing renal function, we are monitoring the effect of radiation on the renal blood vessels. We have used the radioactive renogram for this purpose and have obtained serial readings in pigs where the other, unirradiated, kidney has served as a control (Hopewell and Berry, 1974).

The position of each kidney was identified by intravenous pyelo-

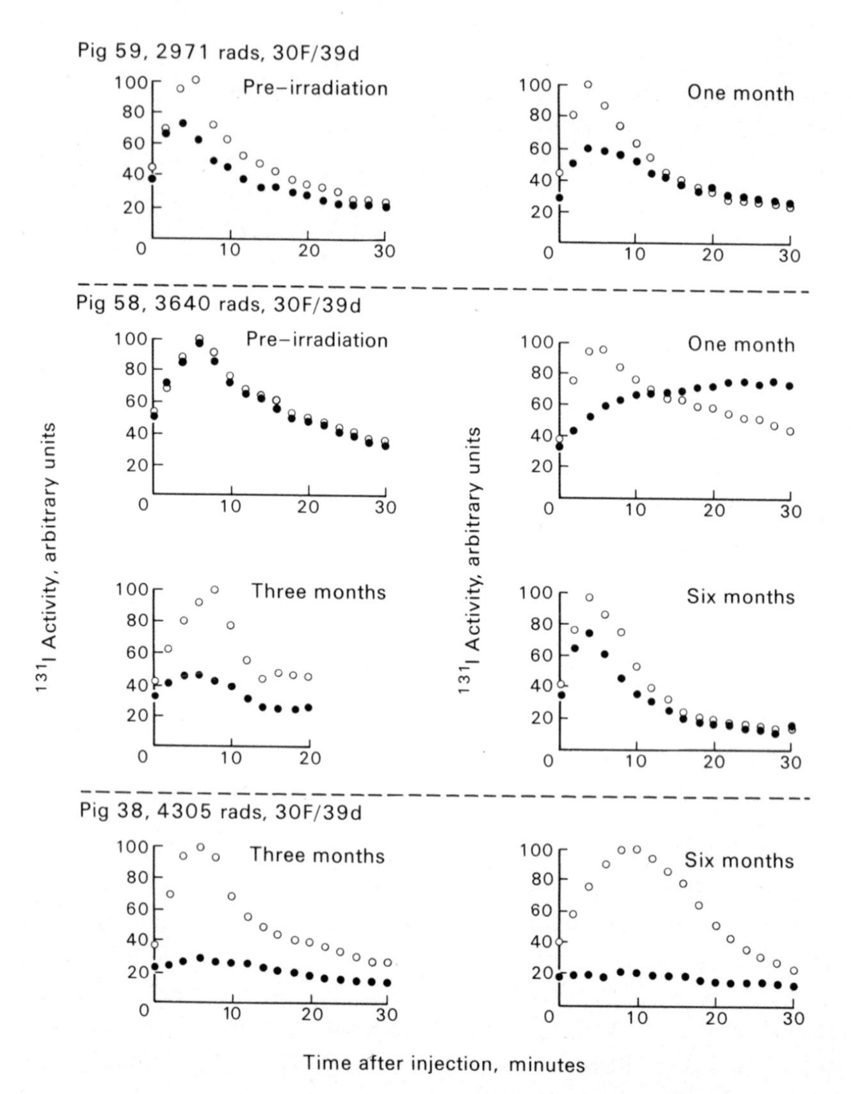

Fig. 2.4. Time-dose modification observed in radioactive renograms. The changes in renal function of Pig 58 have been compared with those of a pig receiving a 15 per cent lower dose in the upper four panels and with a 15 per cent higher dose in the lower four panels.

● right (irradiated) kidney

○ left (control) kidney

(*British Journal of Radiology* 1974, **47**, 683. Reproduced by permission of the Editors.)

graphy and that of the right kidney located, relative to the surface, by tattooing the skin with a rectangle 8 × 12 cm so that a radiation beam, set at an angle, did not include the left kidney in its path. Régimes of irradiation were employed involving single doses, six fractions in 18 days, and thirty fractions in 39 days. The middle of the kidney received 70 per cent of the surface dose, with a maximum variation in dose of 13 per cent across the kidney. A range of doses, with incremental variations above and below the dose predicted by the NSD formula, was tested.

Renography, with ^{131}I-hippurate, was performed with separate counters over each kidney and over the heart for measurement of the blood background. The scintillation detectors were connected to an electronic analysing system. Functional modifications were observed in all traces following irradiation, when compared with the non-irradiated, contralateral kidney. Each tracing represents a complex mixture of separate components that requires detailed analysis to evaluate. It seems probable that the rate at which peak isotope activity is reached reflects true vascular damage, whereas the total amount of isotope concentrated by the kidney and the rate of excretion probably reflect the functional capacity of the renal cells. Some variations in renogram tracings, related to the dose and the time factors can be seen in Fig. 2.4.

We have noted very poor correlation between the tolerance levels found experimentally and the theoretical prediction of the NSD formula. The radiation damage associated with six fractions given in 18 days is approximately 30 per cent greater than that associated with treatment in thirty fractions given over 39 days, which is exactly the opposite to that which we found in the skin when equivalent doses, based on the NSD formula, were used in both series of experiments. Whether this difference is due to irradiation effects on the blood vessels or on other specialised tissues in these organs needs to be resolved.

Morphological Studies in Pig Kidneys

Late radiation damage in the kidney is associated with a progressive diminution in the size of the affected kidney (Hopewell and Berry, 1974). Histological sections of renal tissue from specimens taken two months after irradiation showed occlusive changes in the small and large arterioles which were due to clones of endothelial cells. This would be in keeping with Hopewell's (1974) 'sausage segments' hypothesis. It has not been possible, so far, to evaluate serial sections in order to confirm the localised nature of these constrictions.

Effects of Irradiation on the Intestine

We have, in the past, been able to establish that damage due to abdominal irradiation can be quantified by analysis of the epithelial cell lining of the jejunum (Wiernik, 1966a, b, c, d, 1968). For technical reasons serial biopsies from the jejunum are difficult to obtain and so we investigated the large intestine in the hope that such specimens, which are much more readily obtainable, would allow us to evaluate different components of irradiation schedules.

Animal Studies

Large White pigs, similar to those used for our various experiments to estimate the radiation effects on blood vessels, were anaesthetised with halothane and serial rectal biopsies were taken. We have examined the influence on the epithelium of the rectal mucosa of such factors as repeated anaesthetics, the stress of enclosure in a hyperbaric oxygen chamber, the effects of a radiosensitising agent, namely hyperbaric oxygen, and the effects of fractionated courses of irradiation given in atmospheric conditions and in hyperbaric oxygen (Perrins and Wiernik, 1973, 1974; Wiernik and Perrins, 1973). We have undertaken cell counts in which we have differentiated between epithelial, goblet and mitotic cells.

We have found that there was no change in this experimental system during the period of growth of these animals from the time that the first biopsy was taken at 18 weeks up to the age of 18 months; nor was a change induced by the stress of repeated anaesthetics or enclosure in the hyperbaric chamber. On the other hand, the effect of hyperbaric oxygen alone was to increase the mitotic rate temporarily. Irradiation in air resulted in a fall in the various parameters with consequent recovery, overshoot and finally return to the pre-treatment levels. Similar irradiation in the presence of hyperbaric oxygen gave rise to qualitative differences, in that there was a persistent increase in the proportion of goblet cells but no quantitative difference was observed, which confirmed that the pig's rectal mucosa responds in a similar manner to that of human rectal mucosa.

We concluded from this that the pig's rectal mucosa would, therefore, be a suitable experimental system in which to investigate fractionation schedules which may have theoretical advantages but which it would be considered unethical to test in patients until confirmation is obtained that they do not cause an unacceptable increase in either acute or late radiation damage.

Clinical Studies

Epithelial Cell System

By analysis of the epithelial cell counts in the serial jejunal biopsy specimens obtained following courses of different fractionation régimes, we have been able to establish the pattern of response to radiation damage of the whole mucosa and of the goblet cells in particular (Wiernik and Plant, 1970, 1971). We were able to show that a single

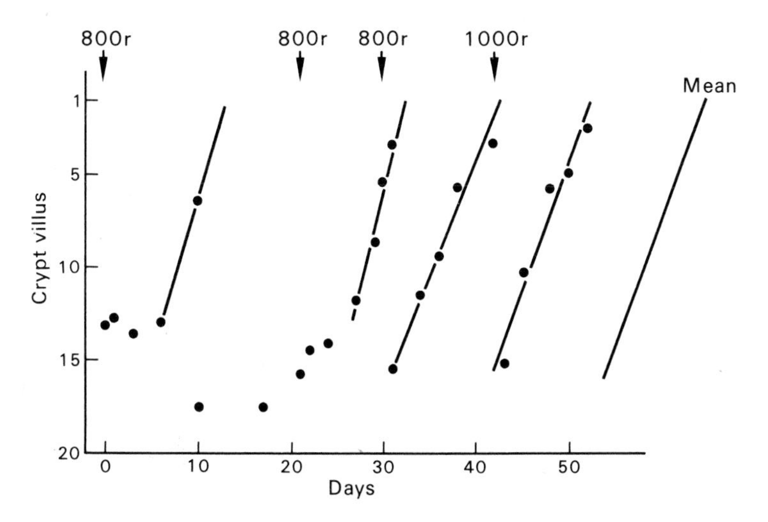

Fig. 2.5. Graph relating the position of the peaks of the cohorts of goblet cells, as they move up the side wall of the jejunal crypt and then the villus, to the time elapsed since irradiation treatment. (*British Journal of Radiology* 1971, **44**, 353. Reproduced by permission of the Editors.)

stem cell system in the crypt gave rise to cells which differentiated into either epithelial or goblet cells and that, following radiation damage, cohorts of goblet cells could be shown to migrate from the crypt up the villus (Fig. 2.5).

One of the questions that has been raised concerning the treatment of patients in a hyperbaric oxygen chamber is whether, under these circumstances, there is more radiation damage to the surrounding normal tissues as well as to the tumour. Many conflicting reports in the literature, based on statistically invalid data, led us to investigate this problem in the patients being treated for advanced carcinoma of the

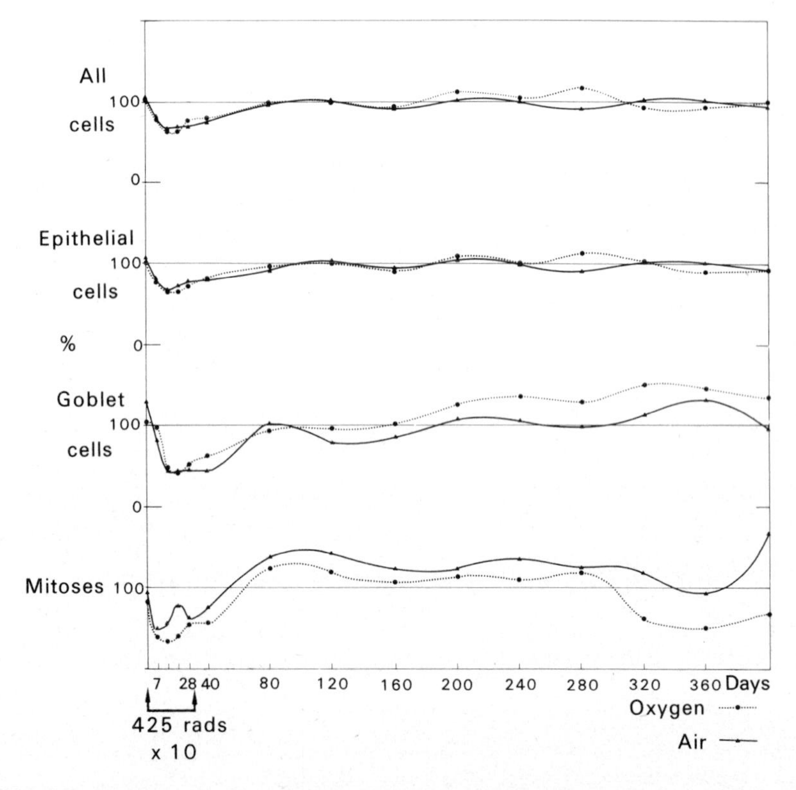

Fig. 2.6. Human rectal mucosal crypt cell counts, expressed as a percentage of the pre-treatment counts, plotted against time elapsed since commencement of irradiation treatment. (*British Journal of Radiology* 1972, **45**, 740. Reproduced by permission of the Editors.)

cervix and bladder in a randomly allocated prospective clinical trial conducted under the auspices of the Medical Research Council (Wiernik and Perrins, 1972). The treatment of the two groups was the same in all respects except that one group was irradiated while breathing air and the other group treated in an atmosphere of pure oxygen at a pressure of 3 ATA (30 psi). All patients had rectal biopsies prior to treatment and then serial rectal biopsies during the succeeding year. We were able to show that there was no quantitative difference between the two groups but only a qualitative difference when the mucosal elements were analysed in a manner similar to that described above (Fig. 2.6).

These patients have now been followed up since the start of the trial in 1968. While the mortality is virtually the same during the first 15 months, the patients treated in hyperbaric oxygen appear to be doing better from 18 months onwards, but the small numbers involved,

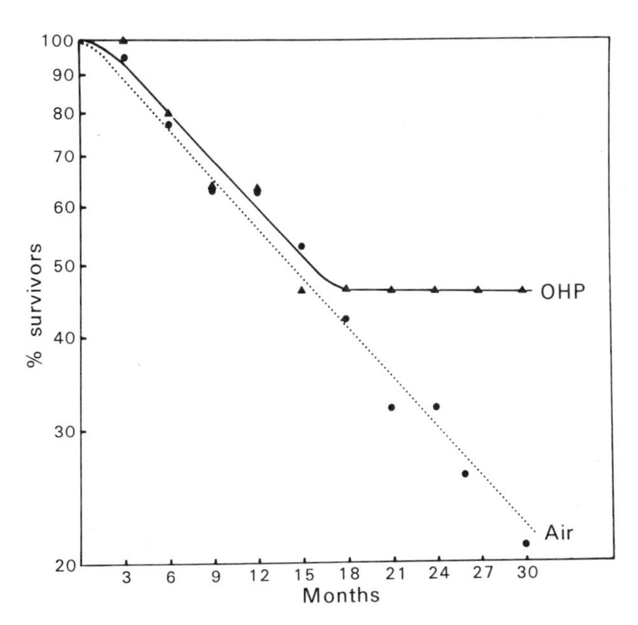

Fig. 2.7. Regression analysis of the logarithm of the proportion surviving versus time in months for patients with advanced carcinoma of the cervix uteri treated in a prospective randomly allocated trial of irradiation treatment in air or in hyperbaric oxygen at 3 ATA. (*Proceedings of the Fifth International Hyperbaric Congress* 1973, **2**, 823. Reproduced by permission of Simon Fraser University.)

thirteen patients in the hyperbaric oxygen group and nineteen patients in the air group, must be borne in mind (Fig. 2.7) (Wiernik and Perrins, 1973).

Mesenchymal Tissues

Following the report in the literature of a pericryptal fibroblast system (Pascal *et al.*, 1968) which could be quantitatively assessed, we re-examined our histological material of the serial rectal biopsies obtained from patients in the MRC hyperbaric oxygen trial and were able to identify this system readily (Fig. 2.8). Perrins devised a graticule for the light microscope with the aid of which we were able to subdivide all rectal crypts into three equal portions and to count the number of pericryptal fibroblasts in each section. Our material allowed us to examine the effects, on this cell system, of fractionated irradiation and of hyperbaric oxygen. Previous authors had claimed that this was a replicating mesenchymal cell system, the cells of which migrated in conjunction with the overlying epithelial cell system. In their studies they used tritiated thymidine to allow them to identify cell replication and movement, though the authors commented on the rarity of mitotic figures in the nuclei of this cell system (Pascal *et al.*, 1968). We have found that the cell kinetics in the pericryptal fibroblast system, following radiation damage, appear to be similar to those of the overlying epithelial cell system and yet, even during the overshoot phase of repair, we have been unable to identify any mitotic figures. Furthermore, at no time have we observed any radiation damage in the nuclei of the pericryptal fibroblasts (Wiernik and Perrins, 1975).

This mesenchymal tissue is of considerable interest as it is the only one, apart from the haemopoietic system, which may be involved in regular replication. Late radiation damage has frequently been ascribed to changes consequent upon damage of the connective tissues but so far there has been no experimental proof for this hypothesis. Further study of this system is planned to try and resolve whether the vascular system, which we are studying in detail already, or possibly the stromal tissues are responsible for the manifestations of late radiation damage with which the clinician is well acquainted, and which limit his ability to eradicate many of the cancers which kill the patient through destruction at the primary site rather than by metastatic spread.

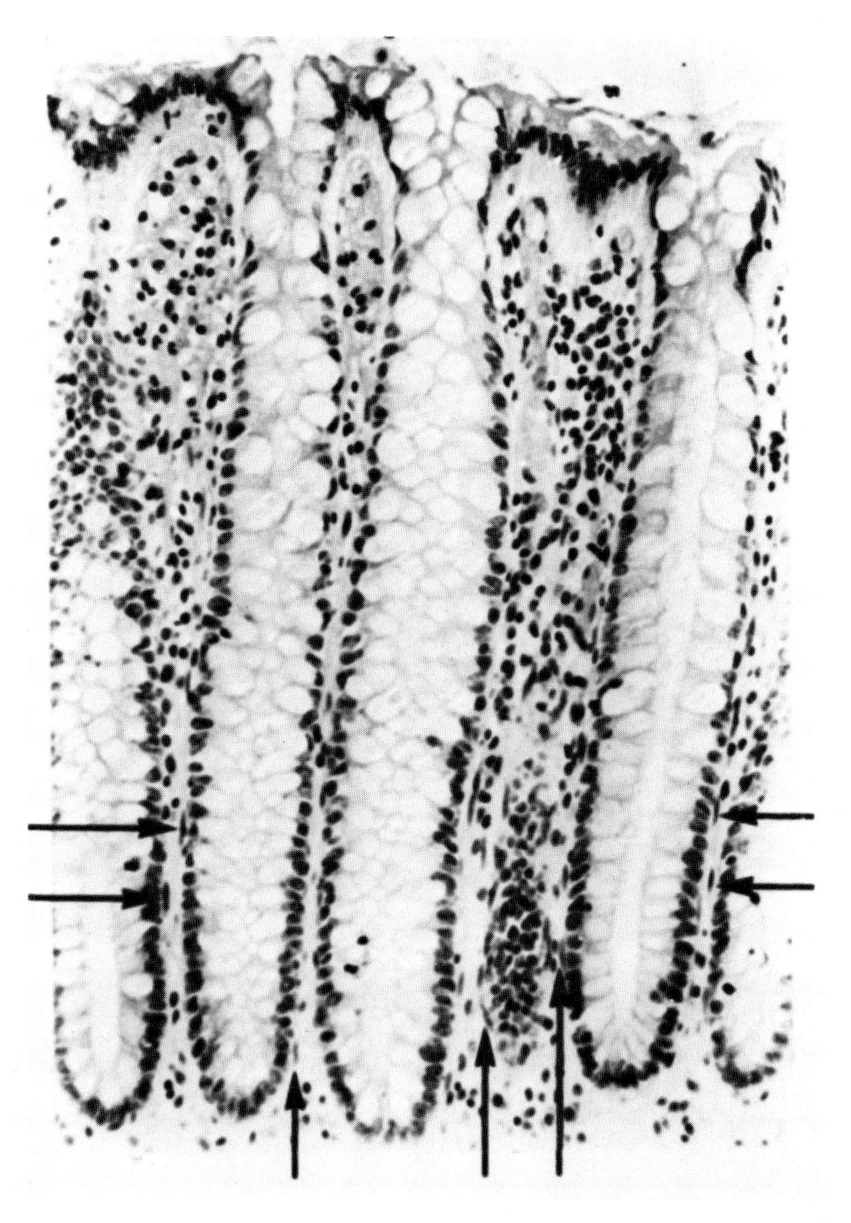

Fig. 2.8. Pericryptal fibroblasts, shown by arrows, forming a sheath round the crypts of human mucosa. (*British Journal of Radiology* 1975, **48**, 382. Reproduced by permission of the Editors.)

I wish to thank all the members of the team who are working at the Churchill Hospital Research Institute, and who are acknowledged as co-authors of papers, for their permission to use our joint work for this chapter. I also wish to express my sincere thanks to the many technicians who have helped with the treatment of the patients, the histological preparations, the animal operations, the animal care, etc., and the secretaries who have helped with the preparation of this chapter.

I am grateful to the Medical Research Council for a long-term grant under which much of this work was performed, also to Tenovus, the University of Oxford, the United Oxford Hospitals and the Department of Health and Social Security, all of whom contributed towards the cost of the Research Institute and some of whom have continued to provide financial aid.

I wish to thank Dr H. G. Frank, Consultant Radiotherapist, and Mr B. Stubbs, Senior Physicist, Regional Radiotherapy Centre, Cookridge Hospital, Leeds, who kindly provided the clinical data on skin tolerance used in their centre and at Manchester and Liverpool.

References

BERRY, R. J., WIERNIK, G. and PATTERSON, T. J. S. (1972) *British Journal of Radiology*, **45**, 793.

BERRY, R. J., WIERNIK, G. and PATTERSON, T. J. S. (1974) *British Journal of Radiology*, **47**, 185–190.

BERRY, R. J., WIERNIK, G., PATTERSON, T. J. S. and HOPEWELL, J. W. (1974) *British Journal of Radiology*, **47**, 277–281.

BEWLEY, D. K., FOWLER, J. F., MORGAN, R. L., SILVESTER, J. A., TURNER, B. A. and THOMLINSON, R. H. (1963) *British Journal of Radiology*, **36**, 107–115.

British Institute of Radiology (1963) *British Journal of Radiology*, **36**, 382–383.

British Institute of Radiology (1972) *British Journal of Radiology*, **45**, 754–756.

BRENNAN, D., YOUNG, C., HOPEWELL, J. W. and WIERNIK, G. (1973) *British Journal of Radiology*, **46**, 649–650.

BRENNAN, D., YOUNG, C. M. A., HOPEWELL, J. W. and WIERNIK, G. (1975) *Clinical Radiology*, in press.

COHEN, L. (1968) *British Journal of Radiology*, **41**, 522–528.

ELLIS, F. (1971) *British Journal of Radiology*, **44**, 101–108.

FIELD, S. B. (1969) *Radiology*, **92**, 381–384.

FOWLER, J, F. (1971) *British Journal of Radiology*, **44**, 81–90.

FOWLER, J. F., MORGAN, R. L., SILVESTER, J. A., BEWLEY, D. K. and TURNER, B. A. (1963) *British Journal of Radiology*, **36**, 188–196.

FOWLER, J. F. and STERN, B. E. (1963) *British Journal of Radiology*, **36**, 163–173.

HAYASHI, S. and SUIT, M. D. (1972) *Radiology*, **103**, 431–437.

HOPEWELL, J. W. (1974) *British Journal of Radiology*, **47**, 157–158.

HOPEWELL, J. W. and BERRY, R. J. (1974) *British Journal of Radiology*, **47**, 679–686.

HOPEWELL, J. W. and WRIGHT, E. A. (1970) *British Journal of Radiology*, **43**, 161–167.

KEYEUX, A., DUNJIC, A., RYOER, E., JOVANOVIC, D. and VAN DE MERCKT, J. (1971) *International Journal of Radiobiology*, **20**, 7–25.

LIVERSAGE, W. E. (1971) *British Journal of Radiology*, **44**, 91–100.

MOUSTAFA, H. and HOPEWELL, J. W. (1974) *Biorheology*, **11**, 208–209.

PASCAL, R. R., KAYE, G. I. and LANE, N. (1968) *Gastroenterology*, **54**, 835–851.

PATTERSON, T. J. S. (1968) *British Journal of Plastic Surgery*, **21**, 113–117.

PATTERSON, T. J. S., BERRY, R. J., HOPEWELL, J. W. and WIERNIK, G. (1974) in *Skin Flaps*, ed. Grabb and Myers. Little, Brown, Boston, Mass.

PATTERSON, T. J. S., BERRY, R. J. and WIERNIK, G. (1972) *British Journal of Plastic Surgery*, **25**, 17–19.

PERRINS, D. J. D. and WIERNIK, G. (1973) *5th International Hyperbaric Congress Proceedings*, ed. Trapp, W. G., Banister, E. W., Davison, A. J. and Trapp, P. A. (1974) Simon Fraser University, Burnaby, BC, **1**, 27–36.

PERRINS, D. J. D. and WIERNIK, G. (1975) *British Journal of Radiology*, in press.

STALLWORTHY, J. A. (1971) *Annals of the Royal College of Surgeons*, **48**, 293–305.

WIERNIK, G. (1966a) *British Journal of Radiology*, **39**, 272–279.

WIERNIK, G. (1966b) *The Journal of Pathology and Bacteriology*, **91**, 389–393.

WIERNIK, G. (1966c) *The Journal of The British Society of Gastroenterology – Gut*, **7**, 149–153.

WIERNIK, G. (1966d) *British Medical Journal*, **2**, 385–387.

WIERNIK, G. (1968) in *Gastrointestinal Radiation Injury*, ed. Sullivan, M. F. Excerpta Medica Foundation, 167–174.

WIERNIK, G. (1973) *British Medical Bulletin*, **29**, 39–43.

WIERNIK, G., BERRY, R. J. and PATTERSON, T. J. S. (1974) *British Journal of Radiology*, **47**, 830–831.

WIERNIK, G., PATTERSON, T. J. S. and BERRY, R. J. (1974) *British Journal of Radiology*, **47**, 343–345.

WIERNIK, G. and PERRINS, D. J. D. (1972) *British Journal of Radiology*, **45**, 737–744.

WIERNIK, G. and PERRINS, D. J. D. (1973) *5th International Hyperbaric Congress Proceedings*, ed. Trapp, W. G., Banister, E. W., Davison, A. J. and Trapp, P. A. (1974) Simon Fraser University, Burnaby, BC, **2**, 820–828.

WIERNIK, G. and PERRINS, D. J. D. (1975) *British Journal of Radiology*, **48**, 382–389.

WIERNIK, G. and PLANT, M. (1970) in *Current Topics in Radiation Research*, **6**, 325–368.

WIERNIK, G. and PLANT, M. (1971) *British Journal of Radiology*, **44**, 348–356.

CHAPTER THREE

Fast Neutron Therapy and the Oxygen Effect: The rationale and early clinical effects

Mary Catterall

Ionising radiations have been used for sterilisation of malignant tumours for about seventy years. They are a highly successful form of treatment for the early stages of several different cancers and are the treatment of choice in some sites, for example, the vocal cord, where a squamous cell carcinoma can be completely ablated with minimal effect on the function of the larynx in more than 75 per cent of cases. Good palliation of ulceration, bleeding and pain can be achieved, often for the remainder of the patient's life, for most primary and secondary tumours, and death from superior mediastinal obstruction need very rarely occur if X-ray or gamma-ray therapy is available. In many cases treatment can be given on an outpatient basis, and with modern machines which deliver sharply cut-off beams of radiation, nausea and sickness are much less troublesome, making a course of palliative radiation worthwhile in the great majority of cases. Nor, with the high energies of beams from modern machines, are skin reactions produced.

Success in radiotherapy depends on delivering a more destructive dose to the tumour than to the adjacent tissues which are unavoidably irradiated. Over the last half century, and particularly in the last twenty years, machines have been developed to deliver gamma rays and higher energy X-rays to achieve this purpose. These developments are described in Chapter 1. It is probable that only relatively minor refinements remain to enhance the delivery of doses of this type of ionising radiation and that progress in the future will be in exploiting and increasing the sensitivity of tumour cells and at the same time increasing the protection of normal cells. In this chapter these methods will briefly be reviewed and the rationale and clinical effects of fast neutrons described.

Among the factors which influence the sensitivity of a tumour to radiation is the degree of oxygenation at the cellular level at the time of radiation. In all cells in which this phenomenon has been investigated – the growing tips of bean roots, bacteria, malignant ascites cells and many others – more radiation is required to kill them when the surrounding oxygen tension is less than that of mixed venous blood, than when it is of the normal value of 20–40 mm Hg. Thus, hypoxia protects cells from the damaging effects and X- and gamma radiation; since many animal tumours can be shown to contain cells which are hypoxic although still able to divide, it is important to consider whether this also applies to human tumours. The work of Thomlinson and Gray (1955) shows that some tumours contain cords of cells, the centres of which are necrotic and non-viable while the peripheries are well-oxygenated, being in close proximity to a blood vessel. Between these two extremes is a zone of cells able to multiply, but in a relatively hypoxic environment and therefore protected from doses of radiation which kill the adjacent well-oxygenated cells.

The breathing of pure oxygen at atmospheric pressure is not effective in oxygenating these cells because the distance between them and the nearest blood vessel is too great for adequate diffusion of the gas; it is necessary to oxygenate the tissues themselves. The technique of giving radiotherapy while the patient is in a tank of pure oxygen at 2–3 atmospheric pressure was therefore developed. The efficacy of this method depends upon there being adequate vascularisation of the tumour by vessels which are patent. Unfortunately, tumours have abnormal and irregular vessels and thromboses are common. The original tank used by Churchill-Davidson and his colleagues was enclosed and of steel, presenting problems of claustrophobia and visualisation for the patient. The modern double-skin Perspex tank is much easier for the patient and reduces many of the technical problems.

This oxygenation technique is also extremely time-consuming, taking up to one hour to treat a patient instead of the usual 5–10 minutes, and therefore requiring extra staff. Some patients cannot tolerate the claustrophobia of the tank and a few suffer from convulsions and headache. There are many technical problems and stringent precautions have to be taken against risk of fire and explosion.

Despite these limitations, it was the opinion of Churchill-Davidson (1967) and van den Brenk (1968) that improved therapeutic results over radiotherapy given in air were obtained. Henk *et al.*, (1970), in a randomised controlled trial of tumours of the head and neck, also showed an advantage to the oxygen-treated patients. However, several other controlled clinical trials, including the first by Cade and McEwen (1967), have shown no such benefit. It is possible that the rapid metabolism of oxygen, which limits its effective distance for diffusion to 150 μm, does not allow adequate oxygenation to many of the cells, especially in the large tumours which are usually the subject of such trials.

Another way of exploiting the oxygen effect is to render the normal tissues hypoxic and deliver to the tumour a very much higher dose of radiation than could have been tolerated if the adjacent tissues had been normally oxygenated. This method is suitable only for tumours, such as sarcomas, situated in the limb, which may be rendered hypoxic by elevation and a tourniquet. However, the difficulty and uncertainty of the degree of hypoxia and the occurrence of unacceptably severe radiation effects on the normal tissues has led Suit and Lindberg (1968) to abandon this technique.

The administration of a course of radiotherapy in daily or thrice weekly treatments for a period of 2–6 weeks, which is the method adopted by the majority of centres, also exploits the beneficial effects of oxygen. In the interval between doses, the inevitably damaged normal tissues undergo some repair, oedema and waste products are removed and blood flow is improved and oxygenates malignant cells which were previously hypoxic, thus rendering them more sensitive to the next dose of radiation. It has been found by Phillips and Hanks (1968) that hypoxic cells are less able to repair sublethal damage than are well-oxygenated ones; this diminished ability is even more marked in chronically hypoxic cells such as are found in the zone surrounding the necrotic centre of a tumour (Suit and Urano, 1969). How far these findings apply to clinical practice is unknown, nor is it known what is the optimum time for each dose in a course of treatment; this probably varies with different types of tumour.

Courses of radiation are sometimes interrupted for a period of about two weeks to allow normal tissues to repair and the oxygenation of the tumour to be improved. Badib and Webster (1969) found an increased effectiveness of the radiation against the tumour on the second part of the course, but clinical trials conducted by Sambrook (1968) and Scanlon (1968) did not show any benefit after such a split course.

There are certain chemical agents which sensitise hypoxic cells to radiation by accepting electrons. One of the most used is synkavit, of which menadione is the active principle. Synkavit has been investigated since 1946 by Mitchell (1968, 1971) and Mitchell *et al.* (1965), but no definite advantages have been demonstrated.

Several chemotherapeutic agents have been used in conjunction with radiotherapy in the hope that they would sensitise the tumour; results in general are disappointing because the normal tissues are also sensitised so that reactions may be increased to an unacceptable degree. The modes of action of the most important of these agents have been reviewed by Bleehan (1973), who suggests that in future more selective sensitisers may be developed for use in sites such as the brain, but that more research is needed on the pharmokinetics of the drug and on the cycle of the malignant cell and the timing of the dose of radiation. The theoretical possibilities of sensitising malignant cells to radiation are great; the mechanisms by which sensitisers act are extremely complicated and have been well reviewed by Adams (1973). He classifies sensitisers which have been used on bacterial systems into five groups: those which suppress the S–H compounds, those that form toxic products such as cuprous ions, those inhibiting repair processes, those which become incorporated with DNA and those which mimic oxygen. He considers that the last-named group, which includes the electron affinic compounds, probably holds out most promise for increasing the effects of X- or gamma radiation in the treatment of patients with cancer.

Gray *et al.* (1953) found that X-rays had much more effect in retarding and inhibiting the growth of cells when they were in an oxygenated rather than a hypoxic environment, but that this protection by hypoxia was significantly less when neutron radiation was used. Therefore, as many animal tumours (and probably also some human tumours) contain hypoxic cells, there is reason to expect greater effects against tumours when neutrons are used. This is the established rationale for the use of fast neutrons.

The Biological Action of Fast Neutrons

Neutrons are heavy, uncharged particles found in the nucleus of the atom; they were discovered by Chadwick in 1932. They are produced with sufficient intensity for radiotherapy when a positively charged atom, for example deuterium, is accelerated by the magnetic field of a cyclotron and is then made to hit a beryllium target. The neutrons so produced can be collimated precisely and used as beams for treating tumours.

Fast neutrons interact with matter in a totally different way from X-rays and gamma rays. The latter interact with atomic electrons; the electron recoils have relatively long ranges and lose energy by producing ionisation rather sparsely along their tracks. Neutrons, on the other hand, interact with atomic nuclei, producing nuclear recoils in the form

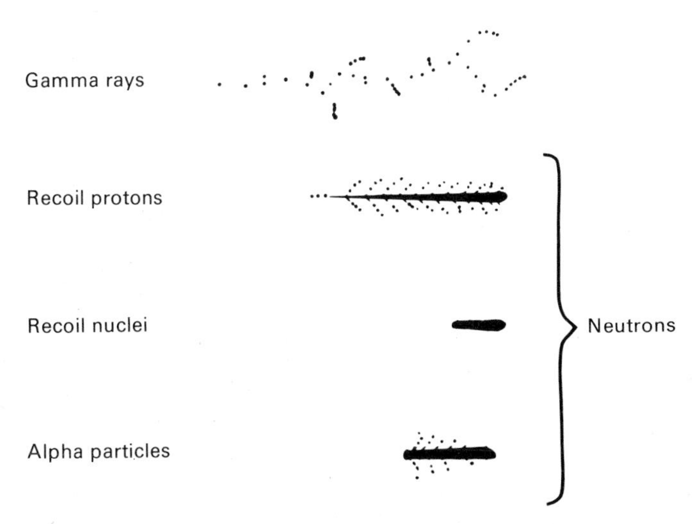

Fig. 3.1. Ionisation tracks of gamma rays (low LET) and of fast neutrons (high LET). Fast neutron radiation also contains some gamma ray ionisation.

of protons, alpha particles and nuclei of carbon and oxygen. These have much shorter ranges and ionise densely along their tracks (see Fig. 3.1). The density of ionisation along the tracks is described as 'linear energy transfer' (LET). X-rays and gamma rays are referred to as 'low LET radiation' and neutrons as 'high LET radiation'. In general, the higher the LET the less marked is the enhancing effect of oxygen and the greater is the relative biological effectiveness (RBE). A great deal of radiobiological work has been done on these phenomena and the literature has been reviewed by Bewley (1973).

Fast neutrons were first used in the treatment of cancer by Stone in 1938, only six years after the discovery of the neutron and before á radiobiological rationale was known. The cyclotron was at Berkeley in California, where he treated more than 200 patients between the years 1938 and 1944 (Stone *et al.*, 1940; Stone and Larkin, 1942; Stone, 1948). Although some cures of extremely advanced tumours were, surprisingly, obtained, the effects on the adjacent normal tissues were too severe to be acceptable. Treatment was therefore abandoned in 1948 and this effectively put an end to further investigation in the USA.

However, in the United Kingdom, the mechanism of the biological action of fast neutrons was being studied experimentally (Gray *et al.*, 1940; Gray and Read, 1942) and differences in the responses of biological systems to fast neutrons compared with X-rays and gamma rays were discovered (Gray and Read, 1944). Mitchell (1946) pointed out that the results of the American clinical investigation could not be regarded as conclusive for several reasons, including unsatisfactory data on the measurement of the doses used and the selection of patients with such advanced disease as to prevent adequate assessment of the effects of fast neutrons. It was suggested that the possible usefulness of fast neutrons in malignant disease should be fully investigated. The Medical Research Council decided to install a cyclotron in Hammersmith Hospital, London, for the exclusive purpose of medical research and the reinvestigation of fast neutrons in the treatment of cancer. The building of this machine was started in 1950.

Ten years of physical and radiobiological research on cells, mice, rats and pigs on the Hammersmith cyclotron preceded any treatment of patients. During that time, differences in the relative biological effects of neutrons and low LET photons were found (Field *et al.*, 1968; Thomlinson, 1968; Field, 1969) and this and other work (Sheline *et al.*, 1971) gave an explanation for the severe effects on normal tissues which Stone had experienced.

It was also found that, following a dose of fast neutrons, much less repair of cellular damage took place than after a dose of X-rays or gamma rays. Extensive work was done to compare the effects of neutrons and X-rays on the skin of pigs (Bewley *et al.*, 1963). Pigs were used because their skin resembles that of man in having fat, hair follicles and sweat glands. It is also pink so that varying degrees of erythema can easily be seen and can be measured objectively. The radiations were given in six fractions, thus mimicking a normal treatment technique. This work showed for the first time that when six fractions of neutrons were used, the effect increased by a factor of 1·3. Stone had used many more fractions than this on his patients and so had effectively overdosed them by at least a factor of 1·3. This work was essential for sufficient understanding of neutrons to allow patients to be treated.

The Development of a Treatment Technique

The present investigation at the Hammersmith Hospital to assess the clinical value of fast neutrons was started in 1969 and since then about 100 patients have been treated each year.

Since 1972, three cyclotrons in the USA have been made available for the treatment of patients. While having the advantage of more energetic and therefore more penetrating beams of neutrons than the Hammersmith cyclotron, none of these machines is situated within a hospital and patients have to travel up to 200 miles for each treatment. However, clinical investigations have begun in all these centres. In the United Kingdom, the Medical Research Council and Cancer Research Council are installing a cyclotron at the Western Hospital in Edinburgh. Two other neutron generators, one at Manchester and one in Glasgow, were installed for the Department of Health and Social Security four and two years ago respectively, but technical difficulties have so far prevented the production of an adequate output of neutrons. Other clinical trials are now being conducted, or planned, in Japan,

East and West Germany, Holland and Belgium. Only preliminary reports are so far available from these centres; thus the clinical results to be discussed here are those from Hammersmith Hospital.

The fast neutron beam from the cyclotron is fixed and horizontal and is therefore technically inferior to modern supervoltage X-ray and gamma ray machines which can rotate completely round a patient who lies supine for treatment. With a fixed horizontal beam, the patient

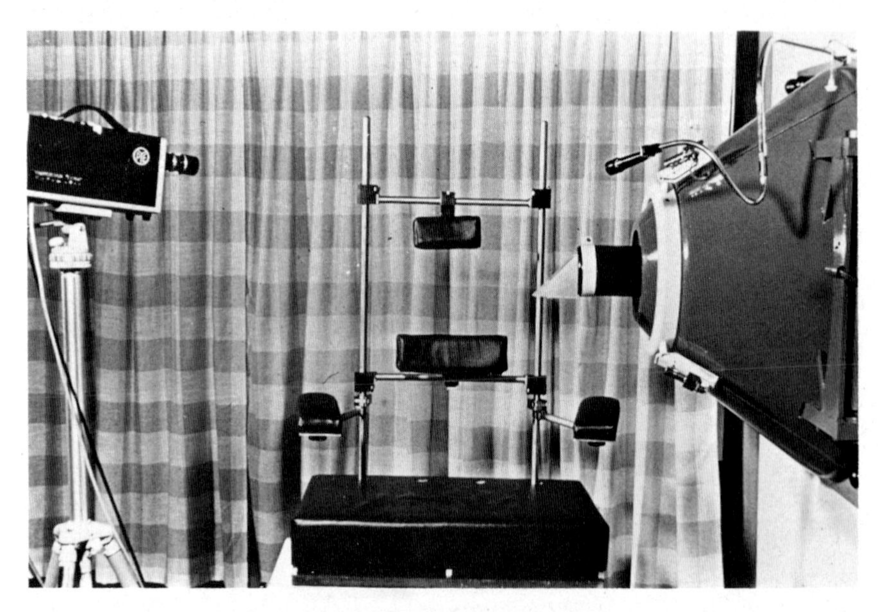

Fig. 3.2. The cone from which a fixed horizontal beam of neutrons is precisely directed to point of entry into the patient's tumour.

usually sits or stands for treatment in a specially constructed support which can be virtually built around each individual to keep him comfortably immobilised in the correct position in the beam (Fig. 3.2). This support is on a pedestal which can be raised or lowered with precision and rotated through 360°, but when necessary the patient can be treated supine or prone on a couch which can be tilted 15° either side of the horizontal. Once special techniques are developed, the fixed horizontal beam, for the majority of patients, is an inconvenience rather than a handicap. It does present difficulties, however, where there are marked anatomical deformities either from kyphosis or from radical surgery such as block dissections of the neck (see Fig. 3.3). Because the output of neutrons is high, treatment times are of the order of four minutes, so the patient does not have to maintain the position for an intolerable time.

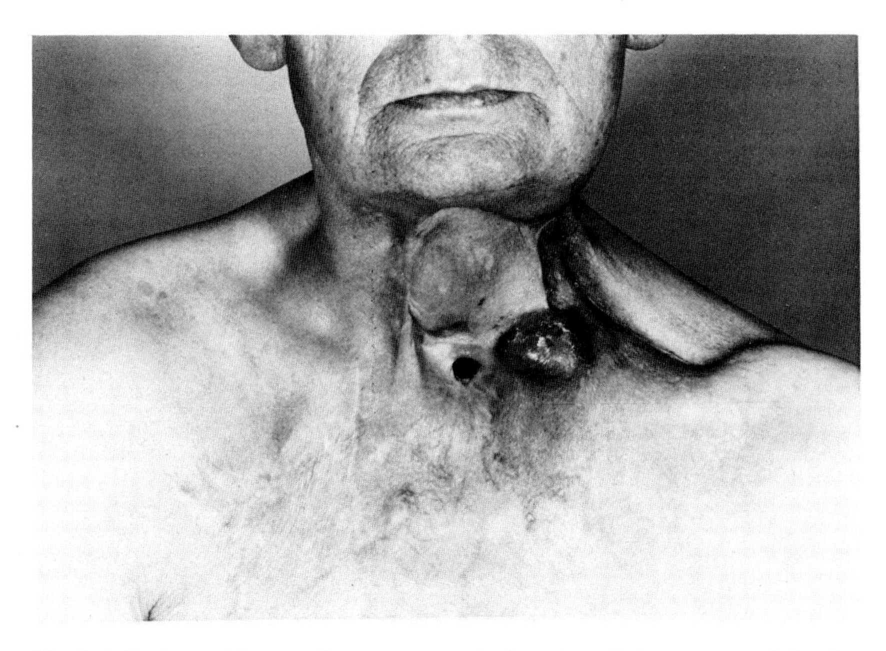

Fig. 3.3. Patient with recurring tumour and distortion of the anatomy following block dissection, causing difficulties in delivering the full dose of neutrons to the tumour.

The greatest disadvantage of the beam is its modal energy of 7·5 MeV neutrons which results in a relatively poor penetration to the tissues. At a depth of 8 cm only 50 per cent of the neutron dose is delivered, compared with 70 per cent from a cobalt source or 80 per cent from a 6 MeV linear accelerator. It is therefore considerably more difficult to deliver a uniformly high dose to tumours, especially where these are large or deeply situated. Even using the convergence of five or six beams, tumours in the abdominal or pelvic cavities cannot be

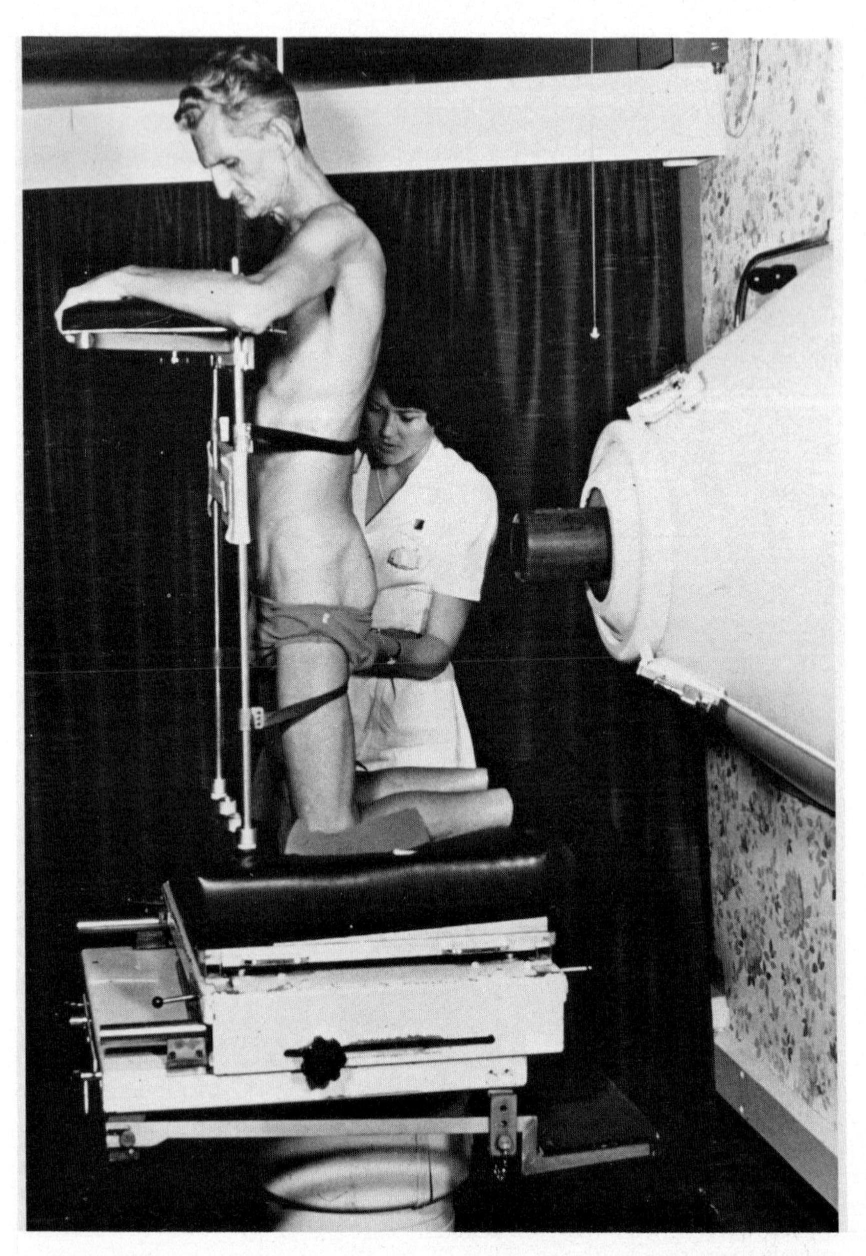

Fig. 3.4. Slim patient with pelvic tumour receiving treatment in the kneeling position.

adequately irradiated except in slim patients and these must be able to stand, kneel or sit for their treatment (Fig. 3.4).

From the radiobiological data, especially the work on pigs' skin, it was known that this beam of neutrons would cause a skin reaction. It thus differs markedly from supervoltage X-rays and gamma rays which, because of their greater penetration, have their maximum effect 1–4 mm below the skin surface and therefore do not produce an erythema, being described as having a 'skin-sparing' effect. The maximum reaction on the skin is produced by 250 kV X-rays, with which a great deal of clinical experience has been obtained so that they provided a useful comparison for the effects of the neutrons. From the radiobiological data, it was known that the relative biological effectiveness of the neutrons for skin was about three times that of 250 kV X-rays.

In view of Stone's experience of necrosis of skin and subcutaneous tissues, it was essential to find a dose of neutrons which would be effective against tumours but would cause a skin reaction from which recovery would be complete. For the investigation of this, patients suffering from multiple metastases were treated with neutrons and with 250 kV X-rays, some nodules receiving neutrons and others X-rays. A total of 35 such patients was treated, having between them 67 areas treated with neutrons and 29 with X-rays. The total neutron dose ranged from 1296 to 1890 rad, and of X-rays from 3000 to 4500 rad, all areas being treated three times weekly for four weeks. Finally, a total neutron dose of 1560 rad was selected; this caused the disappearance of the skin tumours and a skin reaction which healed in all cases (Catterall *et al.*, 1971). This dose is approximately equivalent to 6300 rad gamma rays given in thirty treatments over forty days. Since then all patients have received this standard dose of 1560 rad given in twelve treatments over four weeks. Slight modifications are made if the overall time has to be changed to accommodate the cyclotron's twice-yearly week of maintenance, or because the patient has suffered an intercurrent illness. Four hundred patients have now been treated with this dose so that a great deal of information has been obtained about its effects on a wide variety of tumours and many different normal tissues.

Because this was a new method of treatment with a beam that was technically inferior to megavoltage machines, only patients with very advanced tumours, whose chances of cure by any other means could not be compromised, were treated. This has resulted in many deaths from metastases and a short follow-up in the majority of cases. Most of the data are therefore on the early regression of tumours and the early reactions of normal tissues.

General Review of Response to Treatment

There has been a remarkably consistent regression of large tumours and no histological type has so far failed to respond. Although death from metastases has occurred within six months of treatment in 60 per cent of patients, the tumour had completely disappeared or was shrinking at the time of death in 92 per cent of these. The times taken for regression have been very variable, some poorly-differentiated tumours having completely disappeared before the end of the month's treatment; this is, of course, frequently observed with other forms of radiotherapy. Well-differentiated adenocarcinomas and amelanotic melanomas, on the other hand, have sometimes been extremely slow to regress; where these have been in sites where accurate measurements can be made at frequent intervals, a policy of close observation has been adopted. Some have taken six months to disappear completely, but the completeness of regression of tumours has been one of the most striking findings (Fig. 3.5). There has been failure to cure, leaving residual or recurrent tumours, in 9 per cent of cases treated, but half of these were associated with a low dose.

Regression of the treated tumour has been associated with a consistent relief of pain in all sites and all types of tumour. In only 10 per cent of the very advanced tumours have symptoms not been relieved in the treated area. Half of those who did not have relief of symptoms had tumours in the abdominal or pelvic cavity and it was possible that the symptoms were arising from an untreated part of the growth or from metastases.

Necrosis has occurred in 12 per cent of the treated areas in those patients who lived more than six months after treatment. This is a higher rate than is generally considered acceptable by megavoltage radiation and it is necessary to examine this incidence in detail. In no case was the necrosis unexplained or unexpected and a precipitating factor was present in each case; Stone's experience of severe necrosis

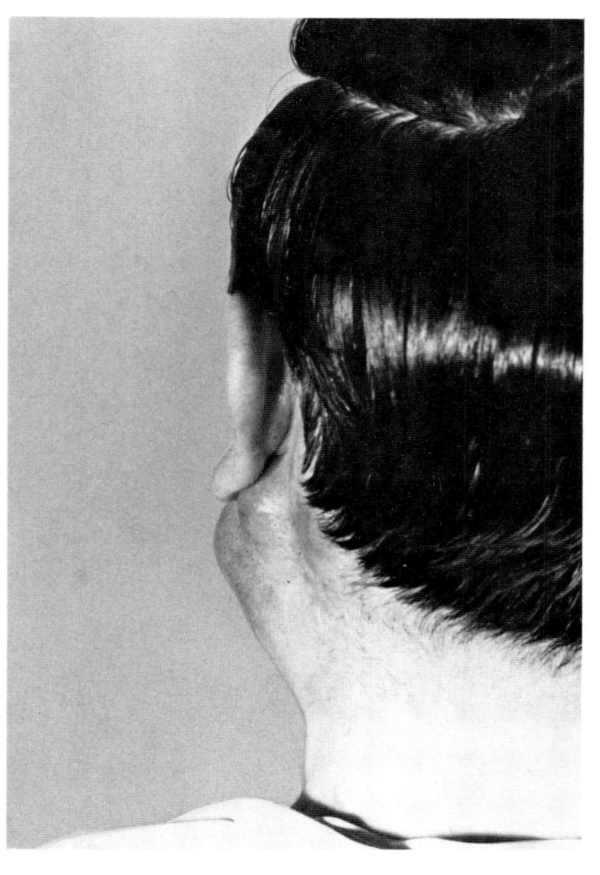

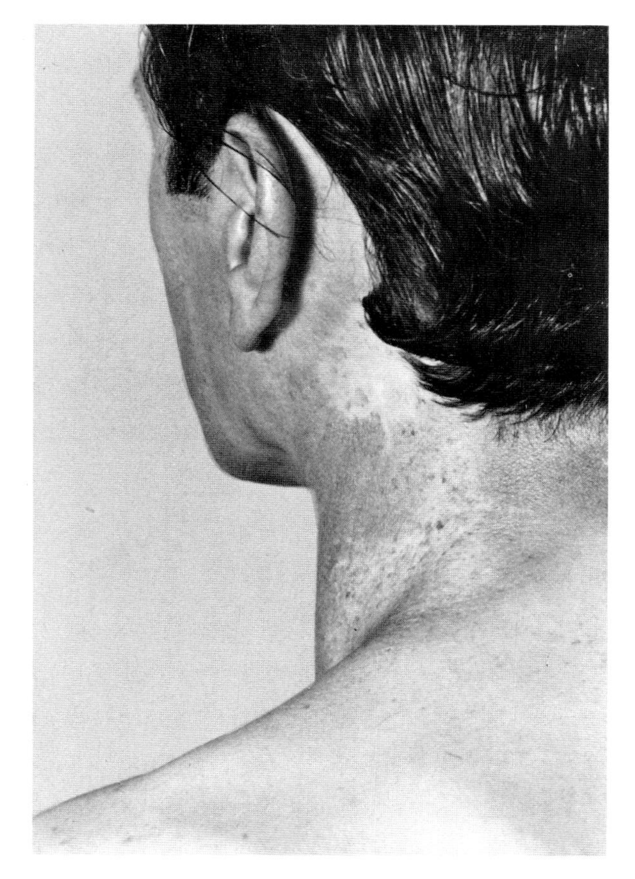

Fig. 3.5. a Patient with fixed mass of glands from a melanotic melanoma initially measuring 12 × 11 × 6 cm. b One year later, no sign of tumour in the treated area but metastases in the lungs and liver.

arising without apparent cause has not been shared. The precipitating factors included: previous irradiation or previous surgery to the area being treated by neutrons; a tumour which was already invading the skin; very large tumours requiring skin areas of 400 cm^2 or more to be treated, resulting in uneven dose-distribution so that some areas received doses of the order of 2000 rad. Lack of care of the skin leading to infection, and trauma by friction from corsets, were also factors which caused breakdown of epithelial surfaces and in some cases necrosis of subcutaneous tissues. When a precipitating factor is present, the patient is seen, before treatment starts, with the plastic surgeon and the probability of a skin graft is explained to him. Three necrotic ulcers, each 10 mm deep, healed with antibiotic ointments, eusol cleaning and breathing of 90 per cent oxygen at atmospheric pressure for about 8 hours each day. An ulcer at the posterior part of the tongue improved markedly after 13 hours in a hyperbaric oxygen tank.

If necrosis seems unavoidable, the site is of critical importance in assessing its acceptability. Skin and subcutaneous necrosis, although painful while infected, can usually be healed or can be covered by plastic surgical repair. But necrosis of even a centimetre of cervical cord is unacceptable because it produces a transverse myelitis. Necrosis of the posterior part of the tongue and epiglottis may result in aspiration of liquids and be very difficult or impossible to heal or to cover.

Effects on Specific Tumours

The numbers of histologically similar tumours which have been treated are relatively small, because the initial policy was to treat and observe a wide spectrum of advanced tumours which had already recurred after radiation, chemotherapy or hormone therapy, or were inoperable and thought unlikely to respond satisfactorily to other forms of radiation. There is no consensus as to which, if any, tumours are resistant to X- and gamma radiation; complete regression is occasionally seen in advanced stages of every histological type. Randomised controlled clinical trials need to be carried out in order to ascertain statistically the optimum treatment for a particular stage and type of tumour. Until the results of such trials are available, comparisons can only be made with previous clinical experiences. Within the limitations of these comparisons, the regressions caused by fast neutrons to advanced tumours in the salivary glands, the buccal cavity and the stomach have been noteworthy. Sarcoma in various sites have all regressed and there has been only one recurrence to date. Invasions of lymphatic glands by adenocarcinoma, melanoma and squamous cell carcinoma have also disappeared completely.

Salivary Gland Tumours

Twelve patients suffered from these tumours, of which five were adenoid cystic, three mucoepidermoid, two adenocarcinoma and two were poorly differentiated carcinoma. One adenocarcinoma had received 5000 rad of gamma rays from ^{60}Co but the tumour recurred and was fungating when neutron therapy was given. All the tumours were fixed deeply and eight were also invading the skin. Eight of the tumours could be contained within two fields of 100 cm^2, but in five the tumours were large and required fields of 170 cm^2. Pain was a dominant symptom in eleven of the patients.

Pain, trismus and fungation when present were relieved in all cases. There had been complete paralysis of the seventh nerve in three patients for more than a year but this was improved in only one. In one patient, where this had been present for only two months, neutron therapy restored this function when the tumour regressed.

There was complete regression of the tumour in every case.

Depilation of the treated skin followed the erythema and dry desquamation of the acute reaction in every case, but there was no necrosis of the skin, bone or subcutaneous tissue. Dry mouth and diminution of taste lasted for about three months after treatment and returned nearly to normal in each case.

None of the tumours has recurred and the follow-up periods since treatment have been 12–40 months. Two patients died of metastases with no sign of tumour in the treated area, one year after treatment, and two others after six months.

The patient whose adenocarcinoma recurred after cobalt treatment died of metastases five months after neutron therapy. Autopsy revealed no tumour in the treated area, to which a skin graft had been successfully applied.

Neutron therapy benefited all the patients treated and there were no unacceptable side-effects. All these salivary gland tumours were inoperable, but their volume was among the smallest of the tumours treated. These tumours usually only respond partially to X-rays and the total regression in each of the twelve treated may be in part due to their relatively small size and their accessibility to the delivery of a uniform dose of neutrons. If this is so, better results might be expected if other tumours of relatively small size were treated or if a beam of neutrons with a higher energy was available so that deep-seated tumours could be irradiated with a uniform dose.

Buccal Cavity and Oropharynx

Tumours in these two sites have rather different responses to treatment, but in the neutron-treated cases the tumours were so large that it was usually impossible to say where they had originated. There were 23 patients and 15 of them also had fixed nodes. The tumours were all squamous-celled carcinomas and 17 were well differentiated.

The patients' symptoms were of marked severity, and the consistent relief of pain, healing of ulceration and resumption of eating were striking. Fourteen were alive with no sign of tumour six months after treatment; nine had died, but five of these had no sign of tumour in the treated area. One year after treatment, nine were still alive and tumour-free. Three others had died but without local tumour being present.

A longer follow-up is required before conclusions can be drawn about recurrence and necrosis rates, but on the present data it appears that fast neutrons should be considered in all cases except very early tumours (Stage T_1), where the results of megavoltage radiation or surgery are good. A report of the first 100 cases of advanced tumours in all sites of the head and neck has been published (Catterall and Vonberg, 1974).

Stomach

Thirty-nine patients with inoperable, recurrent or residual adenocarcinoma of the stomach were treated. Vomiting during treatment to this region with other forms of radiation is usually severe, but it was very rarely observed with fast neutrons and nausea was easily controlled with antiemetics. Symptoms of pain, dysphagia and pyloric obstruction were relieved. An early improvement in appetite later relapsed in most patients. Patients with poorly differentiated tumours and *linitis plastica* died with generalised disease: neutrons, which are a strictly localised treatment, seemed inappropriate for what was, or soon became, a widely disseminated disease.

Tumours of well or moderately well differentiated adenocarcinoma which were palpable on clinical examination disappeared following fast neutron therapy. Barium meals and gastroscopic appearances remained extremely abnormal and diagnostic of recurrent or residual neoplasms. However, autopsy examinations in fourteen cases revealed no macroscopic tumour in ten, and relatively few malignant cells were found microscopically. In the one case where gastrectomy was performed six months after neutron therapy, the anastomoses healed satisfactorily although the tissues had been irradiated. In four of five others who were operated on, healing of the irradiated skin was normal. The irradiated and macroscopically tumour-free stomachs have been anatomically very abnormal with fibrosis and oedema of the walls and submucosal haemorrhages. It was suggested (Catterall and Vonberg, 1974) that a policy of neutron therapy, followed by gastrectomy, be adopted for moderately or well differentiated adenocarcinomas of the stomach where the growth has not metastasised and can be included in the volume covered by converging beams of fast neutrons. The results from this form of management are not yet available.

Sarcomas

Twenty patients with very extensive sarcomas were treated, all of which involved adjacent skin or bone. Five of these tumours were well-differentiated fibrosarcomata, two were leiomyosarcoma, two chondrosarcoma and two osteosarcoma. Three of the patients had tumours which had recurred after a previous full course of megavoltage radiation. Six others had rather poorly-differentiated fibro- or liposarcoma which were extremely large and advanced. In five the sacral area was involved, in two the antra, and in the rest the tumours were in the groin, thigh or leg.

When neutron treatment was started, these patients had no sign of metastases; pain, fungation and large masses were the main symptoms.

None of these twenty tumours failed to regress, but regression was incomplete in four patients who died of metastases less than six months after treatment and whose tumours were reducing in size at this time. Complete clinical regression occurred in sixteen cases and this was confirmed by biopsy in five. One patient's leg was amputated and a few recognisable tumour cells were seen in the bone but there were none in the soft tissues. At autopsy in another case, some residual cells were seen in the bone but not in the soft tissues. Six patients were alive and well 10–30 months after treatment. Pain was relieved completely in every case.

Complications of necrosis of skin and subcutaneous tissues were seen in six patients whose tumours were very large and were infiltrating or frankly ulcerating the skin before treatment. Previous surgery and radiotherapy, or both, had devitalised the tissues in three of these patients. These recurrent tumours disappeared after neutron therapy and skin grafts were successfully applied to two. The patients were well and without cancer, two years later. Twelve patients died of generalised metastases less than one year after neutron therapy. The fact that all these large tumours responded to neutrons, that none has recurred so far and that two regressed completely after previous radiation had failed, compares well with results obtained with chemotherapy. It also suggests that treatment with fast neutrons should be considered before submitting the patient to surgery which, for these tumours, is often mutilating.

Comparison of the Effects of Megavoltage Radiation and Fast Neutrons

The early results of fast neutrons are encouraging and suggest that the advantages indicated by all the experimental animal data are being demonstrated in the treatment of malignant tumours in man. However, to avoid unjustifiable optimism for the future of any treatment in cancer and to analyse its effects on tumours and on normal tissues, it is necessary for comparison to be made as strictly as possible with existing methods.

In comparing the clinical effects of the two modalities under consideration (high and low LET radiation), the treatment of metastatic nodules in the same patient has certain values; for example, the environment of the tumours is the same and so, usually, are the histological appearances. Also, in general, external factors such as drugs and diet will have equal effects on the tumours, leaving differences in regression as due to the treatment administered. However, these patients have a very short prognosis and so cannot be observed long enough for recurrences or necrosis to appear. The tumours most readily seen and measured are in the skin and subcutaneous tissue, do not involve other structures and are easy to irradiate with a uniform dose. Thus they are not representative of the tumours which give rise to the greatest difficulty in radiotherapy treatment and on which data concerning new treatments are required. Nevertheless, they do give some idea of the effect of these two modalities.

Measurements of treated nodules were made on all the early patients in the investigation at Hammersmith and in all cases those treated with neutrons responded as well as or better than those treated with X-rays. The respective measurements, expressed as percentages of the pre-treatment size, of the nodules from an oat-cell carcinoma of the bronchus treated with neutrons and with X-rays are shown in Fig. 3.6.

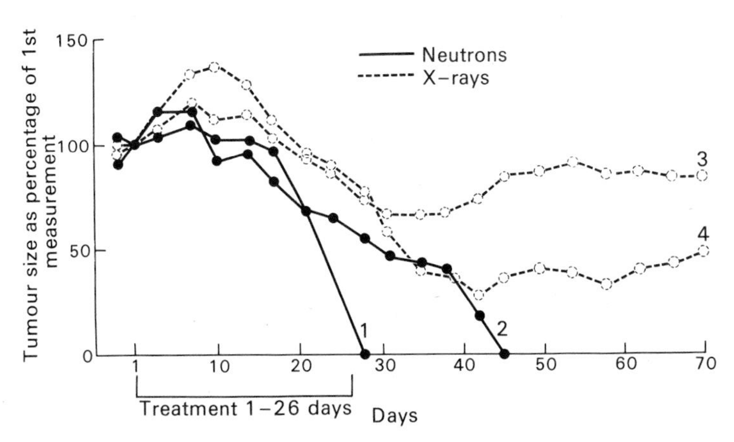

Fig. 3.6. Serial measurements of tumours following treatments show that the neutron-treated tumours disappeared while those treated with X-rays regressed, but were growing again at the patient's death 70 days later.

The neutron-treated tumours regressed completely and did not recur, whereas the X-ray-treated nodules became smaller but did not disappear, and were regrowing at the patient's death 70 days later.

A longer follow-up was obtained in the case shown in Fig. 3.7. This patient's tumours were both cystic basal cell carcinomas measuring

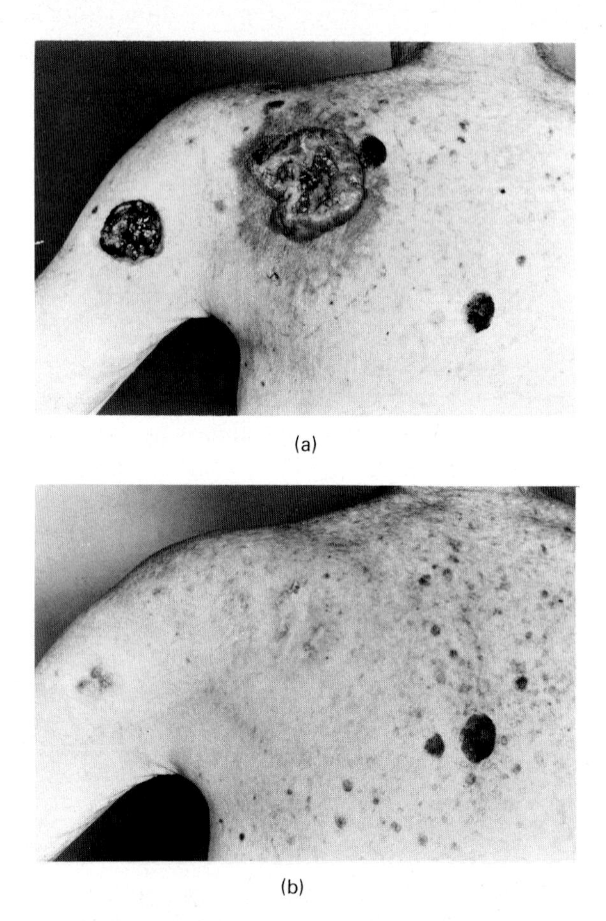

(a)

(b)

Fig. 3.7. a Patient with two large cystic basal cell carcinomas. 5080 rad X-rays given in thirteen fractions over 35 days to the tumour on the arm and 1585 rad neutrons given in twelve fractions over 33 days to the tumour on the scapula produced equivalent skin reactions.
b Eighteen months later, the X-ray treated tumour had recurred but the neutron-treated area had no sign of tumour.

63 × 63 × 3 mm and 40 × 38 × 6 mm; bleeding was a marked feature, necessitating three blood transfusions. The tumour on the left scapula was treated with 1585 rad of neutrons in twelve fractions over 33 days and that on the left arm was treated concurrently with 250 kV X-rays. Because there was less skin reaction after twelve treatments on the X-ray-treated tumour, a thirteenth treatment was given, the total dose being 5080 rad in thirteen treatments over 35 days. The skin reactions were scored and that on the arm was greater than in the neutron-treated area. Both tumours completely disappeared and the patient remained well with no clinical sign of tumour for 19 months. A recurrence was then suspected in the centre of the X-ray-treated area, and a biopsy was positive for cystic basal cell carcinoma. In this case, therefore, there was a clear advantage to the neutron-treated tumour, which was originally the larger of the two; not only had it not recurred when the X-ray-treated tumour had, but the damage to the surrounding normal skin was less.

Because radiotherapists hold different views on the optimum dose for a given tumour, it may be argued by some that the X-ray dose given here was too low; others would, however, think it was high, and yet others would think it was correct. It was undoubtedly within a range that is considered therapeutic. In the context of the comparison with the neutron-treated tumour, the skin reaction produced by the X-rays was at least as great as that produced by the neutrons and yet, for this degree of damage to normal tissues, the treatment to the tumour was less effective.

A randomised clinical trial is being conducted to compare treatments in advanced tumours of the head and neck using megavoltage or neutron therapy. The tumours must be Stage T_3 or T_4 with or without involvement of regional nodes, or Stage T_1 or T_2 with inoperable nodes. This is a multi-centre trial between hospitals in London, Birmingham and South-East England.

The results of the first 100 randomised cases show a statistically significant advantage to the neutron-treated patients in the incidence of complete regression of tumour. This was observed in 31 (62 per cent) of the 50 neutron-treated patients and in 15 (30 per cent) of the 50 supervoltage patients. Using the Peto test, which takes into account the short period observation of some patients, $P = 0{\cdot}001$. Of the fifteen megavoltage patients whose local tumour regressed completely, seven patients later showed recurrence. In contrast, there was no recurrence among the 31 neutron-treated patients whose tumours completely regressed (Catterall *et al.*, 1975).

Despite the local advantages from fast neutrons, there was no long-term gain to these patients because of deaths from metastases and other causes such as cardiovascular accidents. This trial is continuing.

Conclusion

On present evidence it seems unlikely that radiation will be displaced as the major and most useful method of sterilising malignant masses which are not freely mobile and surgically removable, and fast neutrons appear to be an important advance in the treatment of some of these tumours. Stone's words of 1944: 'The general impression . . . is that marked tumour regressions are being produced when they are not expected', remain valid today. They have added importance in view of the techniques and data which have since been acquired and through which the unacceptable side-effects of the American trial are being avoided. More information is required on the long-term effects and this will come from the treatment of earlier cases which have not metastasised, and from the increasing availability of fast neutron sources throughout the world.

References

ADAMS, G. E. (1973) *British Medical Bulletin*, **29**, 48–53.

BADIB, A. O. and WEBSTER, J. H. (1969) *Acta radiologica (Therapy, Physics, Biology)*, **8**, 245–257.

BEWLEY, D. K. (1973) *British Medical Bulletin*, **29**, 7–11.

BEWLEY, D. K., FOWLER, J. F., MORGAN, R. L., SILVESTER, J. A., TURNER, B. A. and THOMLINSON, R. H. (1963) *British Journal of Radiology*, **36**, 107.

BLEEHAN, N. M. (1973) *British Medical Bulletin*, **29**, 54–58.

CADE, I. S. and MCEWEN, J. B. (1967) *Cancer, N.Y.*, **20**, 817–821.

CATTERALL, M., KINGSLEY, D. P. E., LAWRENCE, G., GRAINGER, J. and SPENCER, J. (1975) *Gut*, **16**, 150–156.

CATTERALL, M., ROGERS, C. R., THOMLINSON, R. H. and FIELD, S. B. (1971) *British Journal of Radiology*, **44**, 603.

CATTERALL, M., SUTHERLAND, I. and BEWLEY, D. K. (1975) *British Medical Journal*, **2**, 653–656.

CATTERALL, M. and VONBERG, D. D. (1974) *British Medical Journal*, **3**, 137–143.

CHURCHILL-DAVIDSON, I. (1967) in *Modern Trends in Radiotherapy – I*, ed. Deeley, T. Butterworth, London, 73–92.

FIELD, S. B. (1969) *Radiology*, **92**, 381.

FIELD, S. B., JONES, T. and THOMLINSON, R. H. (1968) *British Journal of Radiology*, **41**, 597.

GRAY, L. H., CONGER, A. D., EBERT, M., HORNSEY, S. and SCOTT, O. C. A. (1953) *British Journal of Radiology*, **XXVI**, 638–648.

GRAY, L. H. and READ, J. (1942) *British Journal of Radiology*, **15**, 72.

GRAY, L. H. and READ, J. (1943) *Nature*, **152**, 53.

GRAY, L. H. and READ, J. (1944) *British Journal of Radiology*, **17**, 271.

GRAY, L. H., MOTTRAM, J. C., READ, J. and SPEAR, F. G. (1940) *British Journal of Radiology*, **13**, 371.

HENK, J. M., KUNKLER, P. B., SHAH, N. K., SMITH, C. W., SUTHERLAND, W. H. and WASSIF, S. B. (1970) *Clinical Radiology*, **21**, 223–231.

MITCHELL, J. S. (1968) *British Journal of Radiology*, **41**, 708–712.

MITCHELL, J. S. (1971) *Cancer: If Curable, Why Not Cured?* Heffer, Cambridge.

MITCHELL, J. S. (1946) Personal communication.

MITCHELL, J. S., BRINKLEY, D. and HAYBITTLE, J. L. (1965) *Acta radiologica* (*Therapy, Physics, Biology*), **3**, 329–341.

PHILLIPS, T. L. and HANKS, G. E. (1968) *Radiation Research*, **33**, 517–532.

SAMBROOK, D. K. (1968) *Frontiers in Radiation and Therapeutic Oncology*, **3**, 180–194.

SCANLON, P. W. (1968) *Frontiers in Radiation and Therapeutic Oncology*, **3**, 195–211.

SHELINE, G. E., PHILLIPS, T. L., FIELD, S. B., BRENNAN, J. T. and RAVENTOS, A. (1971) *American Journal of Roentgenology*, **111**, 31–41.

STONE, R. S. (1948) *American Journal of Roentgenology*, **59**, 771–785.

STONE, R. S. and LARKIN, J. C. (1942) *Radiology*, **39**, 608–620.

STONE, R. S., LAWRENCE, J. H. and AEBERSOLD, P. C. (1940) *Radiology*, **35**, 322–327.

SUIT, H. and LINDBERG, R. (1968) *American Journal of Roentgenology*, **102**, 27–37.

SUIT, H. and URANO, M. (1969) *Radiation Research*, **37**, 423–434.

THOMLINSON, R. H. (1968) *Frontiers in Radiation and Therapeutic Oncology*, **3**, 109.

THOMLINSON, R. H. and GRAY, L. H. (1955) *British Journal of Cancer*, **9**, 539.

VAN DEN BRENK, H. A. S. (1968) *American Journal of Roentgenology*, **102**, 8–26.

CHAPTER FOUR

Malignant Disease of the Nervous System

H. F. Hope-Stone

Tumours of the nervous system may involve the brain, the spinal cord, and the sympathetic nervous system. The primary intracranial tumours comprise about one per cent of deaths coming to autopsy (King, 1970). Metastatic tumours account for about 20 per cent of the total. Spinal cord primary tumours and those of the sympathetic nervous system are much less common, although the latter occur relatively frequently in children. The relative incidence, according to tumour type, will vary somewhat, according to whether one studies autopsy records or those from a neurosurgical department. However, the gliomata are the commonest (about 40 per cent), followed by metastases (20 per cent), meningiomata (12 per cent) and pituitary tumours (5 per cent).

Aetiology

There are no known causative factors in the malignant group to be discussed. Previous injury may light up a known tumour, but there is no convincing evidence of trauma being a causative factor. The fact that the gliomata are more common in men and the meningioma in women suggests a possible hormonal influence.

Pathology

Russell and Rubinstein's classification (1970) is probably the most useful to follow, and can be summarised briefly as follows:

1. Glial tumours
   - Astrocytoma
   - Oligodendroglioma
   - Ependymal (including choroid plexus papillomata)
2. Glioblastoma multiforme
   - Brain
   - Brain stem
   - Optic nerve
3. Pineal tumours
4. Retinal tumours
   - Retinoblastoma
5. Neuronal tumours
   - Medulloblastoma
   - Sympathetic nervous system.

The other tumours to be discussed in this chapter include:

Meningiomas	Pituitary tumours
Haemangioblastomas	Metastatic tumours
Craniopharyngiomas	Spinal cord tumours

It is proposed to discuss each pathological type, but not to include detailed symptomatology and diagnosis, which can be read in the appropriate textbook. With each type the author will outline the role of radiotherapy, the technique to be employed, and the results obtained.

General Effects of Irradiation of the Nervous System

As late as the 1940s it was thought that nervous tissue was relatively radioresistant, and that very high doses of irradiation could do no harm. In 1948 Boden first described the dangers of excessive irradiation dosage to the brain stem and spinal cord. Since then, definite tolerance dose-levels have been worked out for various parts of the nervous system.

Irradiation damage that occurs in the nervous system is first and foremost vascular in nature. It leads to increased capillary permeability, which produces oedema and subsequently discrete damage to the glial cells. Demyelination occurs, but may take up to a year to reach maximum effect. At a later stage, vascular occlusion with proliferation of fibrous connective tissue leads to arteriolar necrosis. The blood–brain barrier may be permanently changed. Finally, the vascular changes lead to cell death and necrosis of the nervous tissue.

Some portions of the nervous system are more sensitive than others; thus the motor areas of the cortex, brain stem and cervical spinal cord are most easily damaged. This increased susceptibility may be related to the fact that these sites have a more vulnerable blood supply. The frontal and occipital lobes of the brain are less sensitive, and the peripheral nerves are relatively radioresistant (Gerstner, 1955). Radiation damage to the latter is secondary to fibrosis in the surrounding tissue, which in turn leads to demyelination – this being well seen in the brachial plexus (Stoll and Andrews, 1966).

Clinically, the effects of exceeding tolerance doses to the nervous system may appear from one to fifteen months after irradiation, the average being nine months. In the brain stem and spinal cord lesion the patient usually complains of numbness and paraesthesiae of the extremities. These symptoms may be transient in nature, and may be made worse by flexion of the neck (known as L'Hermitte's sign). This syndrome was reviewed by Jones (1964); it may be caused by irradiating long sections of the spinal cord, as in the treatment of the reticuloses, and can occur at relatively low dose-levels, in the region of 2500–3000 rad in three to four weeks. Fortunately, permanent damage to the nervous system does not usually follow.

In the more heavily irradiated group, with doses in the region of 4500 rad, permanent spinal cord damage leads to a Brown-Sequard syndrome, due to transverse myelitis. This is often fatal, death being due to broncho-pneumonia or ascending urinary tract infection. The brain may be affected in a similar way, irradiation necrosis leading to permanent damage of vital structures which is likely to lead to death.

In clinical practice there are certain factors of importance. The overall time of administration of irradiation should be taken into account. If a known safe dose is given over five weeks, reducing the time to three weeks may lead to radiation damage. The larger the volume of tissue irradiated, the more likely is radiation damage to occur. Daily fractionation five days a week is much less likely to produce damage than is giving the same tumour-dose in fractions of three times a week; the dose in the latter case is higher per fraction, and would produce a greater radiobiological effect. If it is thought essential to treat a patient on alternate days, then the total dose must be reduced accordingly. Finally, it should be remembered that poor vascularity of the brain may be responsible for excessive irradiation reaction, even though the dose given to the brain is within accepted tolerance levels.

From these observations it is possible to draw up levels of tolerance doses to the nervous system. For large lengths of spinal cord, the maximum safe dose will be in the region of 3500 rad (daily fractionations, five days a week) in seventeen days. For small fields the level will be 4500 rad. In four to five weeks, a more commonly used treatment period, the radiobiological equivalent doses will be 4250–5000 rad.

In the brain itself, vital areas including the brain stem should not receive more than 4500 rad in four weeks (daily fractionations) (Boden, 1950). If treatment is given over six to eight weeks, it has been suggested that 6500–7000 rad can be tolerated with safety (Kramer, 1969). In the rest of the brain, if small fields are used, 5000 rad in four to five weeks is probably safe (Moss, 1969).

The present author feels that 4500 rad in four weeks (or its radiobiological equivalent) should never be exceeded, at any site for any volume treated, as above this level there is always the danger of nervous tissue damage, and there is no convincing evidence that higher doses will necessarily produce a better therapeutic response.

Irradiation Techniques

In general, megavoltage irradiation is to be preferred, as this will ensure the most accurate localisation with small fields, thus sparing the rest of the brain from unnecessary irradiation. Bone absorption will not reduce the intended tumour-dose, and the skin will be spared unpleasant irradiation reaction. Although epilation will occur, better hair regrowth will be obtained with megavoltage than with orthovoltage (Fig. 4.1). Finally, the treatment time is much faster, and the setting up and treatment of the patient much simpler and better tolerated.

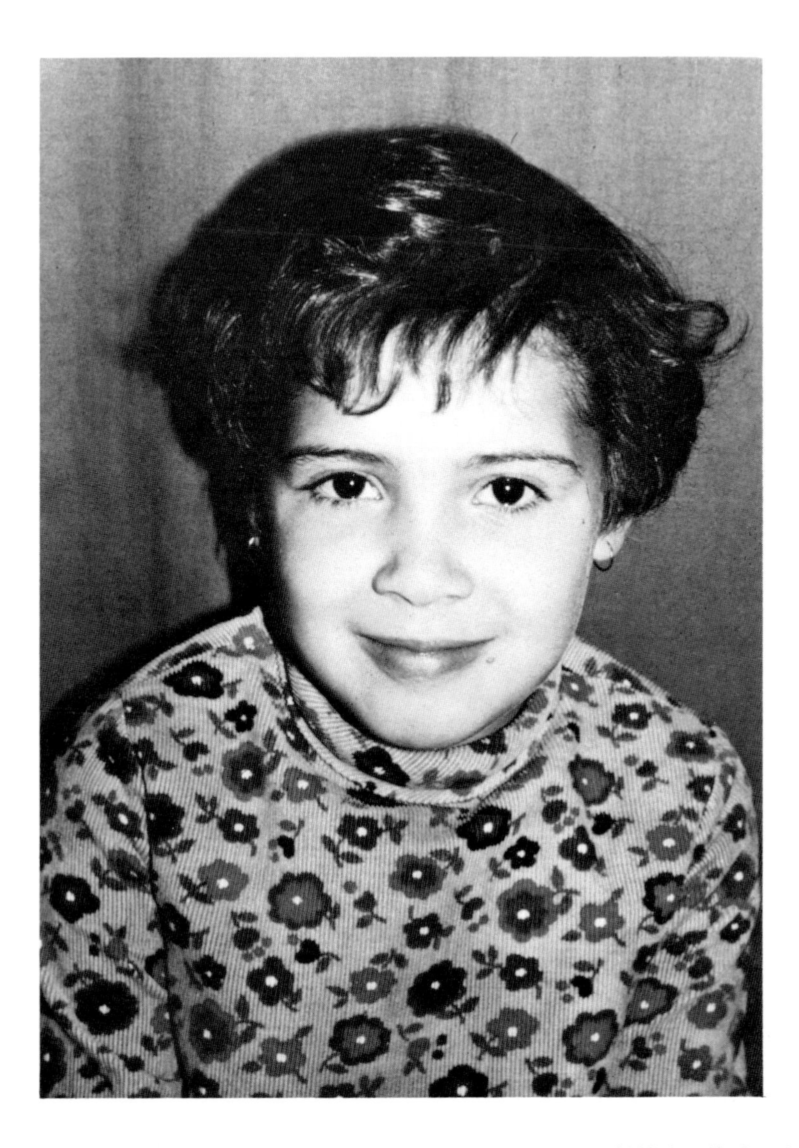

Fig. 4.1. Hair regrowth in a child three years after whole CNS irradiation for medulloblastoma.

The rate at which the irradiation is given and the fractionation of the given dose are both important points. Some years ago it was customary to start with a relatively low dose of irradiation and to increase this slowly over the next few days, in order to minimise the danger of producing cerebral oedema. This risk seems to have been over-stressed, and providing the fractionation is not too large (i.e. the daily tumour dose does not exceed 225 rad), the risk is very small indeed, and the

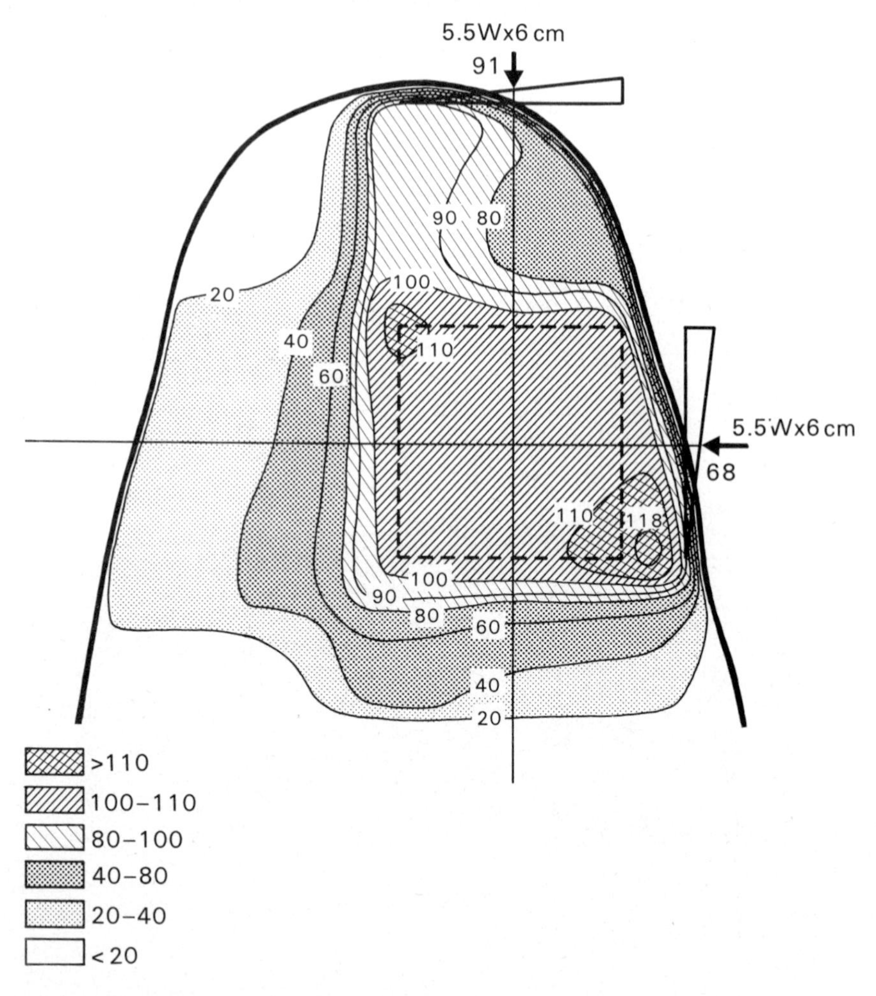

Fig. 4.2. Wedge field technique for localised irradiation to the brain.

maximum daily dose can be given from the first day of treatment. If cerebral oedema is present before the start of treatment it may be reduced by the use of steroids.

To treat the whole brain is relatively easy, as two lateral parallel and opposed fields will give homogeneous irradiation throughout the organ. Smaller tumours, particularly if unilateral or lying in the posterior cranial fossa, are best treated with a wedge technique, which will give homogeneous irradiation without affecting the rest of the brain (Fig. 4.2). Very small fields can be used to treat the pituitary fossa – a 3 cm circle can be set up with two parallel and opposed fields. The slight

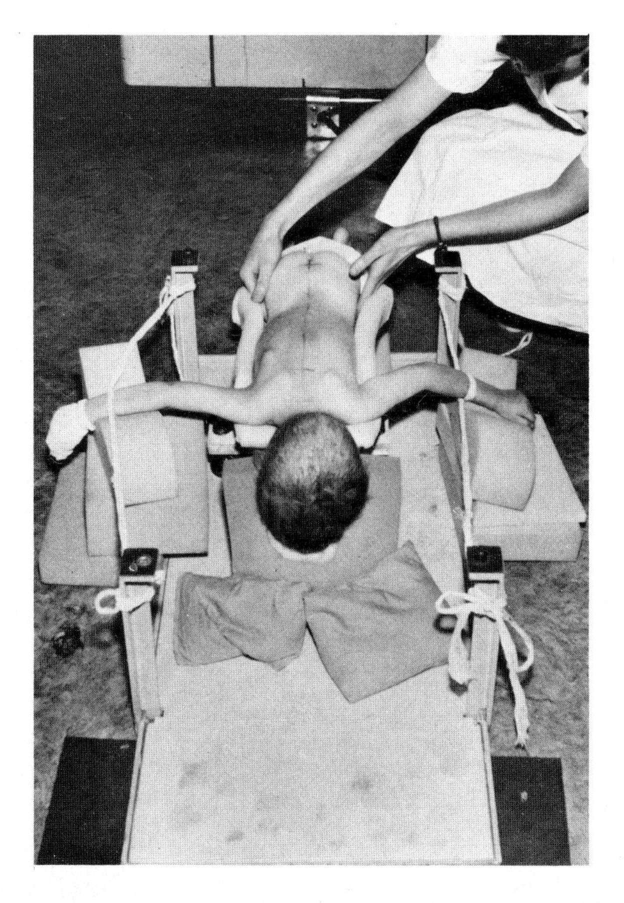

Fig. 4.3. a Child in plaster cast used to treat spinal field – whole CNS irradiation.

disadvantage to this technique is that both temporal lobes will receive the maximum tumour-dose. One way of overcoming this problem is to use a rotation technique, whereby the X-ray machine moves continuously through an area of 300° around the circumference of the skull, avoiding the eyes. This will reduce the dose to any given point in the brain other than the target area, but it will also mean unnecessarily irradiating very much more normal brain tissue than was described in the first technique.

Irradiation to the whole central nervous system is best carried out by the technique first described by Patterson and Farr (1953), and subsequently modified to the more elegant London Hospital method described by Bottrill *et al.* (1965). With this technique one large spade-shaped posterior field is used to treat the whole spinal cord and posterior brain. The brain-dose is raised to the correct level by an additional direct field from the front, using the telecobalt unit. Special care is taken with this latter field so as to avoid irradiating the lens and thus producing a cataract. The spinal cord is given a homogeneous dose

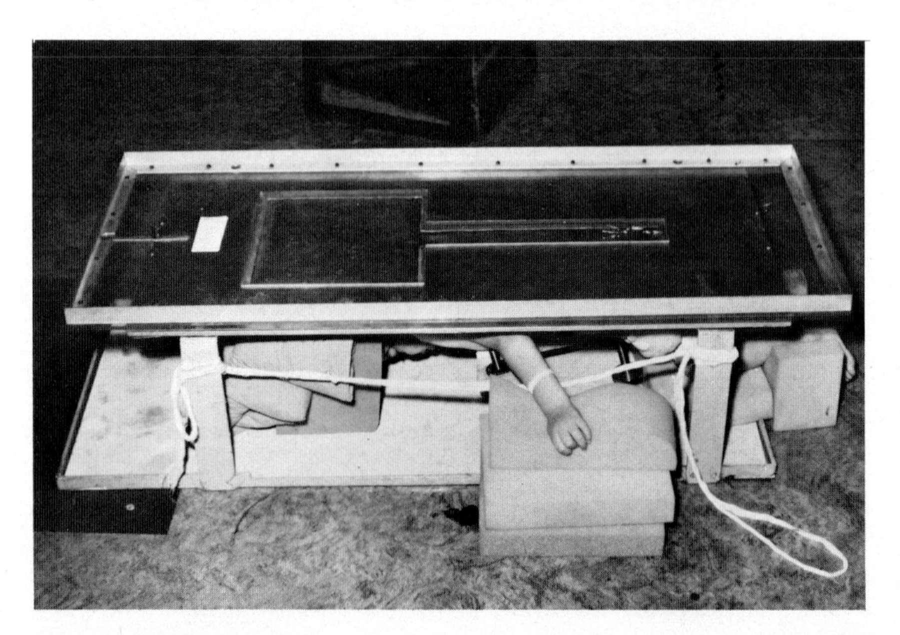

Fig. 4.3. b Orthovoltage filter in position over the child's spine during whole CNS irradiation.

of irradiation by filtering the X-rays of an orthovoltage machine in such a way as to compensate for the varying depth of the cord. A special plaster cast is made so as to allow the patient (usually a child) to lie face down while the posterior field is being irradiated (Fig. 4.3a and b). The latter field may take up to 45 minutes each day to give the required tumour-dose, thus the co-operation of the child and/or adequate sedation is necessary.

Management Problems with Irradiation

Since cerebral oedema is not the problem it was once thought to be, normal daily fractions of irradiation can be given for a period of four to five weeks, even if there is a rise of intracranial pressure. Dexamethasone 4 mg q.d.s. can always be given to reduce the possibility of oedema and to prevent the necessity for further surgery. In the case of whole CNS irradiation it is probably wise to start slowly and to increase the daily dose to a maximum over a few days. This method will also help to increase the tolerance of the bone marrow, which is always likely to be damaged by such wide-field treatment, although only rarely will treatment need to be interrupted for more than a day or two on this account.

Irradiation sickness is rarely a problem when small portions of the brain are being treated, and even when the whole brain or CNS is being irradiated it does not present undue difficulties. Torecan 10 mg t.d.s. or Maxalon 10 mg t.d.s. is extremely effective in preventing this distressing side-effect.

The main difficulty lies with those patients with severe cerebral irritability who are unable to lie still for their treatment. In adults this rarely occurs, but ordinary sedation can deal with the problem if it does. In children, however, particularly under the age of six, adequate co-operation is often difficult to achieve, and if the treatment time is prolonged to 30–40 minutes sedation will usually be required.

If there is any doubt it is usually better to ask an anaesthetist to see the patient before the treatment is started, so that a definite plan of sedation can be followed. At the London Hospital we have found that full anaesthesia from the very beginning is often the best way of solving the problem. Ketalar is an excellent anaesthetic for the purpose, since it does not depress the pharyngeal reflexes and no pre-medication is required. The drug can be given intramuscularly, intubation is not required, and the child is conscious and able to eat and play within two hours of finishing treatment. We have usually found that by the second week of treatment the anaesthetic can be dispensed with, and possibly only mild sedation or even none at all will be required (Hope-Stone, 1970).

Since complete epilation always occurs on the scalp, a wig should be provided. Good hair regrowth will take place within six to nine months.

Skin reactions are not usually a problem. Mild dry desquamation and erythema can be dealt with locally by hydrocortisone ointment.

Long-term brain damage should not occur if the known tolerance levels are adhered to. Children who survive for ten or more years will not be adversely affected, and no abnormal mental changes should occur. Residual brain damage is usually due to the original effects of the tumour and not to the subsequent irradiation.

General Policy of Irradiation

Most patients will have had some surgical treatment, involving at least partial removal and/or biopsy of the tumour, with an adequate decompression. In general, they should be allowed to recover completely from surgery before irradiation is started. Exceptions are cases of extremely radiosensitive tumours, such as the medulloblastoma and the occasional rapidly-growing glioma in a young adult. Patients in this last group may be very ill at the start of treatment, but nevertheless should begin irradiation as soon as possible. Before treatment is planned the referring neurosurgeon should be asked to mark out on the appropriate X-ray films the site and size of the tumour.

Patients whose tumours have already produced irreversible neurological damage and who therefore are unlikely ever to live useful lives should not be considered for routine post-operative radiotherapy.

All patients should start their treatment while in hospital. Adult patients, if fit enough, and with the consent of the neurosurgeon, can attend as outpatients if not travelling long distances. Children should always remain in hospital, but there is no reason why they should not spend the weekends at home if their general condition is good enough.

Re-treatment

Once a full, radical course of irradiation has been given to the brain, it is doubtful whether further treatment should be given if recurrence takes place within the next two or three years. After this time has elapsed, irradiation can again be considered. There are two problems to be dealt with: firstly, it is absolutely essential that true recurrence is present, as the same symptoms and signs can be produced by irradiation necrosis, and further treatment would prove to be disastrous; secondly, if another course of irradiation is given then the neurosurgeon and the radiotherapist must accept that there is a major risk of radiation damage to the brain. If the alternative is death due to spread of the tumour then the risk can be accepted, but if the tumour is slow-growing and not producing symptoms it may be better to leave things well alone.

Irradiation for Special Tumours of the Brain

Gliomata

Astrocytoma

Cerebellar astrocytomas in children are best treated by surgical extirpation. The results are excellent, and some would say that they are really benign tumours. German (1961) reported a 53 per cent twenty-year survival rate. There is no place for routine irradiation, but if the tumour has not been completely excised it would seem reasonable to give a radical course of post-operative irradiation. Using a wedge field technique the posterior cranial fossa can be treated to a tumour-dose of 4000 rad in four weeks, without damage to the child. Patterson (1952) reported a 40 per cent five-year survival rate with this method.

The cerebral astrocytomas are much more malignant. They fall into two main groups: Grades I and II, which probably do not benefit from irradiation, and the more malignant Grades III and IV, which should probably receive treatment after surgery. Marsa *et al.* (1973) described 37 cases in which there was a 72 per cent five-year survival in fifteen cerebral cases, but only 20 per cent survival in a similar number of brain stem lesions. Bouchard and Pierre (1960) showed an increase in the five-year survival from 38 to 49 per cent if irradiation were given.

Moderately large irradiation fields should be used, treating with a parallel opposed technique or wedged fields, to a tumour-dose of 4500 rad in four weeks.

Oligodendroglioma

These tumours are the least common of the gliomas, and occur mainly in the cerebral hemispheres, growing relatively slowly. It is difficult to know the value of irradiation; Sheline *et al.* (1964) report a 31 per cent five-year survival for those treated by surgery alone, but 85 per cent with added irradiation. Thus, it would seem wise to give all patients the benefit of the doubt and to use post-operative irradiation in all cases.

Ependymoma and Choroid Plexus Tumours

Since these tumours occur in or near the ventricles they are difficult, if not impossible, to remove surgically. They are radiosensitive, thus treatment is almost obligatory. McWhirter (1955) stated that seedling metastases, via the cerebrospinal fluid, can occur, and are most likely if the tumour is an ependymoblastoma. Moss (1969) states that the infratentorial tumours certainly behave in this way, and both these authors advocate total CNS irradiation, particularly in children. Other authors doubt that leptomeningeal spread is such a common occurrence and advise only local irradiation. Kricheff *et al.* (1964) quote a 28 per cent survival figure using this latter method. Since the evidence for metastases is slight, and since whole CNS irradiation is such a time-consuming and tedious technique, the present author agrees that only local irradiation need be given. A tumour dose of 4000 rad in four weeks (daily fractionation) should be adequate. The ependymoblastoma should receive whole CNS irradiation.

Glioblastoma Multiforme

Brain

The role of radiotherapy in these highly malignant tumours is still debatable. The prognosis in the short term seems to be improved by irradiation. Taveras *et al.* (1962) showed a 4 per cent one-year survival with surgery only, and a 32 per cent survival if irradiation was added; yet at five years the total survival rate was almost negligible. A two-year survival figure of 8 per cent has been reported by Arrizpizibal (1971). Bloom *et al.* (1973) are more optimistic, and think that a 5 per cent five-year survival can be achieved.

Since these tumours are very malignant and spread diffusely through the brain, some authors suggest that very large irradiation fields should be used, or even the whole brain treated (Kramer, 1969). The results of this latter author were no better than those of Legre *et al.* (1969), who had a two-year survival figure of 9 per cent using moderately large fields, and Arrizpizibal (1971) using only localised fields. Dose-levels of 4500–5500 rad in four to five weeks were used in these series, but even higher doses (5280 in four weeks) have been advocated, and might produce better short-term results than surgery alone (Ramsay and Brund, 1973); but at these dose-levels the hazard of irradiation necrosis must then be taken into consideration.

One can conclude that, provided the patient is fit, post-operative irradiation should always be considered. Relatively large fields, though not necessarily to the whole brain, should be used to give a tumour-dose in the region of 4500 rad in four weeks.

Brainstem

The problem here may be the inability to make a definite histological diagnosis, due to the danger of even attempting a biopsy. If there is sufficient clinical and radiological evidence of tumour, then irradiation should be considered. Relatively small fields can be used, and Bouchard and Pierre (1960) have reported a 30–40 per cent five-year survival figure in their cases. The present author has seen excellent short- and long-term survival following localised irradiation to these sites, but one is always suspicious of the original diagnosis if histological proof is lacking.

Optic Nerve

These tumours are found most commonly in children, and present with visual failure and proptosis. Eventually both eyes may be affected. The tumour grows slowly and insidiously, and severe damage may occur before the disease is diagnosed. Treatment at an early stage is by surgery, and may achieve cure. Clintorian *et al.* (1964) reported 21 out of 24 patients alive and well at 24 years. If surgery is incomplete or impossible, then irradiation should always be tried. With a careful technique the lens can be avoided and good vision retained. Beam-directed megavoltage wedge fields can achieve a good dose-distribution (Fig. 4.4a). As with all brain tumours, the head is best held fixed for treatment, and if the child is irritable anaesthesia may be required (Fig. 4.4b).

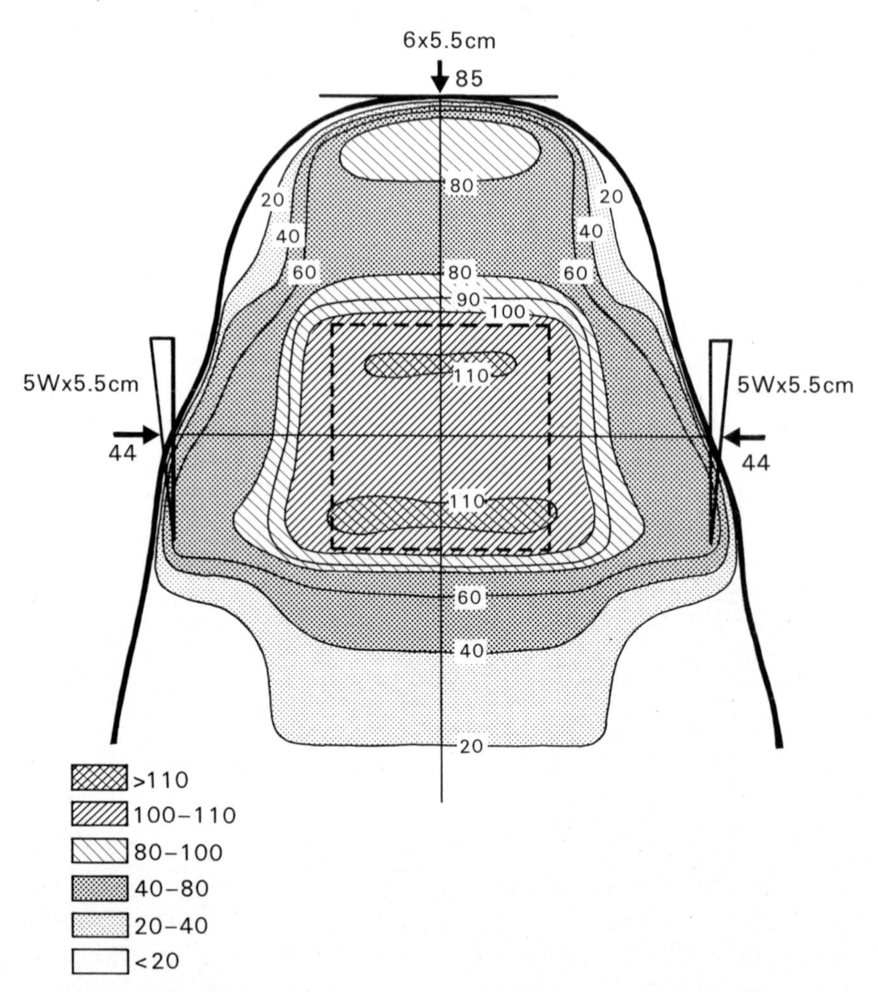

Fig. 4.4. a Wedge field technique for optic glioma.

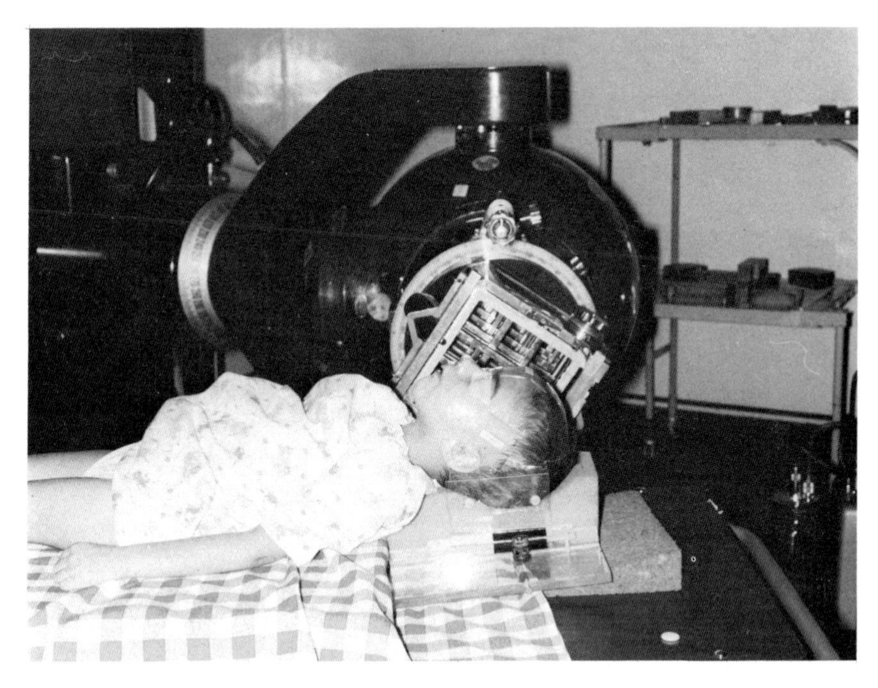

Fig. 4.4. b Set-up for treating optic glioma: the child's head is fixed in a Perspex jig.

Pineal Tumours

Pineal tumours are relatively rare, the commonest being a pinealoma, or atypical teratoma. Spread may occur by seedling metastases, particularly if the tumour is a pinealoblastoma. They occur in the first two decades of life, and may present with hydrocephalus, visual disturbances, or hypothalmic upsets including diabetes insipidus and/or pubertus praecox. Treatment consists of relief of the hydrocephalus, since any attempt at radical surgery may be disastrous (Northfield, 1973). Irradiation should always be given; usually in the more benign type of tumour a pair of parallel and opposed, relatively small fields can be used to give a tumour-dose of 4500 rad in four weeks. If the histology suggests pinealoblastoma, whole CNS irradiation is required. Results are difficult to assess, since most reports consist of a few cases each. Northfield (1973), in a survey of the literature, suggests that a 20 per cent four-year survival figure may be obtained with irradiation.

Retinal Tumours

Retinoblastoma

This is the commonest intra-ocular tumour of childhood. It can occur from birth up to the age of 7 years. The disease may be sporadic (in about 96 per cent) or is inherited as an irregular Mendelian dominant trait. Some sporadic cases may be familial, but the majority are not, and the chance of a second child having the same disease is less than 6 per cent (Duke Elder and Dobree, 1967). The familial type is bilateral in 20–35 per cent of cases. The chance of a patient of this group being cured of the disease and then producing children who develop the same tumour is in the region of 30 per cent; thus genetic counselling may be required.

The tumour grows insidiously; the first sign may be the classical 'yellow cats-eye'; fungation and haemorrhage occur later. X-rays show calcification of the tumour in 70 per cent of cases.

Treatment can be by surgery, radiotherapy, or chemotherapy, or a combination of the three. Enucleation of the eye for early unilateral disease can cure about 50 per cent of cases. If, after surgery, there is evidence of tumour in the cut end of the optic nerve, irradiation should be considered. This can be given with a ^{60}Co mould to the orbital cavity, or by external megavoltage irradiation, giving tumour-doses in the region of 3500–4000 rad in three to four weeks.

If the tumours are bilateral but relatively early, then vision in both eyes may be saved by irradiation alone. Stallard (1966) has over the years modified and improved the technique whereby a ^{60}Co disc in a platinum applicator is stitched to the sclera. It is kept in place for six or seven days, and then removed. The dose to the base of the tumour is 19 000 rad, but at the apex nearest the lens it falls to 3500 rad. This dose is sufficient to eradicate the tumour without permanently damaging the lens. The problem of irradiation-induced cataract is difficult, since it is known that the lens may be damaged with doses as low as 800–1200 rad. Williams (1967) describes two categories, the first being a stippled opacity which does not progress and does not require treatment, the second a progressive opacity which will require surgical extraction at a later date.

If the disease is bilateral but too advanced to be treated by the ^{60}Co disc method, external irradiation can be given (Williams, 1972). A direct megavoltage field (3 × 4 cm) can be used; the child must keep its eyes open during treatment, as this will diminish the irradiation reaction to the conjunctiva and cornea. A tumour-dose of 3400 rad in 28 days is well tolerated. Cataract occurs in 100 per cent of cases, but only in about 20 per cent is vision affected and these can be treated and improved by surgical means. Williams (1967) described 46 bilateral cases treated with a combination of enucleation of the less-affected eye and external irradiation of the other – 35 were alive and well with good vision at five years.

Chemotherapy has been used as an adjuvant to irradiation. Tapley (1964) used the akylating agent tetramine, and claimed good results, and since the irradiation dosage was lowered there was less damage to the lens. Williams (1967) prefers cyclophosphamide.

Neuronal Tumours

Medulloblastoma

These are rare tumours affecting mostly children, but they can occur in young adults. The incidence in Great Britain is about 80 per year. Surgery will always be required both for diagnostic purposes and to remove enough tumour to achieve an adequate decompression.

Since these tumours are the most radiosensitive of all brain neoplasms, radical surgery need not be attempted; even palliative removal carries a very high mortality rate, and there is no justification for taking surgical risks. If the intracranial pressure is very high, the surgeon should not be tempted to carry out a by-pass operation into the venous circulation, since this would remove any chance of eradicating the neoplasm. The craniotomy will serve as an adequate decompression and steroids can be added if need be. Irradiation should be begun as soon as the child is fit enough to tolerate treatment, usually the day the sutures are removed. Treatment by surgery alone produces no long-term survivals, but over the past two decades the results by irradiation have steadily improved from 16 per cent (Lampe and McIntrey, 1954) to 33 per cent (Bloom, 1969).

The most important advance has been the use of homogeneous irradiation of the whole of the central nervous system, giving a minimum tumour-dose of 3000 rad to the spinal cord and a maximum dose to the brain of 4000 rads (Hope-Stone, 1970). This has produced very good results at the London Hospital, as the following results show:

Time period	*Number of cases*	*Type of X-ray treatment*	*5-year survivals Number*	*%*
1943–50	16	Partial or matched	1	6
1950–68	24	Homogeneous	14	59

In this series there are as yet not many ten-year survivals, but of thirteen cases available for study ten are alive and well; four of these patients have survived for twenty years; no case has recurred five years after treatment. All of these long-term survivors are perfectly fit and able, both physically and mentally; no severe irradiation stigmata are seen. Neither marked growth retardation nor kyphoscoliosis have occurred. Thyroid carcinoma and leukaemia have not been seen. The older female patients are all menstruating normally. Pregnancy can occur, and normal children are produced (Hope-Stone, 1970).

Recurrence of the tumour, if it occurs, is usually within two or three years. I do not think that further irradiation should ever be given, but chemotherapy could be considered. Metastases usually occur if a by-pass operation was performed before irradiation was given, and may involve the skeletal system. Symptomatic improvement may be achieved in these latter cases by irradiation or chemotherapy; if the latter is used, vincristine might be a drug worth trying. However, it should be remembered that in both groups such treatment can only be palliative in nature, and should not be persevered with at the cost of upsetting the patient.

Since recurrence is rare after four years, the five-year survival rate is a good indication of cure, and this should be achieved in 50 per cent of cases if the irradiation technique outlined above is used.

Sympathetic Nervous System Tumours

These tumours are derived from the ganglion cells of the peripheral nervous system, and their precursors. They consist of neuroblastoma, ganglioneuroblastoma, and ganglioneuromata.

Neuroblastoma. These occur mainly in early infancy, the commonest site of origin being the adrenal gland; other sites include the retroperitoneal sympathetic chain in the pelvis, the posterior mediastinum, and the neck. A rare but interesting tumour is found arising from the olfactory mucosa. Histologically they are recognised by their tendency to rosette formation. The tumour spreads by direct invasion and by lymphatic and venous channels, involving the liver, lymph nodes and skeleton. Intra-cerebral metastases are rare, but may be secondary to a primary mediastinal tumour (Hope-Stone, 1974). Neuronal maturation may take place in both the primary and the metastases; thus spontaneous regression may occur, leading to disappearance of the tumour, or a change to the more benign ganglioneuroma (Kissane and Ackerman, 1955).

The primary adrenal tumour presents with painless abdominal swellings, malaise and anorexia. Bone pain from metastases is a common presenting symptom. The extra-adrenal lesion may be asymptomatic in the mediastinum, or may present with cough and chest pain. Spinal cord involvement can occur early at this and other sites, giving rise to spinal cord compression or even paraplegia (Hope-Stone, 1961). Radiological calcification is a pathognomonic sign (Fig. 4.5), but a soft tissue mass may also be seen. Biochemical investigation of the urine shows raised levels of catecholamines (homovanyllic acid (HVA) and vanillylmandelic acid (VMA)) in 95 per cent of cases (Bell, 1968).

Surgery should always be attempted, both to establish the diagnosis and to remove as much tumour as possible. Since complete removal of the tumour is usually impossible, post-operative irradiation should always be given. These tumours are relatively radiosensitive. The area to be treated should include the tumour bed and the immediate lymphatic drainage areas. In the abdomen, large parallel opposed fields can be used. An IVP localisation film is used to outline the opposite kidney, which should be shielded to avoid irradiation nephritis, although the midline should be crossed so as to treat as much of the lymphatic

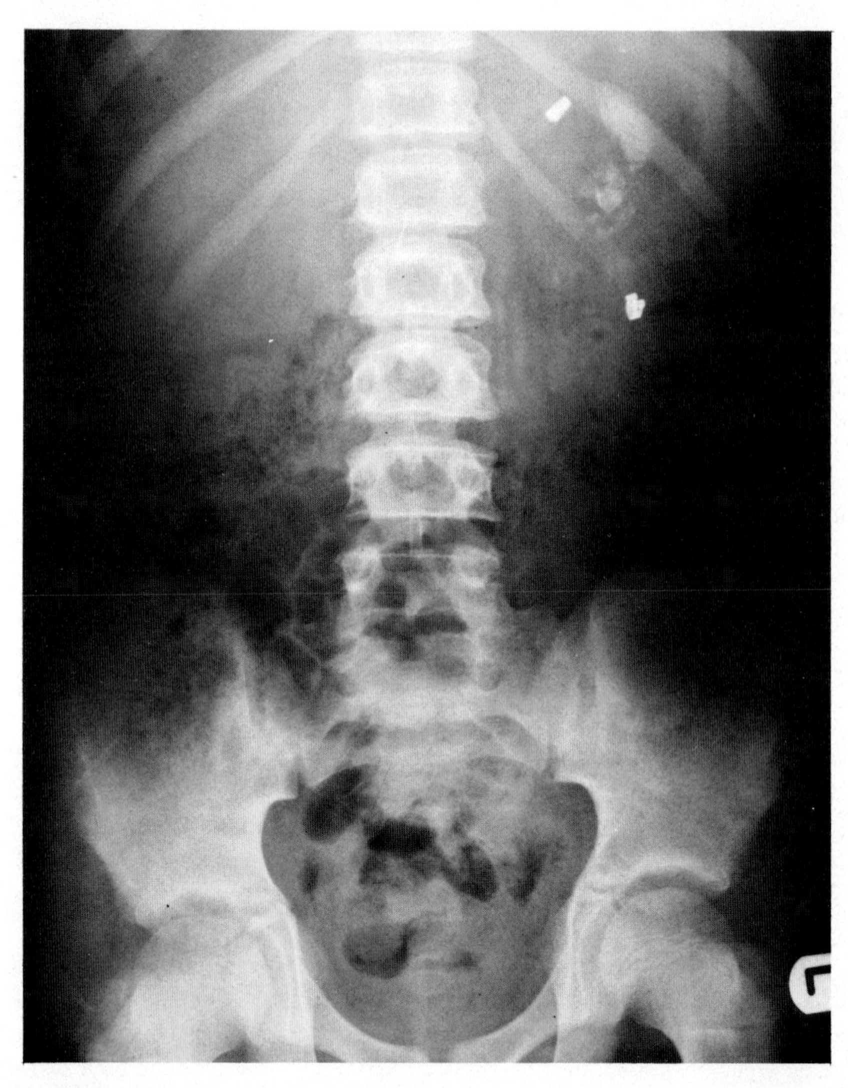

Fig. 4.5. Classification in neuroblastoma.

drainage as possible. If the tumour is more extensive and the opposite kidney has to be included in the treatment area, then shielding to the latter should be used if the dose exceeds 2250 rad, which is tolerance level for this organ (Kunkler *et al.*, 1952). (See Chapter 11.)

A tumour-dose of 3000 rad in twenty treatments over 28 days is usually adequate, and at this dose-level there should be little systemic upset. Very young children will require sedation or an anaesthetic. If the pelvis is the site of origin of the tumour, the same dose can be given, although consideration may need to be given to lifting the ovaries out of the pelvis temporarily in order to prevent genetic damage or sterility (Toft and Wittenberg, 1968).

In the mediastinum, although large opposed fields can be used, in young females this may lead to long-term side-effects, as shown in one of the author's cases – a patient treated at the age of three, and who seventeen years later had almost complete failure of breast growth (Hope-Stone, 1974). This can be avoided if large wedge fields are used and the patient treated through the posterior mediastinum.

A wedge technique can be used to treat tumours in the head and neck region, and was used recently in treating an olfactory neuroblastoma with good result, following the giving of a tumour-dose of 3000 rad in three weeks (Fig. 4.6).

The results of treating early cases with these methods is to produce an overall five-year survival figure of 20 per cent. The best results occur in young children and the extra-adrenal primary sites. Young *et al.* (1970) reported a five-year survival figure of 50 per cent in eighteen such cases.

Many tumours are inoperable, but they should always receive irradiation, as not only may good remission be obtained but cure has been claimed using relatively low tumour-dose-levels to large areas (Stella *et al.*, 1970). Some inoperable tumours may be rendered operable by primary irradiation to dose-levels of the order of 2500 rad (Saenger and Dorst, 1968).

Palliative irradiation may be required for advanced tumours if chemotherapy has failed to control the disease. Single doses of 800 rad or five daily treatments to give a dose of 2500 rad may be given to sites such as the bone, subcutaneous and periorbital deposits. If there is spinal cord involvement, laminectomy and irradiation will produce a

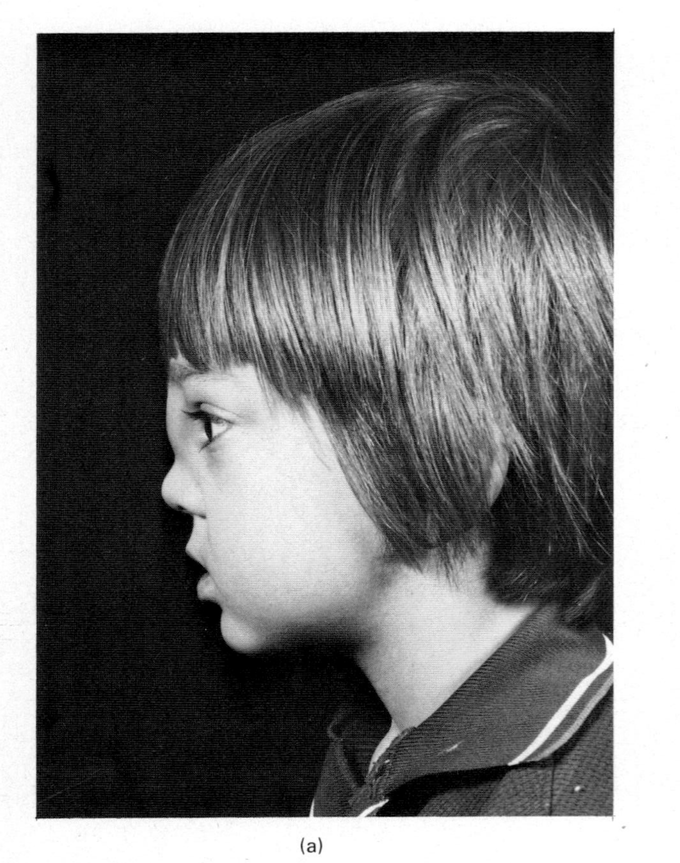

(a)

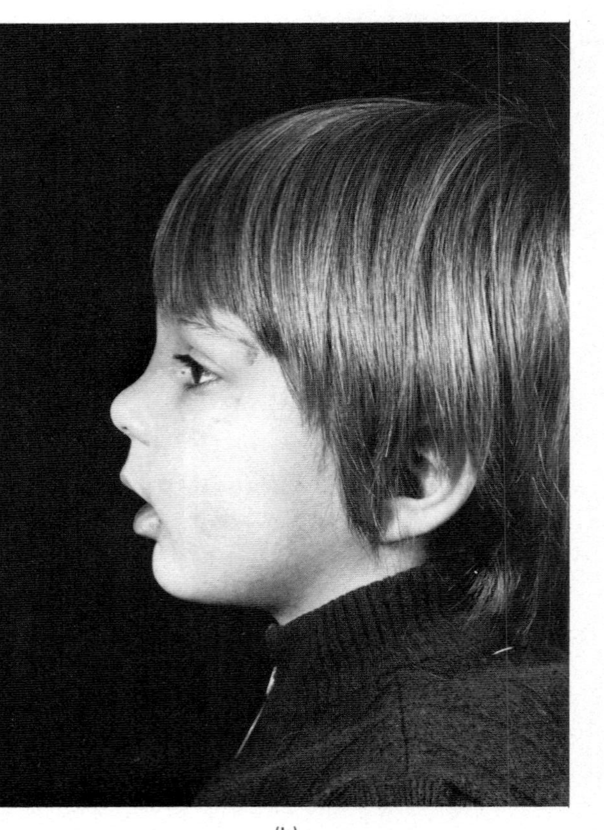

(b)

Fig. 4.6 Olfactory neuroblastoma (a) before and (b) after irradiation

more rapid response than drug therapy. An incident dose of 2000 rad in one week to the spine should be effective.

Ganglioneuroblastoma. This is quite rare in comparison with the turn-over described above; it occurs mainly in the retroperitoneal and mediastinal regions. Although less malignant and therefore more slow-growing, it can metastasise, and treatment again should be by a combination of surgery and radiotherapy. Stowens (1957) described eight of seventeen cases alive and well at two years or more.

Ganglioneuroma. This is a benign tumour, and should be treated by surgery alone or even left *in situ* if not causing symptoms.

Meningioma

Since the majority of these tumours are benign and can be adequately dealt with by surgery, routine post-operative irradiation is not required. Occasionally these tumours are very vascular, having a high mitotic index, and may even be sarcomatous in appearance. This would suggest that local recurrence is likely. In the small group of these latter cases which are inoperable, if the cavenous sinus is involved or recurrence cannot be dealt with surgically, irradiation should be considered. Since they are really benign tumours no risks should be taken, and therefore brain tolerance should not be exceeded; a wedged field technique to a tumour-dose of 4500 rad in four weeks should be adequate.

Haemangioblastoma

The great majority of these tumours are satisfactorily treated by surgery (Northfield, 1973). If they are very large and highly vascular, surgery might be considered too dangerous, and irradiation could be considered. Moderate tumour-doses, in the region of 3500–4000 rad in three to four weeks should do no harm in this relatively benign condition, and might even sclerose the blood vessels sufficiently to produce tumour regression. Complete ablation of the tumour by this method is most unlikely.

Craniopharyngioma

These epidermoid tumours are thought to arise from epithelial remnants of Rathke's pouch, and are uncommon. They usually occur before the age of twenty, grow slowly and produce their effects by pressure on surrounding organs. Clinically they are characterised by raised intracranial pressure, endocrine disturbances, particularly hypopituitarism, and mental impairment. Surgery is the treatment of choice, but is fraught with many difficulties unless the tumour is entirely intrasellar (Northfield, 1973).

In all cases where surgery has been incomplete, post-operative irradiation should be considered. A tumour-dose of 4500 rad, given with small parallel and opposed fields, may be sufficient. If the tumour is completely inoperable, Kramer *et al.* (1961) advocate a much higher dose: 5500 rad in five weeks; by using very small carefully localised fields, brain-damage may be avoided. They claim very good results, nine out of ten cases being alive at six years. A recent report by Sharma *et al.* (1974) showed an 80 per cent two-year survival; but since these tumours are very slow-growing one would need to know the ten- and fifteen-year survival figures before talking of cure.

Pituitary Tumours

These comprise three main histological groups: eosinophil, chromophobe, and basophil; occasionally carcinoma may occur. The total incidence is about 5 per cent of all intracranial tumours.

Eosinophil Adenoma

Comprising about 37 per cent of pituitary tumours, these present classically with gigantism in children and acromegaly in adults. In the latter group both endocrine and visual disturbances may be produced. In many cases the patient may be quite unaware of the disease, or may complain of headaches and paraesthesiae. In both groups the real danger to the patient lies in side-effects, namely diabetes, and hypertension leading to heart failure. These effects will certainly shorten the patient's life, and active treatment is required. Although the diagnosis can be made clinically and radiologically, confirmation can be obtained by estimation of the growth-hormone level, which can also be used to monitor the progress of the disease and effectiveness of treatment.

Surgery alone can be quite effective, and at the end of ten years in Cushing's series 57 per cent were still alive (Northfield, 1973). Although surgery, either by transfrontal craniotomy or the trans-sphenoidal approach, has become much less dangerous, the advantage of irradiation, at least by external methods, is that it does not require operation and so eliminates both the morbidity and the mortality. Unless the diagnosis is in doubt, irradiation may well be the treatment of choice.

External irradiation has been used for many years. It was not initially a satisfactory form of treatment, since when only orthovoltage equipment was available many fields had to be used in order to achieve a satisfactory tumour-dose. This was not only time-consuming and relatively inaccurate, but produced a great deal of epilation. The maximum tumour-dose given was in the range of 2500–3000 rad and, although this produced some arrest of the tumour growth, regression of the signs of acromegaly was not always achieved.

These difficulties are easily overcome, however, by megavoltage therapy. A homogeneous tumour-dose of 4000–4500 rad in three to four weeks (daily fractionation) can easily be given with a pair of parallel and opposed fields (about 4 × 4 cm) which can be accurately localised to the pituitary fossa with marker films (Fig. 4.7). An alternative method is to rotate the machine around the skull through an arc of 300°, thus reducing the total dose to the temporal lobes of the brain; this will also reduce the dose to the hypothalamus, which may be very vulnerable to irradiation. However, it has been suggested that irradiation of this latter organ might be beneficial since the hypothalamus may be responsible for producing and releasing factors which encourage the growth of eosinophil adenoma, and irradiation might suppress the activity of these factors (Lawrence *et al.*, 1972). One of these factors has been described as a growth-hormone-inhibiting agent, deficiency of which might lead to acromegaly (Bessner *et al.*, 1974).

The results of external irradiation can be assessed both by the clinical improvement and by measurement of growth-hormone levels. Thus in Lawrence's series (1972) nine out of twelve cases showed reduced hormone levels, and 21 of 28 cases achieved good clinical response.

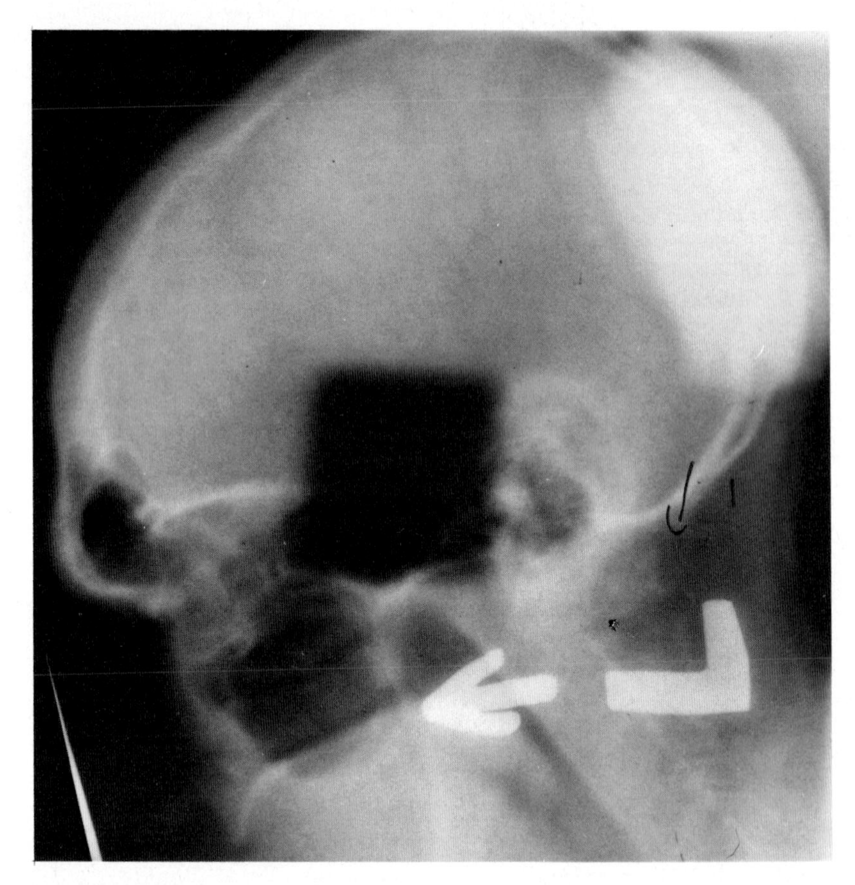

Fig. 4.7. Marker localisation film taken on ^{60}Co.

If it is thought necessary to ablate the pituitary completely in order to achieve the appropriate result, a very high dose of irradiation will be required. This can only be achieved by an interstitial implant of radioactive isotope, or by proton or π-meson irradiation. The first method has been well described by Wright *et al.* (1970) using ^{90}Y. Seeds can be placed in the pituitary fossa, using a trans-nasal approach through the sphenoid bone. A trocar and cannula can be inserted through the bone under direct vision, using a two-plane image-intensifier. The radioactive seeds can be screwed into position, thus reducing the chance of a CSF leak. Dosages in the region of 50 000 rad are given. The whole procedure can be carried out in about half an hour under a light anaesthetic.

This technique is not without problems, however. In the first place, the sphenoid bone must be well pneumatised, in order to allow the passage of the trocar. CSF rhinorrhoea occurred in about 13 per cent of Wright's series (1970), and had to be dealt with by muscle graft. Twelve per cent developed meningeal infection. Optic nerve damage did not occur in Wright's series, but it is always a potential hazard, as was shown in the original series reported by the same group in 1961 (Joplin *et al.*). Even though the operation is relatively easy, hospital admission is required.

Finally, at least 50 per cent of these cases subsequently developed pan-hypopituitarism, and required replacement therapy for the rest of their lives. The only real advantage of this method is that the patients have a much better regression of soft tissue and bony overgrowth. This may please the clinician, but since the patients are usually unaware of their original physical disability they are not necessarily impressed by such an improvement of their appearance. Wright's series (1970) showed a 53 per cent satisfactory response-rate.

Proton irradiation is of great theoretical interest to the radiotherapist, but requires a highly sophisticated and expensive apparatus, namely the 900 MV synchrocyclotron (available in only a few centres in the world). This machine can deliver a very high dose (4000–9000 rad) of proton irradiation to a very localised area, sparing the rest of the brain from irradiation. Lawrence *et al.* (1962) describe sixteen cases so treated, thirteen of whom were alive and well twenty months later; four of these required replacement therapy. In Massachusetts Kjellberg and Kliman (1974) have used this technique to give a single tumour-dose of 7000 rad. This is given through twelve portals, taking $1\frac{1}{2}$–2 hours to carry out. In 254 acromegalic cases they claim a 56 per cent complete and an 85 per cent partial remission. There was some morbidity, particularly in relation to visual disturbances, but these were described as only temporary phenomena.

The results of both these techniques are no better than external irradiation. The potential morbidity is greater, and the problem of replacement therapy is always present. Thus this author does not see the necessity in most cases of using these more complicated techniques when a simpler one will suffice.

Chromophobe Adenoma

These comprise about 50 per cent of pituitary tumours. The commonest presenting symptom is a defect of the visual fields, with the classical bitemporal hemianopia occurring in about 65 per cent of cases. Pressure effects on the pituitary itself may lead to pan-hypopituitarism, causing amenorrhoea in women and loss of libido in men.

The choice of treatment lies, again, between surgery and irradiation. If the diagnosis is confirmed both clinically and radiologically, irradiation can be used as the primary method of treatment in the majority of cases. If there is no improvement of the visual fields within six weeks of starting treatment, operation should be performed forthwith (Northfield, 1973).

Irradiation is given by the same simple method of opposed fields to a tumour-dose of 4000–4500 rad in three to four weeks. The size of the fields will obviously depend on the size of the tumour. Air encephalography is often useful in outlining the tumour, particularly if there is suprasellar extension. Treatment is easily done on an outpatient basis. Dramatic improvement of the visual fields may be seen within a few days. Occasionally the visual fields suddenly deteriorate, but this does not necessarily mean that the tumour is growing rapidly; it is more likely that haemorrhage into the necrotic mass has occurred, and the symptoms will soon improve without specific treatment.

Results of treating these tumours to moderate doses of irradiation are very gratifying. Colby and Kearns (1962) reported a good five-year response in 57 per cent of 127 cases. Chang and Pool (1967) reported visual improvement in 78 per cent of 51 cases, using the above dose-levels, but had a recurrence rate of 11 per cent. If symptoms recur, further external irradiation is not advisable but interstitial irradiation or surgery should be considered. Occasionally the diagnosis is in doubt. Surgery should be carried out, but since complete removal is rarely possible, post-operative irradiation should always be considered.

Basophil Adenoma

These comprise about 10 per cent of all pituitary tumours. Some will cause Cushing's syndrome by secretion of ACTH, although of course this may often be produced by a primary adrenal adenoma, and rarely by bronchial carcinoma. Welbourne (1969), in a study of 57 cases of Cushing's syndrome, showed that 37 were pituitary-dependent (twelve having a definite pituitary tumour); another twelve had a primary adrenal tumour, and one a bronchial neoplasm. Occasionally, after bilateral adrenalectomy for the primary tumour, a pituitary basophil adenoma will subsequently develop.

Treatment should be given to the pituitary in those patients in whom evidence of excess cortisol secretion from the gland is present. It is doubtful if surgery is necessary, as the secretion can be controlled by irradiation. Interstitial isotope implants can be used, but are associated with all the hazards outlined previously. Moderate doses of external megavoltage irradiation can produce good results. Orth and Liddle (1971) reported 51 cases treated to tumour-doses of 4000–5000 rad in four to five weeks; ten cases were cured for periods up to fourteen years; thirteen cases were improved, and included five children in whom growth continued at a normal rate; twenty-one were not improved, and required surgery. Seven were lost to follow-up.

Carcinoma

This is rare as a primary growth in the pituitary gland, but it is seen more often as a metastasis, particularly from the breast. The primary tumour should be treated with surgical excision; post-operative irradiation will be required in most cases, as surgery is rarely complete.

Metastatic Tumours of the Brain

These comprise about 20 per cent of all brain tumours (Russell and Rubinstein, 1970). The commonest primary is in the bronchus, followed closely by the breast, and less often by the stomach and kidney. Reticuloses are rare, apart from primary microgliomatosis (see Chapter 7), and the occasional meningeal plaque.

If the lesion is solitary, the question of operation should be considered. Certainly if the kidney is the primary site and there are no metastases elsewhere, surgical excision should always be considered. It is doubtful whether breast metastases should be treated surgically, as there are usually occult metastases in other parts of the body, and irradiation will be able to deal with the brain lesion. Occasionally a metastasis may be associated with an operable primary lesion of the lung; both the secondary and the primary have been successfully removed in such patients (Northfield, 1973). The chief indication for surgery is in those cases where there is a long time-interval between treatment of the primary neoplasm and the presentation of an apparent solitary metastasis, since the diagnosis of metastases may be wrong, and only surgery will reveal the true picture.

Irradiation to both single and multiple metastases may be helpful in controlling symptoms. If the prognosis is very poor, as in carcinoma of the lung, it is doubtful whether treatment is worthwhile. Deeley and Edwards (1968) treated such a group of cases, of which 50 per cent were improved for at least a month.

In carcinoma of the breast with brain secondaries it is worth trying hormone therapy first, particularly using dexamethasone which will at least help to reduce cerebral oedema. Failure to respond to this is an indication for radiotherapy, as the latter should be effective and survival may be increased for months or even years.

The only real indication for irradiation of metastases from other primary sites is the presence of severe intractable headaches, which are unrelieved by adequate analgesics and high doses of dexamethasone.

If the tumour is solitary and unilateral, as may be the case in breast and kidney metastases, a wedge field technique, treating only one side of the brain, can be tried. A tumour-dose of 3000–3500 rad in two or three weeks is well tolerated, and will cause severe epilation only on the treated side of the skull. With other neoplasms the chance of multiple lesions is high; thus the whole brain should be irradiated, giving a maximum tumour-dose of 3000 rad in two weeks. If the patient is very ill, a single dose to the whole brain is remarkably well tolerated: 800 rad can be given with two large opposed fields – the patient should remain in hospital, and be given dexamethasone 4 mg q.d.s.

Spinal Cord Tumours

About 15 per cent of all CNS tumours arise in the spinal cord.

Intra-medullary Tumours

These comprise about 20 per cent of the total and can be divided into three groups:

Astrocytoma. These are the commonest. They grow quite slowly. If the tumour is invasive, surgery is carried out only for diagnostic purposes; if the tumour is expansile it may be possible to carry out complete excision. In both types of tumour, post-operative irradiation should be considered (Northfield, 1973). Only the involved portion of the cord, with a margin of 5 cm above and below, need be treated, using a wedge field technique from the back with the patient in the prone position. A tumour-dose of 4000 rad in the cervical region and up to 4500 rad lower down the cord can be given in four weeks (20 daily fractionations). If the tumour is spilt at the time of the operation then the whole of the spinal cord below the neoplasm may need to be irradiated.

Ependymoma. These are nearly as common as the astrocytoma, and probably occur more frequently in the spinal cord than elsewhere. The cauda equina is frequently the affected site. Radical surgery here is impossible, since too many nerve roots would be damaged (Connolly, 1970). Local irradiation must be given to tolerance levels – 4500 rad in four weeks. Since the ependymoblastoma is likely to produce seedling metastases, whole CNS irradiation will be required.

Glioma. Least common of all the tumours, these are rarely operable, except in the occasional tumour arising in the cervical cord. Irradiation may produce some tumour regression and should be given to tolerance levels, after laminectomy and partial removal of the tumour.

Intra-dural Tumours

Lying outside the spinal cord, these tumours are mostly benign – in particular the meningioma, schwannoma, and blood vessel tumours. Surgery is often quite successful in their management; irradiation may be needed for an inoperable blood vessel tumour.

Extra-dural Tumours

Chordoma. Most commonly found in the sacro-coccygeal region, these are occasionally found in the spheno-occipital area. Surgery should always be attempted first, in order to remove the bulk of the tumour, but complete excision is rare. However, growth of this tumour is slow, and irradiation will slow down the rate of regrowth, even if it cannot eradicate the neoplasm. Unfortunately, chordomas are radioresistant, and high doses need to be given. Kamrin *et al.* (1964) suggest a tumour-dose of 5000 rad or more, and certainly their result of thirteen out of twenty patients alive and well at thirteen years is impressive.

Myeloma. This is usually part of a generalised disease, involving both the soft tissues and vertebrae as well as the rest of the reticulo-endothelial tissue. Spinal cord compression leading to paraplegia can occur rapidly. Treatment should be by a decompression laminectomy, followed by irradiation. Fortunately, myelomas are radiosensitive, so that large fields can safely be used, giving a tumour-dose of 2500 rad in ten treatments. Cytotoxic drug therapy will probably be required for the general manifestations of the disease.

Metastatic Tumours

These are the commonest of all extra-dural tumours. The primary sites most frequently involved are the lungs, breast, prostate and kidney. The reticuloses comprise another large group. In both cases, soft tissue masses and vertebral involvement can lead to spinal cord compression. In the reticuloses, if the diagnosis is known, irradiation can be successfully given without the need for surgery – long fields to a tumour-dose of 2500 rad in two weeks will usually suffice. Since solid tumours tend to be less radiosensitive it is probably better to carry out a laminectomy, which will not only reduce the cord compression very rapidly but will also confirm the diagnosis. Post-operative irradiation will always be required, since only the posterior portion of the tumour can be removed.

It should be stressed that in any patient presenting with incipient paraplegia from suspected metastatic disease, treatment by either method should be started at the earliest possible moment. Procrastination may lead to disaster since, once paraplegia has been present for more than twenty-four hours, improvement following surgery or irradiation is much less likely. If there is any doubt the patient should be transferred to a hospital which has both a neurosurgical and a radiotherapy department.

New Methods of Treating Tumours of the CNS

Combinations of surgery and local cytotoxic drugs into the tumour cavity were suggested by Guardfield and Dayan (1973), but in the small group of cases they reported there was little improvement seen.

Boron capture therapy, using slow neutrons, would appear to have some theoretical advantages, but no useful results have been demonstrated.

Irradiation and cytotoxic drugs in the management of medulloblastoma have been suggested, but again with no positive results.

Immunotherapy plus post-operative irradiation has been tried, using subcutaneous injections of irradiated autologous human tissue cells. Bloom *et al.* (1973) did not find any improvement in the short-term results.

The use of hyperbaric oxygen to increase the sensitivity of poorly-oxygenated tumours has been suggested. No satisfactory trials have yet been carried out which suggest that this is a particularly useful method. It is just possible that oxygenation might even increase the danger of radionecrosis (Van den Brenk *et al.*, 1968). Irradiation under hypothermia, with a view to increasing the oxygen-tension, has not been found to be effective (Bloch *et al.*, 1966).

Conclusion

Treatment of tumours of the nervous system by irradiation is both difficult and usually exceedingly time-consuming. Apart from the pituitary tumours and the very radiosensitive medulloblastoma, the results are not very gratifying. Nevertheless, every case should be considered individually, on its own merits; no hard and fast rules can be laid down for particular neoplasms. It seems to this author that although the initial response is not as obviously satisfactory as in treating, for example, the equally malignant carcinoma of the lung, the occasional excellent long-term results justify the expenditure of time and effort required to treat these tumours.

References

ARRIZPIZIBAL, S. A. (1971) *Radiology*, **101**, 201–202.

BELL, M. (1968) *Journal of American Medical Association*, **265**, 155–156.

BESSNER, G. M., MORTIMER, G. H., CARR, D., SCHULLY, A. V., COY, D. H., EVERED, D., KASTIN, A. J., TUNBRIDGE, W., THORNE, M. and HULL, R. (1974) *British Medical Journal*, **1**, 352–355.

BLOCH, M., BLOOM, H. J. G., PENMAN, J. and WALSH, L. (1966) *British Journal of Cancer*, **20**, 722–728.

BLOOM, H. J. G., PECKHAM, M. J., RICKHARDSON, A. E., ALEXANDER, P. A. and DAYNE, P. M. (1973) *British Journal of Cancer*, **27**, 256–265.

BLOOM, H. J. G. and WALLACE, H. (1969) *American Journal of Roentgenology*, **105**, 43–63.

BODEN, G. (1948) *British Journal of Radiology*, **xxi**, 464–469.

BODEN, G. (1950) *Journal of Faculty of Radiologists*, **2**, 79–94.

BOTTRILL, D., ROGERS, R. T. and HOPE-STONE, H. F. (1965) *British Journal of Radiology*, **38**, 122–130.

BOUCHARD, J. and PIERRE, P. (1960) *American Journal of Roentgenology*, **84**, 610–627.

CHANG, C. H. and POOL, J. L. (1967) *Radiology*, **89**, 1005–1016.

CLINTORIAN, A. M., SCHWARTZ, J. F., EVANS, R. A. and CASTOR, S. (1964) *Neurology*, **14**, 83–87.

COLBY, M. Y. and KEARNS, T. P. (1962) *Proceedings of Staff Meetings, Mayo Clinic*, **37**, 15.

CONNOLLY, R. C. (1970) in *Clinical Surgery*, ed. Gillingham, J., Butterworth, London, 231–233.

DEELEY, T. J. and RICE EDWARDS, J. M. (1968) *Lancet*, **1**, 1209–1212.

DUKE ELDER, S. and DOBREE, S. H. (1967) in *Systems of Ophthalmology*, ed. Duke Elder, S., Kimpton, London, 673–725.

GERMAN, W. J. (1961) *Clinical Neurosurgery*, **7**, 1–9.

GERSTNER, H. B., ORTH, J. S. and RICHEY, E. O. (1955) *American Journal of Physiology*, **180**, 232–236.

GUARDFIELD, J. and DAYAN, A. J. (1973) *Journal of Neurosurgery*, **39**, 315–321.

HOPE-STONE, H. F. (1961) *British Journal of Surgery*, **210**, 424–429.

HOPE-STONE, H. F. (1970) *Journal of Neurosurgery*, **32**, 1, 83–88.

HOPE-STONE, H. F. (1974) in *Recent Advances in Radiotherapy*, ed. Deeley, T., Butterworth, London, 120–150.

JONES, A. (1964) *British Journal of Radiology*, **37**, 727–740.

JOPLIN, G. C., FRASER, R., STEINER, B., LARS, J. and JONES, E. (1961) *Lancet*, **2**, 1277–1280.

KAMRIN, R. P., POTANO, N. R. and POOK, L. (1964) *Journal of Neurosurgery, Neurology and Psychiatry*, **27**, 157–165.

KING, T. T. (1970) in *Clinical Surgery*, ed. Gillingham, J., Butterworth, London, 145–213.

KISSANE, J. M. and ACKERMANN, C. V. (1955) *Journal of Faculty of Radiologists*, **7**, 109–114.

KJELLBERG, N. R. and KLIMAN, B. (1974) *Proceedings of Royal Society of Medicine*, **67**, 32–33.

KRAMER, S. (1969) *Acta radiologica (Therapy, Physics, Biology)*, **8**, 111–117.

KRAMER, S., MCKISSOCK, W. and CONCANNON, J. P. (1961) *Journal of Neurosurgery*, **18**, 217–226.

KRICHEFF, T. I., BEKER, M., SCHNEEK, S. A. and TAVERAS, J. M. (1964) *Journal of Neurosurgery*, **21**, 7–14.

KUNKLER, F. B., FARR, R. F. and LUXTON, N. W. (1952) *British Journal of Radiology*, **25**, 190–200.

LAWRENCE, J. H., TOBIAS, L. A., BORN, J. L., SANGALLI, H., CARLSON, R. R. and LINFOOT, J. A. (1962) *Acta radiologica*, **58**, 337–346.

LAWRENCE, M., PINSKY, S. M. and GOLDFINE, I. D. (1972) *Annals of Internal Medicine*, **128**, 368–377.

LAMPE, L. and MCINTREY, R. S. (1954) *American Journal of Roentgenology*, **71**, 659–668.

LEGRE, J., AMALRIS, R. and PUDART, J. (1969) *Acta radiologica (Therapy, Physics, Biology)*, **8**, 118–123.

MARSA, G. W., PROHART, J. L., RUBINSTEIN, L. H. and BAGSHAWE, A. (1973) *Cancer*, **3**, 646–655.

MCWHIRTER, R. (1955) in *British Practice of Radiology*, ed. Rock Carling, E., Butterworth, London.

MOSS, W. T. (1969) *Therapeutic Radiology*, Mosby, St Louis, Miss., 476.

NORTHFIELD, D. W. C. (1973) *Surgery of the Central Nervous System*, Kimpton, London.

ORTH, D. R. and LIDDLE, G. U. (1971) *New England Journal of Medicine*, **2855**, 244–247.

PATTERSON, E. (1952) *Journal of Faculty of Radiologists*, **4**, 175–179.

PATTERSON, E. and FARR, R. F. (1953) *Acta radiologica*, **39**, 323–336.

RAMSAY, R. G. and BRUND, W. N. (1973) *Journal of Neurosurgery*, **39**, 197–201.

RUSSELL, D. S. and RUBINSTEIN, L. J. (1970) *Pathology of Tumours of the Nervous System*, Arnold, London.

SAENGER, E. L. and DORST, J. P. (1968) *Paediatric Therapy*, ed. Shirley, H. C., Mosby, St Louis, Miss., 925–927.

SHARMA, U., TANDON, P. R., SAXENA, K. K., SINGAL, R. M. and BURUAH, J. D. (1974) *Clinical Radiology*, **25**, 13–17.

SHELINE, G. E., BOLDREY, E., KARLSBERG, P. and PHILLIPS, T. L. (1964) *Radiology*, **82**, 84–89.

STALLARD, H. B. (1966) *Acta ophthalmologica*, **151**, 214–220.

STELLA, J. C., SCHWEISGATH, D. and SCHLIENGER, M. (1970) *American Journal of Roentgenology*, **108**, 324–332.

STOLL, B. A. and ANDREWS, J. J. (1966) *British Medical Journal*, **1**, 834–837.

STOWENS, D. (1957) *Archives of Pathology*, **63**, 451–459.

TAPLEY, N. DU V. (1964) in *Ocular and Adnexal Tumours*, ed. Boniuk, M. Kallmann, St Louis, Miss., 158.

TOFT, M. and WITTENBERG, M. H. (1968) *Journal of American Medical Association*, **205**, 159–160.

TAVERAS, J. M., MOUNT, L. A. and WOOD, E. H. (1956) *Radiology*, **66**, 518–528.

TAVERAS, J. M., THOMPSON, H. G. and POO, J. I. (1962) *American Journal of Roentgenology*, **87**, 473–479.

VAN DEN BRENK, H. A. S., RICHTER, W. and HARLEY, B. H. (1968) *British Journal of Radiology*, **41**, 205–214.

WELBOURNE, R. B. (1969) *Annals of Royal College of Surgeons*, **44**, 182–193.

WILLIAMS, I. G. (1967) *Proceedings of Royal Society of Medicine*, **60**, 189–196.

WILLIAMS, I. G. (1972) *Tumours of Childhood*, Heinemann, London, 111–115.

WRIGHT, A. D., HARTIG, M., PALTER, H., JEVAURWERK, I. G., BOYLE, F. H., ARNOT, R., JOPLIN, G. F. and FRASER, J. R. (1970) *Proceedings of Royal Society of Medicine*, **63**, 220–222.

YOUNG, L. W., RUBIN, P. and HANSON, R. E. (1970) *American Journal of Roentgenology*, **108**, 75–91.

CHAPTER FIVE

Neoplasms of the Head and Neck

J. M. Henk

Malignant tumours of the upper air and food passages and associated structures are termed 'head and neck cancers'. These tumours are relatively uncommon, comprising about 5 per cent of all cancer in Great Britain. Nevertheless, they have been of prime importance to the radiotherapist in the development of the art and science of his specialty.

Head and neck cancers are mainly squamous cell carcinomata, with fairly predictable patterns of behaviour and spread; distant blood-borne metastases occur late in the course of the disease, usually not before involvement of lymph nodes is apparent. It is less usual for a patient to succumb from blood-borne metastases in the absence of local recurrence than with many other types of malignancy. Most lesions are readily accessible to clinical examination by both inspection and palpation, so that regular close observation is possible during the course of treatment and follow-up. Therefore radiation response can be studied and local recurrence diagnosed early and with certainty, so that the local effectiveness of treatment can be assessed accurately.

In the head and neck a wide variety of different normal tissues are to be found in close apposition and therefore must inevitably be irradiated in the course of radiotherapy to malignant neoplasms. These include tissues with such widely differing structure and cell proliferation patterns as skin, mucous membrane, bone, cartilage, mucus glands and central nervous system, all readily available for clinical study of radiopathological effects.

These anatomical and pathological peculiarities have made head and neck cancer the object of much careful study by radiotherapists over the past sixty years. Consequently many of the developments in radiotherapy have stemmed from studies of treatment of these tumours, for example, the principle of prolonged fractionation (Coutard, 1932), determination of optimum dosage for both external beam and interstitial therapy (Paterson, 1952) and the demonstration of the existence of the oxygen effect in human carcinoma (Henk and Smith, 1973). The value of new techniques in radiotherapy, such as neutrons (Chapter 3), concomitant cytotoxic drugs (Gollin *et al.*, 1972) and chemical sensitisers (Krishnamurthi *et al.*, 1967) can often best be tested by controlled trials in treatment of head and neck cancer.

Surgery and/or Radiotherapy

In the majority of patients with head and neck cancer both surgery and radiotherapy hold out possibilities of cure. In some cases, the chances of cure with either method of treatment may be slight, but better hopes can be pinned on a combination of the two. The approach may be primarily a radiotherapeutic one, in which case surgery is reserved for proven residual or recurrent tumour, or primarily surgical, where radiotherapy may be used pre- or post-operatively.

The choice of treatment for the individual patient is often difficult, depending on factors such as the patient's age, general condition, occupation, and mental state, as well as the site and stage of the neoplasm. The best results are obtained where there is close collaboration between surgeon and radiotherapist, preferably in joint consultation clinics where the patient and his disease can be assessed and a treatment strategy devised. This latter usually requires the active participation of the surgeon and radiotherapist and may involve other clinicians such as the oral surgeon and chemotherapist. It is important that the initial decision on the policy of management should be recorded in the patient's notes and adhered to as far as possible subsequently; to this end treatment and follow-up are best conducted at a combined clinic.

Radical Radiotherapy

The aim of radical radiotherapy is the total destruction of all reproductively viable malignant cells, and hence the cure of the patient, by radiation. In order to obtain the greatest possible chance of success, the maximum tolerable dose is delivered. Some degree of morbidity from acute mucosal reactions must be accepted, as must the possibility of an occasional case of necrosis.

Radical radiotherapy may be used where the tumour is inaccessible to surgery, e.g. carcinoma of the nasopharynx, or where the disease is too advanced to be operable, e.g. fixed neck nodes. It may be an alternative treatment to surgery for operable disease, in which case the aim is to preserve intact in the patient the affected organ, e.g. carcinoma of the larynx where surgical treatment involves laryngectomy and consequent loss of voice.

Follow-up after radiotherapy is mandatory. Lymph node metastases may develop and must be detected while they are still amenable to curative treatment. Also there may be evidence of failure of radiotherapy, in the form of persistent neoplasm in the treated volume. Sometimes an inoperable tumour treated by radical radiotherapy, although not cured, may be rendered operable (Buschke and Galante, 1959). Alternatively, a recurrence may appear months or even years later as a result of re-growth from microscopic foci of neoplastic cells which survived irradiation.

Where there is residuum or recurrence, surgical cure may be possible. Such 'salvage' surgery is of course performed on heavily irradiated tissues, and therefore carries a risk of complications consequent upon impaired blood supply, such as delayed wound-healing, fistula formation, wound break-down, and, most catastrophic of all, carotid artery rupture. Radiation changes in small blood vessels develop slowly, so the hazards of salvage surgery tend to increase with time after radiotherapy. The complication rate is lowest when surgery is performed within three months of completion of radiotherapy. However, an accurate clinical and histological assessment of complete tumour regression cannot be obtained until at least two months have elapsed after radiotherapy, so the clinician must beware of being too hasty in diagnosing residual tumour and proceeding to operation.

Elective Surgery

Elective operations are performed on tissues which have not received maximum doses of radiation; they are technically easier than salvage operations and carry much lower complication rates. These considerations, together with the development of improved techniques for reconstruction after extensive resection, have led to renewed enthusiasm for elective surgical treatment of head and neck cancer in recent years, with a consequent trend away from radical radiotherapy. However, it is not clear whether survival rates are being improved as a result, or whether the quality of life of survivors is better.

There is unfortunately a complete lack of evidence on these issues from controlled clinical trials. Retrospective studies, of which there are many in the world literature, will always tend to favour surgery because of selection of younger and fitter patients for this method. The relative merits of policies of radical radiotherapy and elective surgery are particularly difficult to assess in the case of advanced laryngeal carcinoma and will be discussed more fully under this heading later in the chapter.

Radiotherapy is rarely able to control local recurrence after surgery (Deutsch *et al.*, 1971). Consequently, in those cases where the risk of recurrence is high, radiotherapy is best given immediately before or after operation, rather than delayed until recurrence appears.

Pre-operative Radiotherapy

Pre-operative radiotherapy aims to increase the chance of surgical cure. It is based on the concept that local recurrence or metastases result from dissemination at operation of cells derived from the actively-growing periphery of the tumour. These cells have a good blood supply, are well oxygenated and therefore radiosensitive. They can be almost completely eliminated by moderate doses of radiotherapy insufficient to cause normal tissue reaction or to impair wound healing. The more radioresistant poorly-oxygenated cells, which require much larger doses of radiation to eliminate them, are situated towards the centre of the tumour and therefore most likely to be removed at operation without risk of dissemination.

Pre-operative radiotherapy has been tested and found to be effective in a wide variety of rodent tumours. In most experimental animal systems a low dose of radiation administered immediately before excision of the tumour significantly increases survival rates. Usually a dose of about one-third of the LD 50 for the particular tumour is effective pre-operatively; such a dose by itself cannot cure any tumours (Powers and Palmer, 1968).

In clinical practice there are two schools of thought on pre-operative radiotherapy, the low dose and the high dose. The low-dose technique consists of giving up to 2000 rad in one week or less, and operating immediately before any vaso-dilatation from acute radiation response occurs. Two prospective controlled trials have so far been reported, both of which show a reduced local recurrence rate as a result of pre-operative radiotherapy, but no improvement in survival. Strong (1969) reported a trial of radical neck dissection with and without 2000 rad in five treatments pre-operatively; local recurrence in the operated side of the neck was 33 and 54 per cent respectively, significant at the 5 per cent level. Lawrence *et al.* (1974) reported a similar trial in patients undergoing surgery for oral cavity carcinoma, using a dose of 1400 rad in two fractions; the local recurrence rate was 13 per cent lower in the irradiated group, but the difference did not reach statistical significance. In neither trial was there any increase in post-operative complications or delay in wound healing.

The high-dose method consists of giving about 80 per cent of a radical tumour-dose, i.e. 4000 to 5000 rad in 4–5 weeks; there must then be a delay before surgery of a further three or four weeks to allow the acute radiation reaction and vaso-dilatation to subside. No prospective controlled trials of this method have so far been reported, but in retrospective series improved results have been claimed, e.g. Goldman *et al.* (1972); Constable *et al.* (1972). Advocates of high pre-operative doses consider that the larger the number of cells that can be killed by radiation, the greater the chance of cure. However, dosage should not be raised to the levels used in radical radiotherapy as there will then be a significant increase in post-operative complications (Roswitt *et al.*, 1972; Rafla, 1972). The patient who has a full radical dose of radiotherapy followed within a few weeks by elective surgery has 'the worst of both worlds'; he suffers the discomfort and debilitation of a long course of radiotherapy, he fails to gain the advantage of retaining the affected organ, and in addition is subjected to a high risk of post-operative complications.

Hendrickson and Liebner (1968) compared high- and low-dose radiotherapy for supraglottic carcinoma in a small controlled trial; they found no difference in results between the two. If, as seems likely, the low-dose method can reduce local recurrence rates equally as well as the high-dose method, then the former should be preferred on the grounds of convenience and causing less upset to the patient.

Where the relative merits of the policies of elective surgery with pre-operative radiotherapy, or radical radiotherapy (with salvage surgery where necessary) are in doubt, e.g. in supraglottic carcinoma, a compromise policy is sometimes adopted. Radiotherapy is given to a dose-level similar to that used for high-dose pre-operative treatment, and then the patient is reassessed. If the tumour is regressing well, it is regarded as radioresponsive and further radiotherapy given to make up a full radical dose. If there is little or no regression, surgery is performed. Unfortunately, however, the rate of tumour shrinkage depends on many factors apart from the ultimate radiocurability of the tumour, especially the cell turnover rate and the rate at which dead tumour cells lyse or can be removed by phagocytic activity. Suit *et al.* (1965) were unable to demonstrate any correlation between regression rates and ultimate prognosis in patients irradiated for oropharyngeal cancer. It is probably unwise at the present state of our knowledge to decide upon definitive treatment on the basis of early tumour shrinkage; it is preferable to decide on the treatment strategy initially and adhere to it as far as possible.

Post-operative Radiotherapy

Post-operative radiotherapy has not found general favour in head and neck cancer. It cannot be expected to prevent the development of metastases from tumour cells disseminated at the time of surgery. It can only serve to prevent local recurrence arising from cells left in the operation field; such cells may well be poorly oxygenated in the post-operative period. The operation field which is potentially contaminated with malignant cells is always much larger than the original tumour, so that post-operative radiotherapy necessitates irradiation of a larger volume of normal tissue, limiting the dose which can be given. These theoretical considerations have discouraged both animal experiments and controlled clinical trials. Perez and Olsen (1970), working with a mouse lymphosarcoma, showed that the benefits of post-operative radiotherapy were much less than those of pre-operative radiotherapy.

In head and neck cancer, post-operative radiotherapy is best reserved for those cases where surgery is thought to be incomplete, from the operative findings or from histological examination of the resected specimen. The results reported by Fletcher and Evers (1970) suggest that in these circumstances post-operative radiotherapy given to maximum tolerance doses may control the disease in some cases. Low dose pre-operative radiotherapy does not preclude subsequent post-operative radiotherapy.

Palliative Radiotherapy

Palliative treatment aims to relieve symptoms in patients in whom there is no chance of cure. Where radiotherapy is used palliatively a moderate dosage is normally employed which causes little or no reaction, e.g. 2500 rad in two weeks. This is well below the dose which can give any reasonable chance of complete permanent tumour control, but is sufficient to destroy an appreciable proportion of the tumour to relieve a specific symptom, e.g. pain or bleeding. The patient's downhill progress from disseminated disease continues, but the terminal illness is less distressing.

In the head and neck this approach rarely succeeds. It is unusual, except in the case of some of the less common anaplastic tumours, for local disease to regress after small doses of radiation and for the patient subsequently to die of metastases before the local disease recurs and again gives symptoms. In general, radiotherapy is best used radically or not at all.

Improving the Therapeutic Ratio

There are two approaches to attempting to improve the results of radical radiotherapy. The first is directed at the oxygen effect, discussed in greater detail in Chapter 3. The hypoxic tumour cell is undoubtedly a real problem in squamous carcinoma of the head and neck; several controlled trials have demonstrated that hyperbaric oxygen can improve local clearance rates of head and neck tumours significantly.

The second approach seeks to exploit differences in cell proliferation patterns between tumours and normal tissue. Ultimately, the therapeutic ratio of radiotherapy probably depends on the differential effect between damage to tumour, which in the case of squamous carcinoma has a high rate of cell proliferation and cell loss, and damage to the vasculo-connective tissue with its slow cell turnover rate. Various fractionation schedules have been devised in an attempt to increase this differential effect, but the optimum for head and neck cancer has never been determined; it probably differs for every tumour. A wide variety of fractionation schedules are in current use, with treatment times varying from three to nine weeks, giving between two and five fractions weekly. A six-week treatment time with five fractions weekly is the most popular, but there is no evidence from controlled trials to support the use of any particular scheme.

Chemotherapeutic agents are toxic to actively proliferating cells, but do not affect cells in the resting phase of the cell cycle. They may therefore be expected to enhance the cell-killing effect on the tumour to a greater extent than on the vasculo-connective tissues. Four cytotoxic agents are in fairly widespread use in conjunction with radiotherapy for head and neck cancer; three of them are S-phase specific, namely methotrexate, 5-fluorouracil, and hydroxyurea. The fourth, bleomycin, acts at several points in the cell cycle; its affinity for squamous epithelium makes it a particularly useful agent in squamous carcinoma. All these agents are the subject of controlled clinical trials (Kramer, 1971; Gollin *et al.*, 1972; Richards and Chambers, 1973; Rygard, 1975) and some slight improvement in results from their use is being claimed. However, most of the trials are being conducted in advanced disease where the results of all forms of treatment are poor. Objective assessment of the place of concomitant chemotherapy will have to await the results of further trials, especially in patients with a better prognosis.

Management of Neck Nodes

For many years there was a widely held belief that metastases in lymph nodes were relatively resistant to radiation, and that even where the primary tumour was treated by radiotherapy, lymph node metastases, if present, should be treated surgically. This concept resulted from experience in the management of oral cancer in the 1930s and 1940s, when many of the primary lesions were treated very successfully by radium needle implants, but the only method of irradiation of the neck was by orthovoltage X-rays.

An implant has both physical and biological advantages over external radiotherapy, namely a high dose sharply localised to the tumour-bearing volume, short treatment time to avoid tumour repopulation, and a low dose-rate to overcome the problem of hypoxia; it can give excellent results when performed by a skilled radiotherapist who has plenty of practice at the technique, as was the case when oral cancer was much commoner in Britain. On the other hand, it is very difficult to administer adequate radiotherapy to the neck using either orthovoltage X-rays or interstitial techniques, so results of irradiation of lymph node metastases were poor. Nevertheless, Martin (1950) reported a series of 146 patients with oral cancer in whom the neck nodes were treated by a combination of radium implant and deep X-ray; a five-year survival of 27 per cent was obtained, compared with 25 per cent in a series of 410 similar cases where the nodes were treated by radical neck dissection.

The advent of megavoltage radiotherapy has made it possible to deliver a homogeneous dose to both primary and lymph node metastases *en bloc*. Results of such treatment demonstrate that the concept that a lymph node metastasis is more radioresistant than the primary from which it is derived is no longer tenable. Primary and nodes usually respond alike; it is no more frequent to see a node failure with the primary controlled than is the converse, as is shown by the results given below.

	Hanks et al., 1969	*Wizenburg et al., 1972*	*Henk, 1975*
Number of patients treated	69	113	122
Primary and nodes controlled	42%	52%	31%
Primary and nodes recurrent	43%	26%	39%
Primary controlled nodes recurrent	3%	8%	16%
Primary recurrent nodes controlled	12%	11%	14%

The management of neck nodes will now be discussed according to the TNM system:

Lymph Node Staging

N_0 no palpable nodes
N_{1a} mobile homolateral nodes, not considered to contain growth
N_{1b} mobile homolateral nodes, considered to contain growth
N_{2a} mobile bilateral or contralateral nodes, not considered to contain growth
N_{2b} mobile bilateral or contralateral nodes considered to contain growth
N_3 fixed nodes

Stage N_0, N_{1a}, N_{2a}

The advisability of 'prophylactic' treatment of the regional lymph nodes draining a tumour-bearing area is highly controversial. Undoubtedly in some cases microscopic foci of tumour will be destroyed before they can develop into clinically apparent metastases or spread further. At the same time, many uninvolved nodes will also be removed or irradiated, with the possible disadvantage of impairment of immunological defences against the tumour. The role of regional lymph nodes in tumour immunity is uncertain; animal experiments on the whole tend to suggest that by the time a primary tumour is clinically apparent the clone or clones of specifically sensitised lymphoid cells are either overwhelmed or distributed systemically, so surgery or radiotherapy to the regional nodes will not alter in any way the immunological response of the host to the tumour (Pilch *et al.*, 1971).

Head and neck surgeons hotly debate whether or not routine 'prophylactic' radical neck dissection should be performed, or whether, after treatment to the primary, the patient should be followed up carefully and surgery performed only when nodal metastases appear. The proponents of routine radical neck dissection claim that survival rates are highest where *en bloc* resections of primary and nodes are performed (Southwick, 1971) and point to retrospective studies which suggest that survival is higher after prophylactic than after therapeutic neck dissection (Roux-Berger *et al.*, 1949).

The opponents of the concept (Fayos and Lampe, 1972; Jesse and Lindberg, 1971) argue that less than 25 per cent of patients with head and neck tumours subsequently develop lymph node metastases with a controlled primary lesion. This figure contrasts sharply with reports of histological evidence of lymph node involvement by tumour in up to 60 per cent of patients on whom a prophylactic neck dissection is performed. The finding of foci of cancer cells in lymph nodes apparently does not necessarily indicate that such cells are viable and will cause further trouble. About 75 per cent of metastatic nodes are controlled by surgery, which leaves only a very small proportion of patients (4·5 per cent in the Jesse and Lindberg series) who could possibly have benefited from prophylactic surgery; these authors argue that the remainder would have had unnecessary operations.

Prophylactic neck irradiation is just as effective as prophylactic radical neck dissection, probably more so. It has been practised by some radiotherapists for many years, especially in nasopharyngeal carcinoma. In treatment of oropharyngeal, hypopharyngeal and supraglottic carcinoma the immediate lymphatic drainage is usually included in the fields treating the primary. More recently the value of prophylactic node irradiation in oral cavity carcinoma has been demonstrated (Bagshaw and Thompson, 1971). The dose required to control microscopic foci of tumour is less than that required to cure clinically apparent disease. Approximately 80 per cent of a radical tumour dose, i.e. 5000 rad in five weeks, is an effective 'prophylactic' dose.

In the individual patient a number of factors will influence a decision whether or not to treat the clinically negative neck prophylactically by surgery or radiotherapy. The most important factor is the probability that lymph node metastases will develop subsequently. This depends on:

(*a*) *The site of the primary.* Lymph node metastases are uncommon from carcinomata of the glottis, lip and upper jaw, but common from all parts of the pharynx and the supraglottis.
(*b*) *The size of the primary* which, especially in the mouth, correlates well with the incidence of subsequent lymph node metastases. Lesions above 2 cm in diameter in the mouth are usually recommended for prophylactic lymph node treatment.
(*c*) *Histology.* Lymph node metastases are more common from anaplastic than well-differentiated squamous carcinoma.

Other factors which must be taken into account are the general condition and age of the patient, the likelihood of cure of the primary tumour, and whether or not it will be possible to follow up the patient at regular intervals in order to detect node metastases at an early and potentially curable stage.

Stage N_{1b}

The operation of radical neck dissection has long been considered the treatment of choice for mobile unilateral nodes (Bond and Mansfield, 1959). However, the local recurrence rate after this operation is high, approaching 50 per cent in many reported series. This figure can be reduced considerably by pre-operative radiotherapy (Millburn and Hendrickson, 1967; Strong, 1969). Post-operative radiotherapy may usefully be added, especially in those cases where there is doubt whether surgical clearance has been complete.

There is probably no longer any place for radical neck dissection alone. The choice of treatment for unilateral mobile nodes lies between surgery combined with radiotherapy and radical radiotherapy alone. The objection to the latter is that recurrence after radiotherapy manifests itself as a diffuse infiltration rather than the reappearance of discrete mobile masses, hence salvage surgery in the neck rarely succeeds. The combined approach is probably preferable for node metastases from well-differentiated squamous carcinoma, especially in the mouth and larynx, while radiotherapy alone is adequate for the more anaplastic nodal metastases from the nasopharynx and oropharynx.

Stage N_{2b}

Bilateral radical neck dissection is feasible, but removal of both internal jugular veins is hazardous, while the risk of recurrence is higher if a jugular vein is preserved. Treatment should be by a combination of radiotherapy and surgery, or by radiotherapy alone. The latter is often quite satisfactory, especially as bilateral mobile nodes are most common from the more radiosensitive primary tumours in the nasopharynx and oropharynx. Where bilateral nodes are treated radically by radiotherapy, care must be taken to avoid a high dose to the spinal cord; refined beam-direction techniques are therefore required.

N_3

Fixed nodes are unsuitable for initial surgery. Radiotherapy is the treatment of choice. With careful techniques of beam-direction to ensure a homogeneous dose to the tumour while avoiding vital structures, eradication of fixed node metastases is a possibility. Even where complete regression of nodes is not obtained, radiotherapy may render large masses in the neck amenable to subsequent surgery.

Carcinoma of the Oral Cavity

The oral cavity extends from the lip anteriorly to the anterior faucial pillar posteriorly. The vast majority of malignant tumours at this site are squamous carcinoma, usually well-differentiated and often associated with recognisable pre-malignant changes. They occur mainly in middle-aged and elderly people and are commoner in men than women. The widely differing incidences in various parts of the world suggest an association with dietary habits, economic conditions and social customs.

In the United Kingdom the incidence of mouth cancer is declining rapidly. The number of new cases reported annually fell from approximately 4000 in 1932 to less than 1000 in 1970. This decline in incidence is attributed to rising economic standards with better nutrition, improved dental care, and control of infections. Unfortunately the prognosis for those individuals who do develop the disease is not improving (Binnie *et al.*, 1972). The proportion presenting at an advanced stage is tending to increase, possibly due to the rising age-incidence which always accompanies a decline in total incidence, and the possibility that the type of tumour now seen is biologically more aggressive than the traumatic or chemically-induced tumours which formerly predominated. A contributory factor is the failure of medical and dental practitioners to recognise at an early stage what is now a rare disease.

Carcinoma of the Lip

Carcinomata of the lip are almost always of the well-differentiated squamous variety. Spread to regional lymph nodes is relatively uncommon. About 7 per cent of patients will have lymph nodes involved at the time of presentation, and a further 5 per cent will develop them subsequently (Krantz *et al.*, 1957).

Carcinoma of the lip is highly radio-curable. With small tumours of 2 cm diameter or less, local recurrence after radiotherapy is almost unknown (del Regato and Sela, 1959; Dick, 1962). Radiotherapy failure is rare even with very large lesions. Surgery is equally successful. The choice of treatment between radiotherapy and surgery depends on convenience and the expected cosmetic result. For large lesions, which require extensive reconstructive surgery, radiotherapy is preferable. For smaller lesions the early cosmetic results of radiotherapy are superior but after a few years there may be atrophy and telangectasia so that, in the long term, there may be little to choose between the two methods. Surgery may be preferred for the small lesion on the grounds of being more expeditious.

Where radiotherapy is chosen for carcinoma of the lip it is nowadays nearly always given by external beam. To obtain a really good cosmetic result, fractionation over at least four weeks is desirable. The radium 'sandwich' mould still has its advocates; this method has the disadvantages of requiring the services of a skilled technician, some discomfort to the patient, and radiation hazard to staff; its advantage is that it produces an excellent cosmetic result with an overall treatment time lasting only eight days.

Carcinoma of the Tongue and Floor of Mouth

The oral cavity contains the mobile portion of the tongue in front of the vallate papillae, the so-called 'anterior two-thirds'. Tumours at this site will be considered together with those of the floor of the mouth because of similarity in behaviour, treatment and prognosis. The so called 'base' or 'posterior third' of the tongue belongs anatomically and embryologically to the pharynx; tumours here behave differently from those of the oral cavity, and will be considered under the heading of oropharynx.

Carcinoma of the tongue and floor of mouth carries a much worse prognosis than carcinoma of the lip. The primary tumours are less radiocurable and metastases to regional lymph nodes occur much more readily. The five-year survival rate in Great Britain is less than 30 per cent and has not improved over the past 30 years.

Pre-malignant lesions in the mouth are common; these show dyskeratosis without invasion on histological examination. Clinically they appear as whitish patches known as leukoplakia. However, this appearance may be due merely to hyperkeratosis or lichen planus, so that histological examination is necessary to demonstrate pre-malignant change. Pre-malignant lesions should not be irradiated; radiotherapy may cause the epithelium to revert temporarily to a normal appearance, but recurrence is likely and subsequent frank carcinomatous change is not prevented.

The verrucous carcinoma is a rather rare variety of well-differentiated squamous carcinoma with abundant keratin production. It has been claimed that this tumour is relatively radioresistant, and even that radiotherapy is contra-indicated because of the risk of inducing anaplastic change and more rapid spread (Kraus and Perez-Mesa, 1966). However, in the author's experience this type of lesion can be treated by radiotherapy with good results.

Invasive squamous carcinoma is usually moderately or well-differentiated, although occasional anaplastic varieties occur. It is often claimed that the more anaplastic tumours are more radiosensitive; this is not necessarily true. Certainly they regress more rapidly than the well-differentiated varieties, but they recur more rapidly, and ultimate radiocurability correlates poorly with histological grade. There is better correlation between tumour morphology and radiocurability; the proliferative exophytic type of tumour with minimal infiltration responds well to radiotherapy, whereas the more deeply-infiltrating variety, presumably with a poorer blood supply and high proportion of hypoxic cells, is less likely to be cured. However, the single most important factor determining both the outcome of radiotherapy and the ultimate prognosis is the size of the primary tumour. The larger the primary, the higher the recurrence rate after radiotherapy and the higher the incidence of lymph node metastases. Frazell and Lucas (1962) in their series of 1544 patients with carcinoma of the tongue treated in New York report that where the primary was less than 2 cm in diameter the five-year survival was 61 per cent, whereas with primaries larger than 2 cm the five-year survival was 30 per cent.

The relative merits of surgery and radiotherapy have been controversial for many years, with swings of the pendulum of clinical practice first to one and then to the other. Frazell and Lucas (1962) reported that prior to 1939 at the Memorial Hospital, New York, the primary was treated mainly by radiotherapy with 'unsatisfactory' results, the five-year survival rate being around 25 per cent. There was therefore a change towards more aggressive surgery with a claimed improvement, although the five-year survival rate increased only to 30 per cent. Unfortunately, it now seems that the relative merits of various treatment methods will not be resolved by controlled trials in the foreseeable future. For the individual patient the best treatment must be determined by joint consultation in a combined cancer clinic, taking into account the patient, his lesion, and the facilities and clinical skills available.

Pre-malignant areas and very small carcinomata, especially on the tip of the tongue, are best excised. For the larger T_2 or T_3 primary, radical radiotherapy can give a better cosmetic and functional result than surgery, which is best reserved for the radiotherapy failures (Fig. 5.1).

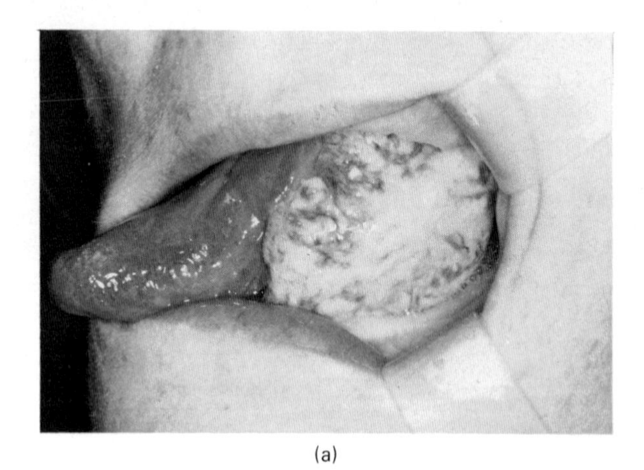

(a)

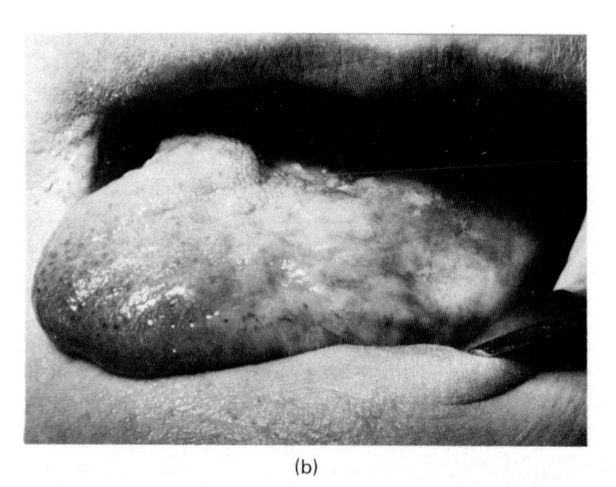

(b)

Fig. 5.1. a Carcinoma of the lateral border of the tongue, invading floor of mouth, in a 40-year-old woman.
b Appearance four years after treatment by external beam radiotherapy. The patient is well with no evidence of tumour.

Irradiation of oral cancer is now most commonly done by external beam using a megavoltage machine. Moulds and superficial X-ray applicators for intra-oral use are now very rarely used, but may still have a place for the treatment of very superficial lesions. In the pre-megavoltage era radium needle implants were used extensively because the only external beam treatment plants available were in the orthovoltage range, which gave an inadequate depth-dose and a high incidence of bone necrosis. Radium needle implants are less favoured now because they require skill and practice on the part of the radiotherapist and present radiation hazards to staff; they are only really suitable for smaller lesions clear of bone, particularly in the anterior two-thirds of the tongue and the buccal mucosa.

The introduction of radioactive iridium wires after-loaded into fine polythene cannulae has overcome many of the geometrical and protection problems of interstitial therapy in the mouth. This technique enables very accurate positioning of the sources, avoiding underdosed areas, and also has the advantage that the wires can be placed much closer to bone than can radium needles. Pierquin *et al.* (1970) reported a local recurrence rate of 3 per cent using iridium, compared with 32 per cent using radium. Pierquin *et al.* (1971) reported a 95 per cent local tumour control at four years of tumours of the tongue and floor of mouth less than 4 cm in diameter. This is far higher than any previously reported cure rates from any form of radiation therapy, but was obtained at the expense of an 18 per cent necrosis rate. Clinical evidence of a better therapeutic ratio from the newer interstitial techniques compared with megavoltage external radiotherapy is therefore still lacking.

Larger lesions, especially those involving bone and where there is lymph node involvement, are probably best treated where possible by *en bloc* resection of primary and nodes, combined with pre- or post-operative radiotherapy, where the age and general condition of the patient permits. Nevertheless, where the suitability of the patient for major surgery is in doubt, it must be remembered that radical radiotherapy can control large tumours and metastatic neck nodes in an appreciable proportion of cases and should not be withheld.

Carcinoma of the Lower Jaw

Carcinoma of the lower alveolus has a similar aetiology and prognosis to that of the tongue and floor of mouth. Early involvement of bone is the rule. The alleged increased radioresistance of carcinoma invading bone, and the high risk of necrosis of the involved mandible, has led to

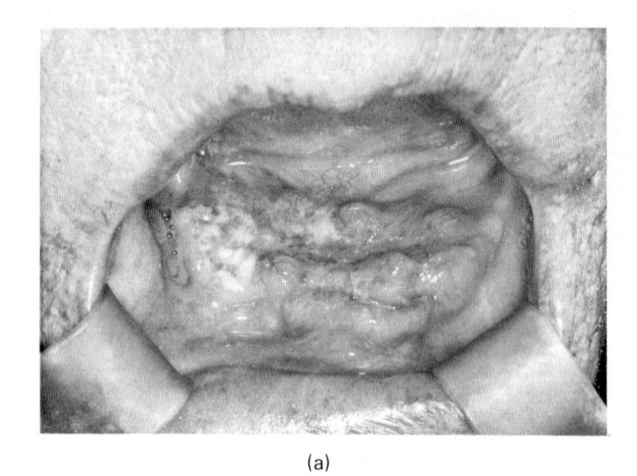

(a)

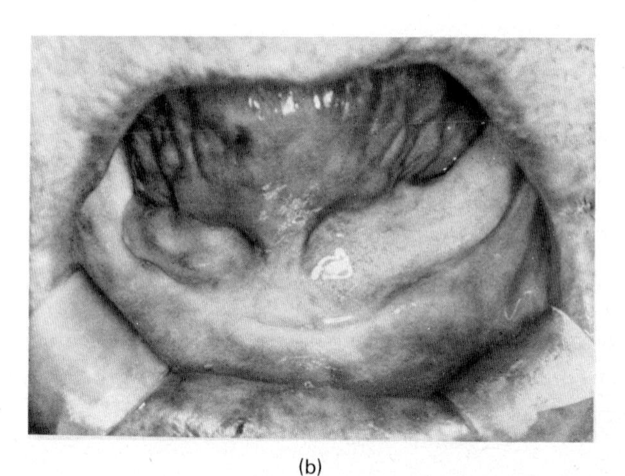

(b)

Fig. 5.2. a Carcinoma of the lower alveolus in a 72-year-old man. There was radiological evidence of bone destruction.
b Complete healing six months after external beam radiotherapy. Bone necrosis did not occur; the patient subsequently developed involved lymph nodes in the neck which were not controlled by a combination of surgery and radiotherapy, and he succumbed two years after the initial treatment.

a general preference for surgery over radiotherapy for cancer at this site. However, hemi-mandibulectomy inevitably leads to some deformity, and rehabilitation, especially in elderly people, is not always easy. Cure by radiotherapy without necrosis is a possibility, so a policy of radical radiotherapy and salvage surgery is reasonable for earlier tumours of the lower alveolus, and for all cases in older people (Fig. 5.2).

Osteoradionecrosis is still a fairly common complication of radiotherapy. It occurs in the mandible but is rare in the upper jaw. It is most common where the primary tumour is involving the lower alveolus, but it may also occur after radiotherapy to lesions elsewhere in the oral cavity, oropharynx and neck where the mandible is in the high-dose volume. The main aetiological factors are high radiation dose, previous involvement of the mandible by carcinoma, and dental extractions. Other factors contribute, such as local trauma from dentures, smoking, poor nutrition, and infection. High dosage to bone was a frequent problem in the days when the only external beam radiation available was in the orthovoltage range; with megavoltage radiation, bone dose can be kept within the tolerance range.

The management of teeth in the patient receiving radiation to the mouth remains controversial. Dental decay occurs rapidly after radiotherapy, more because of diminished salivary flow than from any direct effect on the teeth or their blood supply. Extraction of a tooth from a part of the mandible which has received maximum doses of radiation carries a very high risk of bone necrosis: the trauma of the extraction acts as a mitotic stimulus to the osteoblast, which is normally a resting cell. A proportion of the osteoblasts will have been lethally irradiated and will die when they attempt to divide. Infection and diminished blood supply also compromise healing at the extraction site. Consequently, it became standard practice in radiotherapy to extract all teeth in the path of the beam before starting treatment (Fig. 5.3).

Daly *et al.* (1972) showed, however, that pre-radiotherapy extraction is also a predisposing factor to osteoradionecrosis, and the advisability of routine extraction is now questioned. Insistence on extractions adds further to the patient's distress and in some cases may even lead to refusal to undergo treatment. It is now possible to reduce the incidence of post-irradiation dental caries considerably by the local

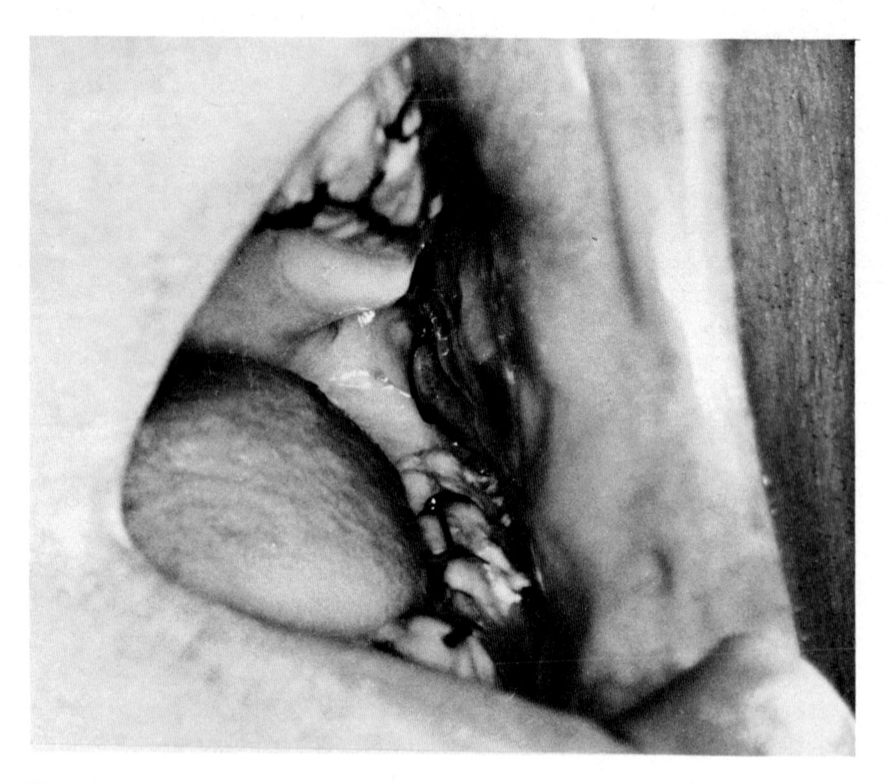

Fig. 5.3. Carcinoma of the upper retro-molar area in a man of 39, before starting radical radiotherapy. All teeth in the vicinity of the tumour have been removed and the gums sutured.

application of sodium fluoride gel using a carrier (Daly *et al.*, 1972), or by covering the teeth with acrylic splints (Coffin, 1973). Solomon *et al.* (1968) have shown that it is possible to extract teeth from an irradiated mandible without causing necrosis provided the patient is hospitalised and appropriate precautions taken. It now seems advisable to adopt a more conservative approach and limit pre-radiotherapy extractions to the more severely diseased teeth.

Carcinoma of the Nasopharynx

Carcinoma of the nasopharynx is a relatively rare tumour in the Western world, representing less than 0·3 per cent of all malignancies

(Hara, 1969), in sharp contrast to South East China where it is the commonest malignancy, representing more than half the total. The high incidence in Chinese is almost certainly due to an ethnic rather than an environmental factor (Ho, 1972). There is a much greater spread of age incidence with carcinoma of the nasopharynx than with other head and neck cancers, and in fact the nasopharynx is the commonest site for a carcinoma below the age of thirty. Occasional cases occur in children and adolescents.

There is a much greater proportion of anaplastic carcinoma than at other head and neck sites; only about 50 per cent of nasopharyngeal carcinoma is of well-differentiated squamous type. Anaplastic carcinoma occurs particularly in the younger age-groups.

The lymphoepithelioma has been the subject of controversy for many years. It is now generally agreed that this is not a separate entity; it is merely an anaplastic carcinoma invading lymphoid tissue and perhaps exciting a lymphocytic reaction. Metastases often lack the lymphoid element, and many pathologists now consider that the term should be discarded altogether and these tumours reported as anaplastic carcinoma (Evans, 1966). There is certainly no justification for regarding lymphoepithelioma as a highly radiosensitive tumour curable by low doses of radiation; it is certainly not as radiosensitive as the lymphomata (Yeh, 1962). Maximum tissue tolerance doses of radiation should always be administered for this type of tumour.

It is doubtful whether there is any difference in prognosis between the different histological types. Anaplastic tumours are less likely to recur locally but more likely to give blood-borne metastases than squamous tumours. Chen and Fletcher (1971) divided their tumours into only two types, lymphoepithelioma and squamous carcinoma; they reported a better local tumour control rate and higher survival rates in the former group. Yeh, on the other hand, failed to find any correlation between histological type and prognosis.

Spread of nasopharyngeal carcinoma occurs rapidly and at an early stage. The lines of spread of the disease and the clinical syndromes so produced are described in detail by Lederman (1961). It is very difficult on clinical and radiological assessment to determine accurately the true extent of the disease, so radiotherapy must always encompass the potential lines of spread including the para-pharyngeal space and base of skull. There is a high incidence of lymph node involvement; in most reported series at least 70 per cent of patients have palpable nodes in the neck when first seen; a lump in the neck is often the presenting symptom. The first nodes to be involved are usually the lateral pharyngeal and posterior deep cervical, which should always be included in the treatment volume. Blood-borne spread to lungs, bone, liver, etc., occurs earlier and more frequently than in other head and neck carcinomas and is rather frequently seen in the absence of local recurrence (Fletcher and Million, 1965).

Since surgery is impossible, treatment is almost entirely by external beam radiotherapy. Interstitial and intracavitary radiation techniques have been tried but are not popular. A high incidence of lymph node secondaries makes irradiation of both sides of the neck from base of skull to clavicle advisable in all patients whether or not nodes are palpable at presentation, the highest survival rate reported being obtained by this approach. Most recently reported five-year survival rates are between 30 and 40 per cent (Moench and Phillips, 1972; Wang and Meyer, 1971; Chen and Fletcher, 1971).

Surprisingly, lymph node involvement seems to make very little difference to prognosis, especially in the case of anaplastic tumours, until the nodes become fixed or involve the supraclavicular region. Failure is commoner at the primary site than in the nodes, so radical neck dissection is rarely needed (Perez *et al.*, 1969). The high incidence of failure at the primary site is due in part to the frequent use of too low a dosage, as the simultaneous use of prophylactic neck irradiation and consequent large fields may lead the radiotherapist to give a below-optimum dose to the primary. A dose of at least 6000 rad in six weeks is needed to give the best chance of tumour control. Failure may also be due to under-estimation of the spread of the disease, especially to the base of skull and lateral pharyngeal nodes, so that the fields of radiation fail to include all the malignancy.

Carcinoma of the Oropharynx

The oropharynx, or mesopharynx, extends from the level of the palate above to the hyoid bone below. It includes the tonsillar fossae, posterior third of tongue and vallecula. The majority of malignant tumours at this site are of epithelial origin, although lymphomata occasionally occur. As in the case of the nasopharynx there is a high proportion of more anaplastic carcinoma. Approximately 80 per cent of patients with oropharyngeal carcinoma have involvement of lymph nodes at presentation or develop them subsequently; lymph node involvement is bilateral in at least 50 per cent.

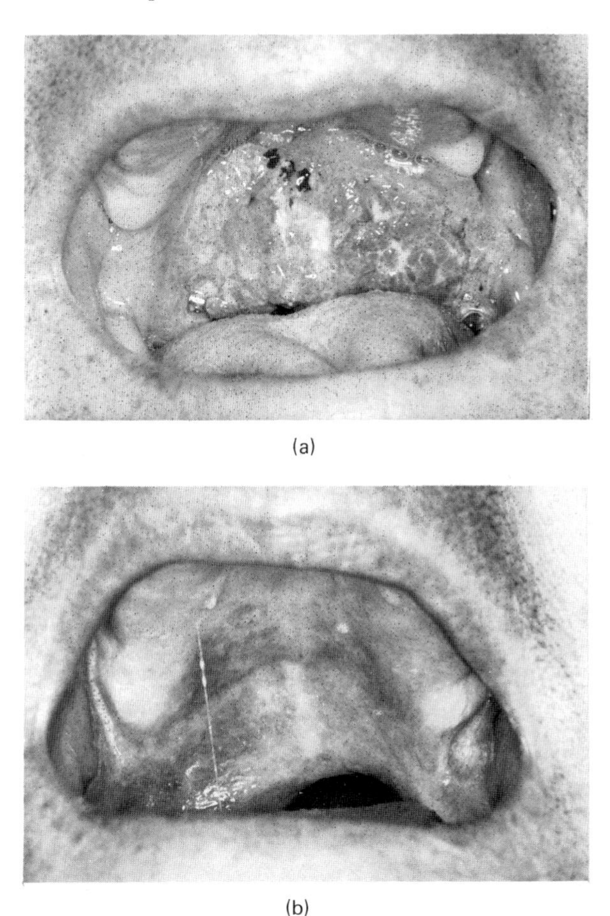

(a)

(b)

Fig. 5.4. a Extensive carcinoma involving soft palate and both tonsillar fossae in a 61-year-old man.
b Complete regression and healing after external beam radiotherapy. Patient survived seven years, eventually succumbing to a new primary carcinoma of the lower oesophagus.

Relatively few carcinomata of the oropharynx are suitable for surgery, then only by extensive operations. The majority are treated solely by radiotherapy. In most cases appropriate technique consists of parallel opposed lateral fields which cover the primary tumour and the immediate lymphatic drainage on both sides. Where there is obvious lymph node involvement it is advisable to treat the neck nodes down to the level of the clavicle 'prophylactically'. It is uncommon for radiotherapy to control the primary while failing to control lymph nodes, so there is probably little place for radical neck dissection, except perhaps in the well-lateralised, better-differentiated tumours of the tonsil.

Five-year survival rates for oropharyngeal carcinoma are similar to those of oral cavity carcinoma, i.e. 30–40 per cent overall. However, the control rate of both primary and nodes by radiotherapy is considerably higher than in the case of oral cancer, and a high proportion of patients who die do so free from disease above the clavicle (Fig. 5.4). There is an appreciable mortality from metastases without local recurrence, and also a large proportion of intercurrent deaths, because many of the cases occur in elderly people, or in association with chronic alcoholism and heavy smoking (Fletcher *et al.*, 1967).

Carcinoma of the Larynx

Carcinoma of the larynx in general carries a better prognosis than most head and neck cancers. It is a rewarding disease to treat, and good results can be obtained by a variety of treatment methods. As a result, there has been a tendency for a competitive spirit to develop between surgeon and radiotherapist. This is unfortunate because the best results are undoubtedly obtained where there is close collaboration between the two disciplines.

In any disease where results are tolerably good there is a reluctance on the part of clinicians to test their treatment methods by prospective controlled trials. Carcinoma of the larynx is no exception. Consequently there is a lack of good objective evidence of which methods of treatment provide the highest survival rates for carcinoma at various sites and stages within the larynx. There are many retrospective series of cases reported in the world literature, with a startling variety of results. For example, radiotherapy for T_2 glottic carcinoma was reported to give a five-year survival rate of 18 per cent by Marchetta *et al.* (1968) and 100 per cent by Hibbs *et al.* (1969). Such differences are accounted for mainly by selection of cases for various methods of treatment, which will differ between centres, and by staging which is not always comparable. In many patients it is impossible to be absolutely certain of the true extent of the disease; some laryngologists will tend to understage, while others overstage.

Against this background of doubt and controversy, the surgeon and the radiotherapist faced with the patient with laryngeal cancer must together try and determine the best treatment for that individual. They must consider not only the chances of survival but also the quality of life. If laryngectomy is contemplated, the patient's chance of developing a means of communication adequate to his needs must be considered; this will depend upon age, sex, occupation and social habits. It may be preferable in some advanced cases to use radical radiotherapy initially in an attempt to preserve the voice, even though the chance of survival may be considered to be 10 or even 20 per cent higher if laryngectomy be performed electively. Not all doctors or patients would agree with Harrison (1969) that on no occasion must preservation of the voice be allowed to jeopardise effective eradication of disease.

Carcinoma of the *true vocal cord* is the most benign of all head and neck cancers. Its growth rate is slow, it spreads late, the incidence of lymph node metastases at presentation being only about 4 per cent, and it soon gives rise to the symptom of persistent hoarseness so that early diagnosis and effective treatment are possible. For the early case there is little argument that initial radiotherapy is the treatment of choice, reserving surgery for recurrence. A small recurrence confined to the vocal cord can be dealt with satisfactorily by laryngo-fissure; more extensive disease requires laryngectomy. Where the tumour is confined to one cord with full mobility the survival rate is scarcely lower than that of the normal population of the same age-group, and less than 10 per cent of cases require salvage surgery. Involvement of the anterior commissure reduces the local control and survival rates by only a few per cent, and should not in itself be regarded as an indication for surgery (Jesse *et al.*, 1971).

For more advanced disease where there is fixation of the cord or extension supra- or subglottically, some authorities prefer immediate laryngectomy; however, many reported series suggest that, even in these cases, initial radical radiotherapy is often successful. There is at least a strong suggestion in the world literature that a policy of radical radiotherapy with salvage surgery is able to preserve the larynx in at least half of all patients with advanced glottic cancer, and gives survival rates similar to those of initial laryngectomy. As mentioned above, there are no results available from controlled trials; the only comparison within one centre, that of Marshall *et al.* (1972), failed to show any difference in survival between treatment by laryngectomy alone, laryngectomy with pre-operative radiotherapy and radical radiotherapy with salvage surgery, but the majority of the survivors of the last-named policy retained the larynx. Survival and local tumour control rates

Table 5.1. Glottic Carcinoma treated by Radical Radiotherapy, Cardiff 1960–1966

Stage	*Number treated*	*Died of cancer*	*Died of intercurrent disease*	*Determinate 5-year survival*	*Tumour control probability at 5 years*
T_1 (one cord involved, full mobility)	49	3	9	93%	92%
T_2 (both cords and/or anterior commissure involved	24	2	9	87%	83%
T_2 (confined to glottis, cord fixed)	13	4	3	60%	61%
T_3 (spread beyond glottis)	53	16	8	63%	58%

obtained in Cardiff between 1960 and 1966 are shown in Table 5.1. Cardiff is a fairly typical regional centre, seeing a high proportion of more advanced disease and where a policy of radical radiotherapy has been generally preferred. The figures are typical of results quoted in the world literature from a number of centres throughout Europe and North America who adopt the same policy.

The *supraglottic* region comprises the ventricle, false cord, posterior surface of epiglottis, aryepiglottic fold and arytenoid. Carcinomata at this site grow and spread more rapidly than those arising on the vocal cord. Involvement of lymph nodes occurs in at least 50 per cent of cases. Presentation is late because a tumour needs to grow to a fairly large size before producing any symptoms such as pain, dysphagia, dyspnoea or hoarseness. Consequently the prognosis is much worse, and five-year survival rates are about 40 per cent on average, varying between over 70 per cent for Stage I to under 10 per cent for Stage IV.

In the early case treatment is either radical radiotherapy or a horizontal partial laryngectomy. The latter operation has not found general favour in Britain where the number of patients with supraglottic carcinoma seen at an early stage remains disappointingly low. The procedure requires considerable skill and experience; the voice is preserved, but swallowing problems are common and rehabilitation can be exceedingly difficult. Radical radiotherapy is therefore preferred generally and control rates are high, approaching 90 per cent for T_1 and 66 per cent for T_2 (Wang, 1973). The disadvantage of radiotherapy is that conservation surgery is difficult in the irradiated larynx, so where radiotherapy fails a total laryngectomy is usually required.

For more advanced supraglottic carcinoma the highest survival rates have been reported from a policy of laryngectomy and block dissection, with pre-operative radiotherapy, e.g. Goldman *et al.* (1972). However, good results have also been published for radical radiotherapy with salvage surgery (Bataini *et al.*, 1971). A controlled trial is urgently needed for this disease to find out whether a policy aimed at preservation of the larynx can be adopted without significantly prejudicing survival rates.

Hypopharynx

Carcinomata occur at three sites in the hypopharynx, namely the pyriform fossa, the 'post-cricoid' and the posterior wall. These all carry a poor prognosis but vary considerably in their natural history and response to treatment.

Carcinoma of the *pyriform fossa* is a disease predominantly of middle-aged and elderly men. Early tumours at this site produce minimal symptoms, therefore late presentation is the rule. Involved lymph nodes are palpable in at least 70 per cent of all patients at presentation. Pyriform fossa carcinoma poses similar therapeutic problems to advanced supraglottic cancer; in fact many large tumours involve both the pyriform fossa and the supraglottis, and the exact site of origin is difficult to determine. Reported five-year survival with radiotherapy varies between 10 and 20 per cent. Surgical series tend to claim slightly higher survival rates, but only a minority of patients are fit and suitable for surgery.

The term '*post-cricoid carcinoma*' is a confusing one because it is used to describe two quite different entities. The post-cricoid plate forms the posterior wall of the larynx and the anterior wall of the hypopharynx. Carcinoma arising at this site is rare. It occurs mainly in men and has a similar aetiological pattern and behaviour to carcinoma of the pyriform fossa. However, in Britain the term 'post-cricoid carcinoma' usually describes a tumour involving the crico-pharyngeal region and the upper cervical oesophagus, usually annular; the more accurate descriptive term 'epi-oesophageal' has been suggested by Lederman (1967). This disease is commoner in females than males. Its highest incidence is in the northern parts of North America and Europe. It is particularly prevalent in Wales where some 35 per cent of cases are associated with the Paterson–Kelly syndrome (Richards *et al.*, 1971).

The prognosis with all forms of treatment is very poor. The primary lesion is usually very extensive at presentation and early involvement of lymph nodes in both sides of the neck and in the mediastinum occurs. For the early case without palpable lymph nodes radical radiotherapy by a double wedge technique, as described by Garrett (1971), may sometimes be successful, and in fact survival rates of up to 25 per cent at five years have been reported. Still higher survival rates in selected cases have been claimed for the operation of pharyngo-laryngectomy, but at the expense of a high operative mortality and morbidity. Later cases, especially where there is lymph node involvement, have an almost 100 per cent mortality. The first nodes to become palpable are usually in the posterior upper deep cervical group, often bilaterally. Where these nodes are involved, the technical problem of treating the primary and nodes in continuity without giving a dangerously high dose to the spinal cord is insurmountable. Patients with lymph node involvement are unsuitable for any form of attemptive curative treatment by either radiotherapy or surgery and there seems little point in attempting anything other than minimal palliation.

Carcinoma of the *posterior pharyngeal wall* is rare. It has a better prognosis than carcinoma of the pyriform fossa or post-cricoid region and is best treated by radiotherapy; cure rates of 30 to 40 per cent can be expected.

Carcinoma of Maxillary Antrum

Carcinoma of the maxillary antrum is an uncommon disease, mainly of middle-aged and elderly people. Ninety per cent of cases are well-differentiated squamous carcinoma, usually slow-growing, with a low metastatic potential. Nevertheless, results of treatment are disappointing, and the mortality is high. This is because late presentation is the rule; symptoms do not normally occur until the tumour has spread beyond the confines of the antrum, by which time there is a very large mass of malignancy present. The incidence of lymph node metastases is relatively low considering the extent of the primary tumours; Wille (1947) reported that 30 per cent of cases had nodes at presentation and a further 5 per cent developed them subsequently. Most other authors have reported a rather lower figure.

Nearly all patients who die with maxillary antral carcinoma have uncontrolled disease at the primary site. Consequently, increasingly aggressive local treatment is being employed. Spread of the tumour may occur downwards into the mouth, forwards into the substance of the cheek, medially to the nasal fossa, upwards to the orbit, or posteriorly into the pterygoid fossa. The adjacent ethmoid and sphenoid sinuses are often involved. It is not possible to remove all the potential tumour-bearing areas in one adequate surgical operation, therefore all cases should receive radical radiotherapy. The value of surgery after radiotherapy is not clear; a post-radiotherapy maxillectomy probably does reduce the risk of local recurrence in patients with moderately advanced disease and is usually performed where possible. Surgical healing after full-dose radiotherapy at this site is not a problem, and as surgery is always incomplete the principle of pre-operative radiotherapy does not apply here; radical dosage should be given.

There are no useful comparisons of the combined method and radiotherapy alone. Retrospective surveys such as those of Hamberger *et al.* (1967) and Badib *et al.* (1969) compare the results of radiotherapy for advanced inoperable cases with a combined method for earlier cases, and therefore no conclusions can be drawn. Similarly, the place of chemotherapy has not been established; pre-radiotherapy intra-arterial infusion has often been employed for antral carcinoma but is fraught with complications. In a small controlled trial Shigematsu *et al.* (1971) showed a significant improvement in one-year recurrence-free rates from the use of intra-arterial fluorouracil.

Radiotherapy is normally by external beam. Before embarking on treatment, the extent of the disease must be defined as far as possible by clinical examination, endoscopy, and radiography. If there is evidence of infection, it is important to control this and to establish drainage of the antral cavity by a palatal fenestration or Caldwell Luc procedure. The pterygoid and ethmoid regions should always be included in the high-dose volume, because involvement of these structures is difficult to ascertain. It is usual to attempt to preserve the ipsilateral eye provided the orbit is not involved by tumour, hence the cornea and lens are shielded from the radiation beams. Where the orbit is involved it is not possible to offer any hope of cure without loss of the eye, so shielding which may result in under-dosage of tumour should not be attempted.

Intra-cavitary radiation is useful after maxillectomy if there is evidence of residual tumour or recurrence on the walls of the cavity. An obturator is made to fit the cavity and loaded with radium. Primary treatment by an intra-cavitary technique, either with a single central source or with a mould, is not recommended because of the inhomogenity of tumour dose and difficulty in treating areas of potential spread adequately, especially to the ethmoid and pterygoid regions.

Carcinoma of the Middle Ear

Carcinoma of the middle ear is another disease characterised by late presentation. It occurs in middle-aged individuals who have a life-long history of chronic otitis media. The first symptoms of malignancy are an insidious increase in pain and discharge from the ear, which may not lead the patient to seek medical advice for many months. Fortunately it is a rare disease representing only about one in 1500 of all malignancies. Involvement of the temporal bone occurs at an early stage. Surgical extirpation of the disease is extremely difficult or impossible. Radical radiotherapy alone produces results as good as those of surgery (Holmes, 1960) but, even so, survival rates are low, below 25 per cent in most series.

The glomus jugulare tumour is one of the few benign conditions where radiotherapy has an unquestioned place in management. This is one of the family of non-chromaffin paragangliomata arising from chemoreceptors in the jugular bulb. It involves the petrous bone and often the middle ear also. It is a rare tumour occurring more often in women, usually in the fourth and fifth decade. It causes deafness, tinnitus, and cranial nerve lesions. It is a highly vascular tumour; consequently, surgical removal is very hazardous. On the other hand, the results of radiotherapy are good. Regression of the tumour with relief of symptoms occurs and is maintained for many years in most cases, although the clinical signs and angiographic features usually persist (Maruyama *et al.*, 1971).

I would like to thank Mr R. Toogood for his help in producing the clinical photographs.

References

BADIB, A. O., KUROHARA, S. S. and WEBSTER, J. H. (1969) *Cancer*, **23**, 533–537.

BAGSHAW, M. A. and THOMPSON, R. W. (1971) *Journal of the American Medical Association*, **217**, 456–458.

BATAINI, J. P., ENNUYER, A. and PONCET, P. (1971) *Annales d'Oto-laryngologie et de Chirurgie Cervico-Faciale* (Paris), **88**, 555–568.

BINNIE, W. H., CAWSON, R. A., HILL, G. D. and SOAPER, A. E. (1972) *Studies on Medical and Population Subjects*, **23**.

BOND, W. H. and MANSFIELD, O. T. (1959) in *Treatment of Cancer in Clinical Practice*, ed. Kunkler, P. B. and Rains, A. J. H. Livingstone, Edinburgh, 263–307.

BUSCHKE, F. and GALANTE, M. (1959) *Radiology*, **73**, 845–847.

CHEN, K. Y. and FLETCHER, G. H. (1971) *Radiology*, **99**, 165–171.

COFFIN, F. (1973) *British Journal of Radiology*, **46**, 365–368.

CONSTABLE, W. C., MARKS, R. D., ROBBINS, J. P. and FITZHUGH, G. S. (1972) *Laryngoscope*, **82**, 1861–1868.

COUTARD, H. (1932) *American Journal of Roentgenology*, **28**, 313–331.

DALY, T. E., DRANE, J. B. and MACCOMB, W. S. (1972) *American Journal of Surgery*, **124**, 539–542.

DEL REGATO, J. A. and SELA, J. W. (1959) *Radiology*, **73**, 839–845.

DEUTSCH, M., LEEN, R., PARSONS, J. A. and MERCADO, R. (1971) *Archives of Otolaryngology*, **98**, 316–318.

DICK, D. A. L. (1962) *Clinical Radiology*, **13**, 304–312.

EVANS, R. W. (1966) *Histological Appearances of Tumours*, 2nd edn, Livingstone, Edinburgh, 945–946.

FAYOS, J. V. and LAMPE, I. (1972) *American Journal of Roentgenology*, **114**, 65–75.

FLETCHER, G. H. and EVERS, W. T. (1970) *Radiology*, **95**, 185–188.

FLETCHER, G. H., MACCOMB, W. S. and LINDBERG, R. D. (1967) in *Cancer of the Head and Neck*, ed. Conley, J., Butterworth, London, 317–323.

FLETCHER, G. H. and MILLION, R. R. (1965) *American Journal of Roentgenology*, **93**, 44–55.

FRAZELL, E. L. and LUCAS, J. C. (1962) *Cancer*, **15**, 1085–1099.

GARRETT, M. J. (1971) *Clinical Radiology*, **22**, 136–138.

GOLDMAN, J. L., SILVERSTONE, S. M., ROFFMAN, J. D. and BIRKEN, E. A. (1972) *Laryngoscope*, **82**, 1869–1882.

GOLLIN, F. F., ANSFIELD, F. J., BRANDENBERG, J. H., RAMIREZ, G. and VERMUND, H. (1972) *American Journal of Roentgenology*, **114**, 83–88.

HAMBERGER, C. A., MARTENSSON, G. and SJÖGREN, H. A. (1967) in *Cancer of the Head and Neck*, ed. Conley, J., Butterworth, London, 224–229.

HANKS, G. E., BAGSHAW, M. A. and KAPLAN, H. S. (1969) *American Journal of Roentgenology*, **105**, 74–82.

HARA, H. J. (1969) *Laryngoscope*, **79**, 1315–1329.

HARRISON, D. F. N. (1969) *British Medical Journal*, **2**, 615–618.

HENDRICKSON, F. R. and LIEBNER, E. (1968) *Annals of Otology, Rhinology and Laryngology*, **77**, 222–229.

HENK, J. M. (1975) *Proceedings of the Royal Society of Medicine*, **68**, 85–86.

HENK, J. M. and SMITH, C. W. (1973) *British Journal of Radiology*, **46**, 146.

HIBBS, G. C., YING, D. and HENDRICKSON, F. R. (1969) *Annals of Otology, Rhinology and Laryngology*, **78**, 319–325.

HO, J. H. C. (1972) *Advances in Cancer Research*, **15**, 57–92.

HOLMES, K. S. (1960) *Proceedings of the Royal Society of Medicine*, **53**, 242–244.

JESSE, R. H. and LINDBERG, R. D. (1971) *Journal of the American Medical Association*, **217**, 453.

JESSE, R. H., LINDBERG, R. D. and HARIOT, J. C. (1971) *American Journal of Surgery*, **122**, 437–439.

KRAMER, S. (1971) *Journal of the American Medical Association*, **217**, 946–947.

KRANTZ, S., BERGER, L. R. and BROWN, P. F. (1957) *American Journal of Roentgenology*, **78**, 780–789.

KRAUS, F. T. and PEREZ-MESA, C. (1966) *Cancer*, **19**, 26–38.

KRISHNAMURTHI, S., SHANTA, V. and MAIR. M. K. (1967) *Cancer*, **20**, 822–825.

LAWRENCE, W., TERZ, J. J., ROGERS, C., KING, R. E., WOLF, J. S. and KING, E. R. (1974) *Cancer*, **33**, 318–323.

LEDERMAN, M. (1961) *Cancer of the Nasopharynx*, Thomas, Springfield, Ill.

LEDERMAN, M. (1967) in *Cancer of the Head and Neck*, ed. Conley, J., Butterworth, London, 347–356.

MARUYAMA, Y., GOLD, L. H. A. and KIEFFER, S. A. (1971) *Acta radiologica*, **10**, 239–247.

MARCHETTA, F. C., SAKO, K. and MATTICK, W. L. (1968) *American Journal of Surgery*, **116**, 491–493.

MARSHALL, H. F., MARK, A., BRYCE, D. P. and RIDER, W. D. (1972) *Journal of Laryngology and Otology*, **86**, 309–315.

MARTIN, C. L. (1950) *Radiology*, **55**, 62–67.

MILLBURN, L. F. and HENDRICKSON, F. R. (1967) *Radiology*, **89**, 123–126.

MOENCH, H. C. and PHILLIPS, T. L. (1972) *American Journal of Surgery*, **124**, 515–518.

PATERSON, R. (1952) *British Journal of Radiology*, **25**, 505–516.

PEREZ, C. A., ACKERMAN, L. V., MILL, W. B., OGURA, J. H. and POWERS, W. E. (1969) *Cancer*, **24**, 1–7.

PEREZ, C. A. and OLSON, J. (1970) *American Journal of Roentgenology*, **108**, 396–404.

PIERQUIN, B., CHASSAGNE, D., BAILLET, F. and CASTRO, J. R. (1971) *Journal of the American Medical Association*, **215**, 961–963.

PIERQUIN, B., CHASSAGNE, D., CACHIN, Y., BAILLET, F. and FOURNELLE LE BUIS, F. (1970) *Acta radiologica*, **9**, 465–480.

PILCH, Y. H., BARD, D. S. and RAMMING, K. P. (1971) *American Journal of Roentgenology*, **111**, 48–55.

POWERS, W. E. and PALMER, L. A. (1968) *American Journal of Roentgenology*, **102**, 176–192.

RAFLA, S. (1972) *American Journal of Roentgenology*, **114**, 131–135.

RICHARDS, G. J. and CHAMBERS, R. G. (1973) *American Journal of Surgery*, **126**, 513–518.

RICHARDS, S. H., KILBY, D. and SHAW, J. D. (1971) *Journal of Laryngology and Otology*, **85**, 141–152.

ROSWIT, B., SPIRO, R. H., KOLSON, H. and PO YOUNG LIN (1972) *American Journal of Roentgenology*, **114**, 59–64.

ROUX-BERGER, J. L., BAUD, J. and COURTIAL, J. (1949) *Mémoires de l'Académie de Chirurgie*, **75**, 120–126.

RYGARD, J. (1975) in press.

SHIGEMATSU, Y., SAKAI, S. and FUCHIHATA, H. (1971) *Acta otolaryngologica*, **71**, 63–70.

SOLOMON, H., MARCHETTA, F. C., WILSON, R. O., MILLER, R. A. and DETOLLA, H. W. (1968) *American Journal of Surgery*, **115**, 349–351.

SOUTHWICK, H. W. (1971) *Journal of the American Medical Association*, **217**, 454–455.

STRONG, E. W. (1969) *Surgical Clinics of North America*, **49**, 271–276.

SUIT, H., LINDBERG, R. and FLETCHER, G. H. (1965) *Radiology*, **84**, 1100–1107.

WANG, C. C. (1973) *Radiology*, **109**, 183–186.

WANG, C. C. and MEYER, J. E. (1971) *Cancer*, **28**, 566–570.

WILLE, C. (1947) *Acta otolaryngologica*, supp. 65, 1–58.

WIZENBURG, M. J., BLOEDORN, F. G., WEINER, S. and GRACIA, J. (1972) *Cancer*, **29**, 1455–1462.

YEH, S. (1962) *Cancer*, **15**, 895–920.

CHAPTER SIX

Tumours of the Chest and Mediastinum

B. S. Mantell

Bronchial Carcinoma

Bronchial carcinoma is epidemic in the Western world. It caused nearly 31 000 deaths in England and Wales in 1971 and its manifestations are seen in every branch of medical practice. A small proportion of the patients are amenable to curative treatment, and some may indeed be cured, but the great majority are not so fortunate. All too often the clinician sees the illness in the final stages of its natural history, and for most patients the diagnosis of lung cancer is a sentence of death.

The mainstay of curative treatment is surgery, but radical radiotherapy also has its successes. In most cases bronchial carcinoma presents with locally advanced disease and occult metastases. The life expectancy is of the order of months, and treatment must be given with the aim of relieving symptoms and improving the quality of what life remains, rather than as a desperate attempt at cure.

For practical purposes the clinician generally considers his cases in the following groups:

Squamous Cell Carcinomas

(*a*) well differentiated and keratinising

(*b*) moderately differentiated
(*c*) poorly differentiated

Undifferentiated Carcinomas
(*a*) anaplastic
(*b*) oat cell

Adenocarcinomas
(*a*) bronchogenic
(*b*) alveolar cell

Curative Treatment of Lung Cancer

The most frequent curative approach is surgical. Only about 20 per cent of patients investigated are considered suitable for surgery. The operative mortality is of the order of 8 per cent for pneumonectomy and 4 per cent for lobectomy (Belcher, 1974), and about 30 per cent of those who survive the operation live for five years. The selection of patients for surgery requires the rejection not only of those with identifiable distant metastases but also of those who have involvement of the mediastinal structures. Thus patients with phrenic or recurrent laryngeal nerve palsies, oesophageal or superior vena caval obstruction and large or bloodstained pleural effusions are all inoperable. A cardiac arrhythmia of recent onset may also mean extensive mediastinal disease.

Tomography in coronal, sagittal and transverse axial planes may afford evidence of enlarged mediastinal lymph nodes, as may bronchoscopy and mediastinoscopy which may also enable a biopsy to be obtained. The fact that two-thirds of the patients operated upon are dead within five years suggests that occult metastatic disease is often present at the time of operation.

Even a small localised carcinoma is often rejected for operation if it involves the trachea or the first centimetre or so of a main bronchus. The patient must also have sufficient respiratory reserve to tolerate the pneumonectomy or lobectomy envisaged. Excision of the right lung carries a particularly great risk of rendering the patient a respiratory cripple. Many surgeons are wary of operating on patients over 70 years of age, who have an increased operative mortality.

There is therefore a group of patients with relatively small localised tumours who are rejected for surgery because of these factors, or who refuse surgery. Such patients may be considered for radical radiotherapy.

The Problems of Radiotherapy as a Curative Treatment for Bronchial Carcinoma

The dose of radiation required to cure an epidermoid carcinoma is of the order of 5500 rad in twenty fractions over four weeks or its radiobiological equivalent. Such a dose is tolerated by a target volume of 500 cc of tissue, but if the volume exceeds about 1000 cc the incidence of complications becomes unacceptable. Curative radiotherapy therefore requires selection of patients in whom the entire tumour mass with a surrounding margin of normal tissue may be enclosed in a volume of 500 cc or at most 1000 cc. This volume must be capable of receiving the full dose while keeping the radiation to the spinal cord within the range this organ will tolerate, i.e. up to 3500 or 4000 rad. Since radiation pneumonitis may develop when lung tissue receives more than about 2500 rad, the total volume of lung encompassed by the treatment beams must be limited.

Thus, just as in selection of patients for surgery, not only distant metastases but also extensive mediastinal disease must be excluded before radical radiotherapy may be recommended. The patient's respiratory reserve must again be taken into account, but with careful planning the volume of lung tissue damaged is minimised. Many patients whose lung function is too poor to tolerate resection may still be treatable by radical radiotherapy.

However, even when the criteria described are satisfied, the tumour itself may be a bulky mass containing a proportion of anoxic cells which are radioresistant.

Before planning treatment the limits of the tumour must be accurately defined, since if any part of the growth escapes the high dose zone, failure will result. Determination of the extent of a lung cancer, even after the investigations described above, may be very difficult. Every thoracic surgeon is familiar with the apparently operable tumour which is revealed at thoracotomy to have involved extensively the mediastinal structures.

In spite of all these difficulties, radical radiotherapy can produce results comparable with those of surgery (Smart, 1966).

Technique of Radical Radiotherapy

It seems an unfortunate characteristic of much writing upon cancer treatment that 'radiotherapy' is often referred to as if it were a single and uniform entity. The reader is informed that 'radiotherapy was given', and perhaps a dosage figure, e.g. '6000 rad', is added. To be at all meaningful a description of a radiation treatment must include not only an estimate of the tumour-dose given, the number and frequency of the fractions and the overall time taken by the course, but should also indicate the size and anatomical contents of the volume irradiated.

The precise meaning of 'radical radiotherapy' is still to some extent a matter of personal philosophy and opinion. In the author's view this implies a régime of irradiation which might be expected to sterilise the tumour in question, for example a dose of 5500 rad megavoltage given in twenty fractions over a period of four weeks. Such treatment can be given only to a limited volume, such as that encompassed by fields of up to 100 cm^2. The treated volume must include the tumour with a margin of about 2 cm of apparently normal tissue in all directions and must be so planned that sensitive structures such as the spinal cord and lung tissue are not irradiated beyond their tolerance. Two, three or four beams are arranged to cross at the treated volume.

Although radical radiotherapy has in the past been given with success in lung cancer using orthovoltage radiations, there is now no place for such treatment other than with megavoltage.

Identification of the treatment volume and its relation to marks on the patient's skin requires the production of radiographs with the patient in the treatment position. These radiographs are best taken on a 'simulator' – a diagnostic X-ray set on a therapy mounting which can simulate the set-up of the megavoltage unit. The patient's position must be reproduced exactly at each treatment session.

An outline of the patient's 'treatment section' is obtained at the level of the tumour. Using the data from the planning radiographs, the volume to be treated, the lung tissue and the position of the spinal cord are marked on the outline. The isodose curves of two, three, or four beams are applied to the outline, making due allowance for oblique incidence and diminished absorption in lung tissue. The aim is to deliver a dose of 5500 rad to the tumour while keeping the dose to the spinal cord below 4000 rad, and exceeding 2500 rad in as little uninvolved lung tissue as possible (Fig. 6.1).

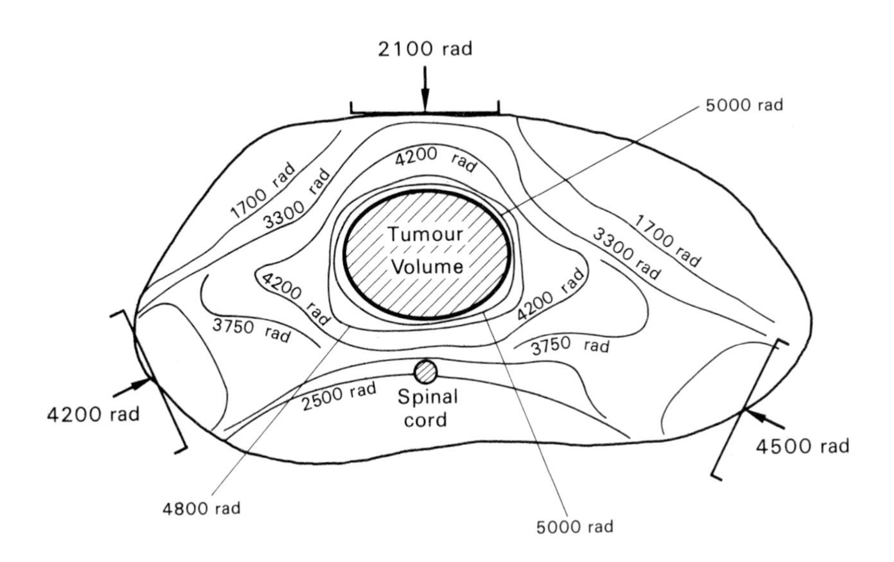

Fig. 6.1. Plan for the radical radiotherapy of bronchial carcinoma.

A course of twenty treatments, five times a week over four weeks as an outpatient is perhaps tedious but is usually well tolerated provided the patient is able to lie comfortably in the position required. Nausea is not usually a complaint, but dysphagia due to radiation reaction in the oesophagus may occur after two or three weeks' treatment. Skin reactions are negligible with high-energy radiation.

The Influence of Histology on Curative Radiotherapy

A histological diagnosis should ideally be made in every case before treatment. Bronchoscopy may yield biopsy material or, failing this, bronchial aspirations for cytology. Percutaneous needle and drill biopsies may be hazardous in lesions close to the mediastinum but for peripheral masses they are safe in spite of an incidence of pneumothorax of about 26 per cent (Steel, 1971).

Evidence of malignancy with an indication of cell type may often be obtained by cytological examination of the sputum. It is desirable that specimens be taken before bronchoscopy as difficulty of interpretation may occur after this investigation.

The majority of patients receiving radical radiotherapy are likely to have squamous cell growths. Tumours of the undifferentiated group are usually too advanced at presentation for an attempt at curative treatment. Adenocarcinomas are often regarded as peculiarly resistant to radiation, but this view is possibly more a tradition than an established fact.

Results of Radical Radiotherapy

The results of radical irradiation for a group of operable lung cancers were reported by Smart and Hilton (1956). Of 33 cases treated, 33 per cent survived five years. Smart (1966) also reported a series of 40 such cases of whom nine (22·5 per cent) were five-year survivors. A comparative trial of surgery and radical radiotherapy for oat cell carcinomas has been conducted by the Medical Research Council (Fox and Scadding 1973). Of the 71 patients assigned to surgery only 32 actually underwent resection, and of the 73 allotted to radiotherapy 62 received radical irradiation. None of the resected patients survived five years, and only three of the radically irradiated group did so, although all three lived on to ten years. It was therefore concluded that radiotherapy is better than surgery for treatment of operable oat cell carcinoma, although it is perhaps more accurate to say that the results of surgery in this tumour are even more appalling than those of radiotherapy! An earlier prospective trial of surgery against radiotherapy in operable lung cancer was that reported by Morrison *et al.* (1963). Although the results at one year favoured radiotherapy, at four years only 7 per cent of irradiated patients were living compared with 23 per cent of operated patients. The dose of radiation used – 4500 rad in four weeks – was perhaps low and a higher dose might possibly have produced a higher survival figure.

In conclusion, therefore, radical irradiation is indicated in those carcinomas rejected for surgery on medical or technical grounds, and in operable oat cell carcinomas except perhaps in the occasional peripheral oat cell growth which may be amenable to surgery (Lennox *et al.*, 1968).

Combinations of Surgery and Radiotherapy

Pre-operative radiotherapy. Pre-operative irradiation may be used in the hope of sterilising the periphery of the tumour so that transection of viable tumour at surgery and therefore subsequent local recurrence may become less likely. It may also be hoped that the bulk of an inoperable tumour will be reduced and its areas of attachment and invasion sterilised so that it will become operable. It might be expected that the risk of dissemination of viable tumour cells at surgery will be reduced by pre-operative radiotherapy.

A randomised prospective study by Shields *et al.* (1970) showed a poorer survival in patients treated by resection after pre-operative radiotherapy. Paulson (1971) reported the use of modest doses of radiation, for example 3000 rad in ten daily fractions, given three to six weeks before very extensive surgery for superior sulcus carcinomas in 32 patients, and he claimed 12 five-year survivors. Bates *et al.* (1974) described 29 cases of operable oat cell carcinoma in whom an immediate pre-operative dose of 1750 rad was given to the tumour and adjacent lymph nodes in seven fractions over eight days. Twenty-four cases came to pneumonectomy and seven survived a minimum of three years.

Whatever the true significance of these special studies, they apply to only a small proportion of the total number of patients with bronchial carcinoma, for the great majority of whom pre-operative radiotherapy seems to have nothing to offer.

Post-operative radiotherapy. In a randomised prospective trial Paterson and Russell (1962) were unable to demonstrate any improvement in survival when the mediastinum was irradiated after pneumonectomy. Occasionally, when after resection residual tumour is known to be present at the bronchial stump or at the site of adherence to the chest wall, radical post-operative radiotherapy may be given, although the prospects for these cases are poor. Sometimes radical irradiation may be given for an apparently localised recurrence at the bronchial stump months or years after surgery.

The results of radiotherapy for cancer found inoperable at thoracotomy are poor. Guttman (1965) reported only 7·4 per cent five-year survivors where no attempt at resection had been made. Where partial resection had been carried out the results were even worse.

In some centres interstitial radiotherapy using radioactive gold grains implanted at operation into inoperable carcinomas has been tried (Smithers, 1955). The difficulties of dosimetry in such an implant and the medical and technical resources required limit this technique severely.

Palliative Radiotherapy for Lung Cancer

Palliative treatment is intended to relieve symptoms. Occasionally when a complication of lung cancer is life-threatening, e.g. respiratory obstruction, palliative therapy may actually prolong life, but as a general rule there is no evidence that its use affects survival. Its value therefore must be assessed in terms of the quality of subsequent life.

Palliative radiotherapy should not produce any symptoms of its own, and should occupy as little of the patient's remaining life as possible. The dose of radiation used should be limited to that necessary to achieve symptomatic relief. Deeley (1966) reported a clinical trial of two different dose-levels in the treatment of inoperable anaplastic bronchial carcinoma. The mean survival of 51 patients receiving 3000 rad was 9·3 months, while that of 51 receiving 4000 rad was 6 months. There was evidence that the incidence of residual growth in the chest, and of distant metastases, was the same in both groups, and those receiving the higher dose had a greater incidence of radiation fibrosis. Johnson *et al.* (1973) have reported a trial carried out on 100 patients with inoperable bronchial carcinoma. Thirty-three patients received telecobalt therapy to a dose of 4800 rad in twenty fractions over four weeks, and a second group of 33 were treated with telecobalt to a dose of 2800 rad in four fractions over ten days. A third group of 35 patients received the same dose and fractionation as the second, but using a 35 MV electron beam. Survival in all three groups was the same

(30 per cent at one year and 6 per cent at five years), while nearly all patients had relief of symptoms, whichever method of treatment was employed.

If the sole object of palliative radiotherapy is the relief of symptoms, is there any justification for treating those patients whose inoperable disease is asymptomatic? Durrant *et al.* (1971) compared four groups of such patients. The first received no treatment until symptoms appeared, the second received routine palliative radiotherapy, the third received routine treatment with nitrogen mustard and the fourth both palliative radiotherapy and nitrogen mustard. The mean survival of all groups was similar – about $8\frac{1}{2}$ months – and the degree of palliation seemed to be the same. Thus there seems to be no advantage in routine treatment in the absence of symptoms. One does find, however, the occasional patient who seems to be cured by palliative radiotherapy, although in fairness it must be remembered that long survival may on rare occasions be encountered after incomplete resection, or even after no treatment at all.

Technique of Palliative Radiotherapy

Although conventional deep X-ray beams are quite adequate for the palliative treatment of most patients with lung cancer, high-energy radiation such as that from a telecobalt unit or a linear accelerator is to be preferred. This is mainly because the skin-sparing property of megavoltage radiation enables the treatment to be given with no skin reaction at all. The lesser side-scatter from high-energy beams means less radiation outside the tumour area, and therefore usually less systemic upset such as nausea. The high dose-rate obtainable, particularly in the case of the linear accelerator, means a much shorter time to be spent by the patient on the treatment table.

Strictly speaking, it is not necessary to irradiate all the known tumour to achieve palliation. For example, if the patient is complaining of dyspnoea due to a mass of tumour obstructing one main bronchus and causing collapse of one lung, the symptom may be relieved by limiting the radiation to the region of the obstruction. In practice, however, it is simpler to irradiate the whole mediastinum in one block. Anterior and posterior opposed fields of the order of 15 × 10 cm are generally adequate for this purpose, and will include asymptomatic parts of the tumour mass which might otherwise continue to grow. A tumour-dose of 2000 to 2500 rad given in five daily fractions, or 3000 rad in ten, is adequate and well tolerated. If supraclavicular nodes are involved by tumour it is usually possible to extend the fields to include them. In this case, however, it is desirable to shield the larynx and suprasternal region with a lead block to prevent temporary hoarseness of the voice, or dysphagia. Such treatment, with minor variation in the size and position of the fields, is suitable for the relief of symptoms of lung cancer such as cough, haemoptysis, chest pain, dysphagia due to oesophageal obstruction and dyspnoea due to bronchial obstruction with collapse. Symptomatic relief is to be expected in about 70 per cent of the patients treated (Hope-Stone, 1967).

Effect of Histology on Palliative Radiotherapy

In general, the technique and dosage described is suitable irrespective of histology. The less-differentiated growths, especially the oat cell carcinoma, may respond extremely rapidly and may be seen to be shrinking from day to day during the course of irradiation, with rapid improvement in symptoms. This suggests a high 'radiosensitivity', but is probably largely a function of a high mitotic rate, since the tumour cells must pass through at least one mitosis before the effect of radiation is manifested (Alexander, 1965). A well-differentiated tumour may respond more slowly, while adenocarcinomas are sometimes considered to be more 'radioresistant' and to require a higher dose, although this is not the present author's own experience. If a symptom such as haemoptysis has not been relieved by the end of a course of 3000 rad in two weeks, it may be justifiable to continue the treatment for another three or four days to bring the dose up to 4000 rad.

Some Special Problems

Superior Mediastinal Obstruction

This distressing syndrome occurs with tumours in the right upper mediastinal region, and is characterised by venous congestion, cyanosis and oedema in the head, neck and arms with enlarged collateral veins on the chest wall. Usually due to lung cancer, it may occur in the lymphomas, and rarely in non-malignant disease (Chajek and Fainaru,

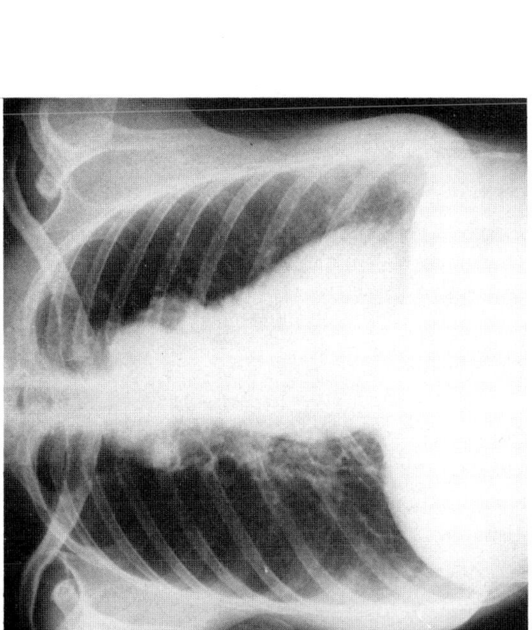

(a)

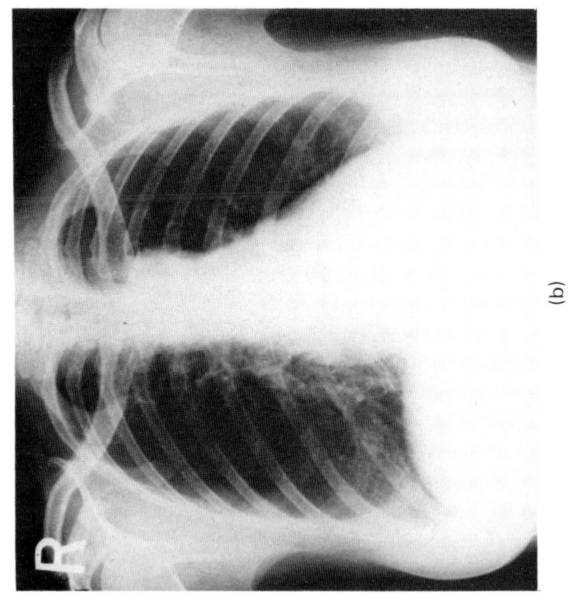

(b)

Fig. 6.2. a Chest X-ray of a case of oat cell carcinoma with superior mediastinal obstruction. b The same case as in (a), after a palliative course of four telecobalt exposures.

1973). Although palliative radiotherapy is usually highly effective in relieving the obstruction (Fig. 6.2.) about 20 per cent of cases may recur (Szur and Bromley, 1956). Such patients may respond to a second course of irradiation.

Hope-Stone and Key (1961) described the use of venography to demonstrate thrombosis in the superior vena caval system in some patients failing to respond to radiotherapy, or subsequently suffering a recurrence of obstruction. These authors found anticoagulant therapy of value in some of these cases.

Respiratory Obstruction

Tumour narrowing the lumen of the trachea or both main bronchi may cause respiratory obstruction which is life-threatening. Although the obstruction may often be relieved by irradiation, the view is widely held that increased oedema caused by the treatment may worsen the condition. There is some objective evidence for this in that Cameron *et al.* (1969) demonstrated a significant reduction in the FEV_1 in the first four days of treatment in many patients before improvement began. These workers later (1972) showed that this effect may be abolished by an intravenous injection of nitrogen mustard before radiotherapy. Also effective was prednisolone given in a dose of 20 mg per day for 24 hours before and 48 hours after the start of radiotherapy. It is the present author's practice to start treatment with nitrogen mustard and then to irradiate cautiously, usually under prednisolone cover. A marked temporary fall in the white blood cell and platelet counts may occur when mustine and radiotherapy are thus combined.

Dysphagia and Hoarseness

Dysphagia may be caused by external compression of the oesophagus by a mass of tumour in the mediastinum, or by direct invasion of the oesophagus by the carcinoma. It is usually worse for solids than for liquids, and may become complete. Relief may be afforded by palliative radiotherapy in more than half the patients (Blanshard, 1955) but some may temporarily require nasogastric or even intravenous feeding and fluids.

A form of dysphagia is often experienced by patients who have developed recurrent laryngeal palsy. Tumour at the left hilum involves the left nerve as it passes under the aortic arch. Occasionally the right nerve may be damaged by metastatic tumour in the root of the neck. The resultant vocal cord paresis gives rise to a hoarse, weak voice and a peculiar 'bovine' cough. These patients often complain of a dysphagia worse for liquids, in that they cough and splutter on attempting to swallow. Recurrent laryngeal palsy is practically never relieved by radiotherapy. Some patients, if surviving long enough, may learn to cope by careful swallowing of fluid in small amounts. Sometimes over-activity of the opposite cord may eventually compensate for the paralysed one, with considerable improvement in both swallowing and voice.

Explosive coughing of fluid immediately after drinking occurs in tracheo-oesophageal fistula. Radiotherapy is of no help, and insertion of a Mousseau-Barbin or Celestin tube is of limited value.

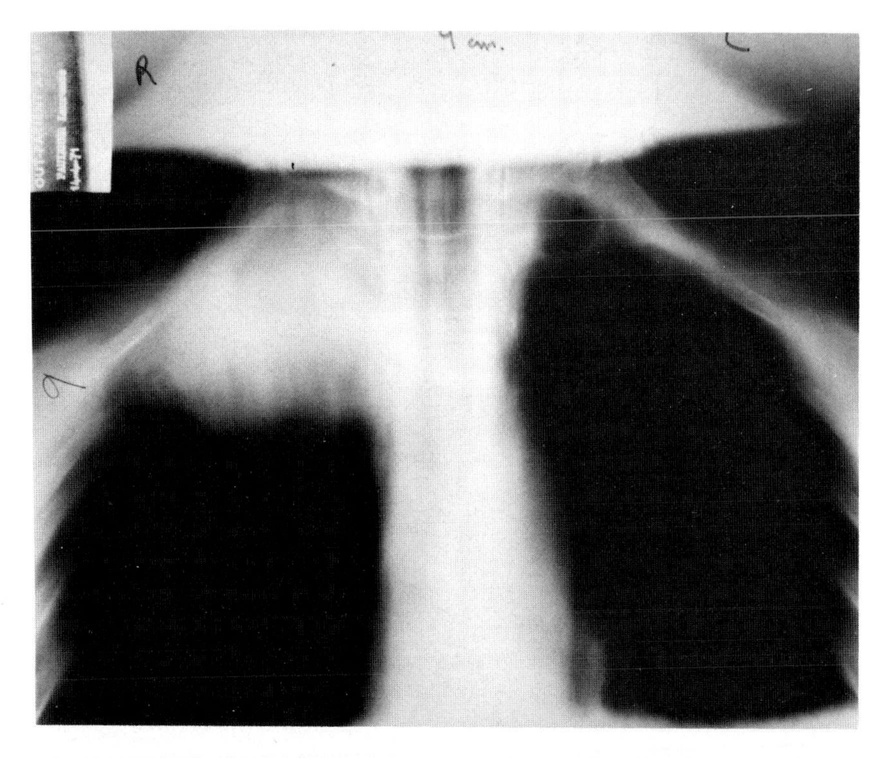

Fig. 6.3. Tomogram in a case of Pancoast syndrome, showing the encroachment of the tumour medially.

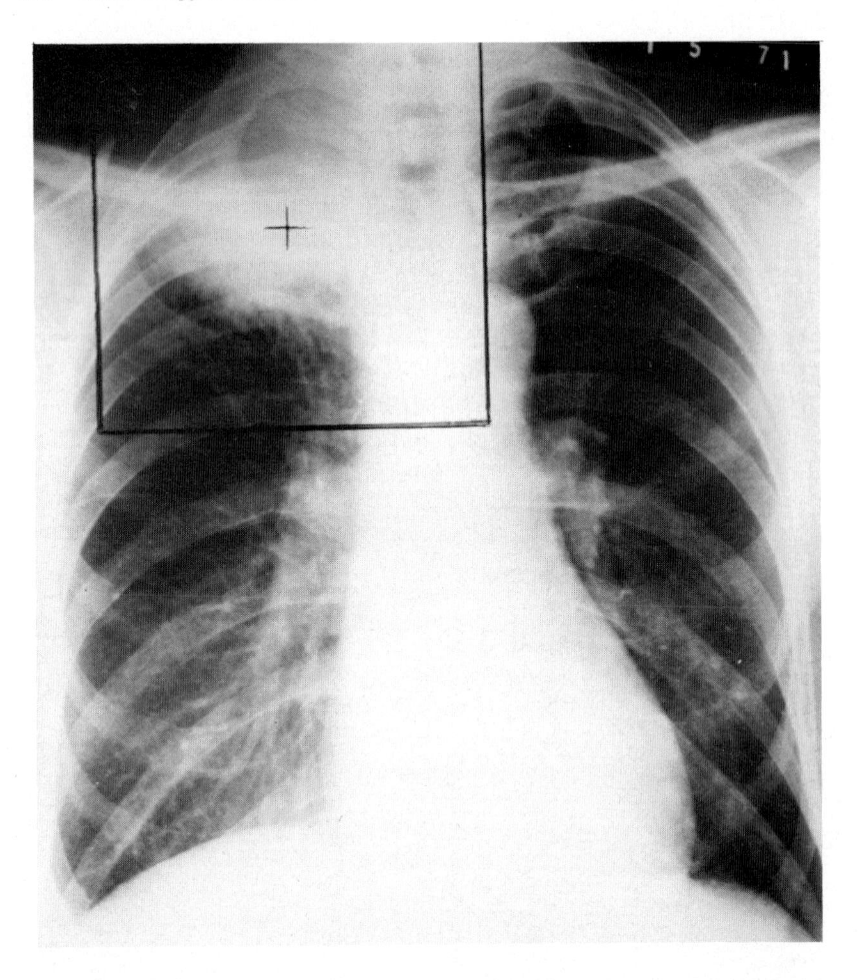

Fig. 6.4. The area to be irradiated in the Pancoast syndrome.

The Pancoast Syndrome (*Figs 6.3 and 6.4*)

This is characterised by pain down the arm with sensory, motor or reflex loss and Horner's syndrome, and is due to a carcinoma at the lung apex. It is named after the American radiologist H. K. Pancoast, who described it in 1932. Such a case with meticulous post mortem findings was described in detail by E. S. Hare (1838) almost a century before Pancoast. The syndrome seems to have acquired an undeserved reputation for intractability to radiotherapy, which may indeed be highly effective in relieving the main symptom of pain. The basis of success lies in a consideration of the morbid anatomy of the apical carcinoma, which not only invades the brachial plexus but penetrates the intervertebral foramina and may reach the spinal cord. The radiation fields used must include this area of infiltration, so they must extend to the midline and preferably beyond. Doses within the tolerance of the spinal cord, for example 3500 rad in two weeks, are quite adequate for palliation (Mantell, 1973). As with any lung cancer, the prospects for survival are generally poor, but some long survivals may be obtained.

Chest Wall Invasion

This common complication of advanced lung cancers, often associated with rib destruction, gives rise to severe pain which is sometimes relieved by radiation. If a dose of 4000 rad in three weeks fails to control the pain, cordotomy may be required.

Pleural Effusion

Although a small exudate may be associated with relatively early tumours, a massive effusion indicates advanced disease usually with extensive pleural deposits of tumour. Such effusions, often blood-stained, cause respiratory embarrassment and may require frequent aspiration. Various agents have been instilled into the pleural cavity in attempts to prevent the re-accumulation of fluid. Radioactive colloidal gold has been largely abandoned on account of the radiation hazard, and 20 milligrams of mustine have been shown to be equally effective (Levison, 1961).

Hickman and Jones (1970) have described the use of mepacrine instilled intrapleurally. Success with this drug appears to depend upon the production of a pleural reaction and subsequent adhesions producing a pleurodesis. Ninety milligrams of mepacrine dissolved in saline are instilled at the first aspiration, 180 mg at the second and 360 mg at any subsequent aspirations. Local pain, and sometimes transient yellow discoloration of the skin, are possible side-effects.

Whichever method is used, it is essential to empty the pleural cavity as completely as possible of fluid (taking care not to replace it by a pneumothorax), before instilling the chosen agent, so that the pleurae may come into contact and adhere together over as wide an area as possible. It may be necessary to use an intercostal catheter with constant suction, and an underwater seal, to achieve this end.

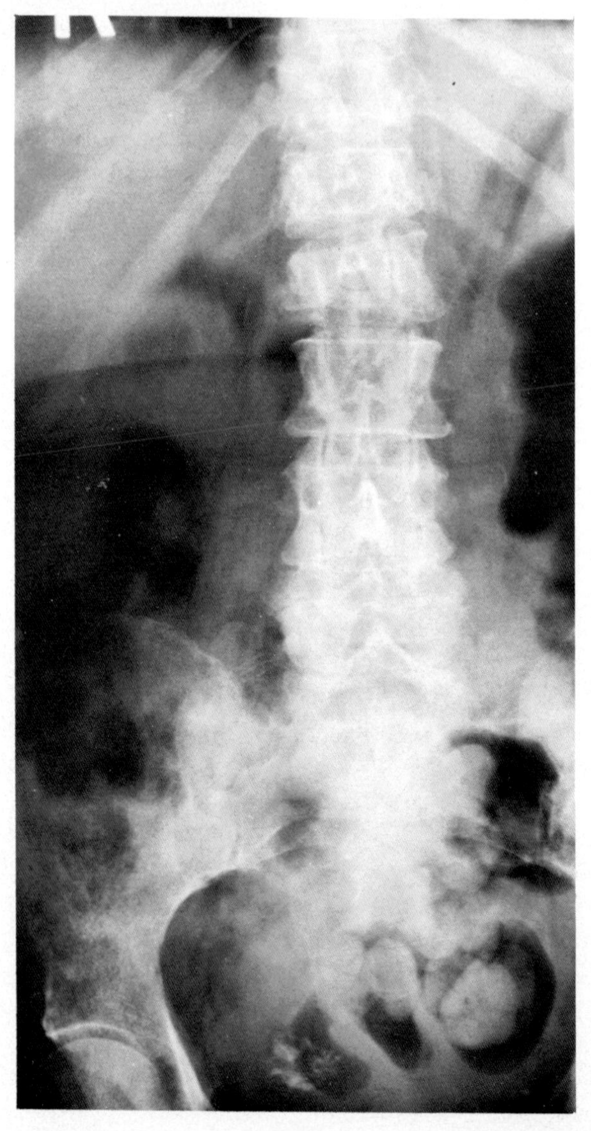

Fig. 6.5. a.

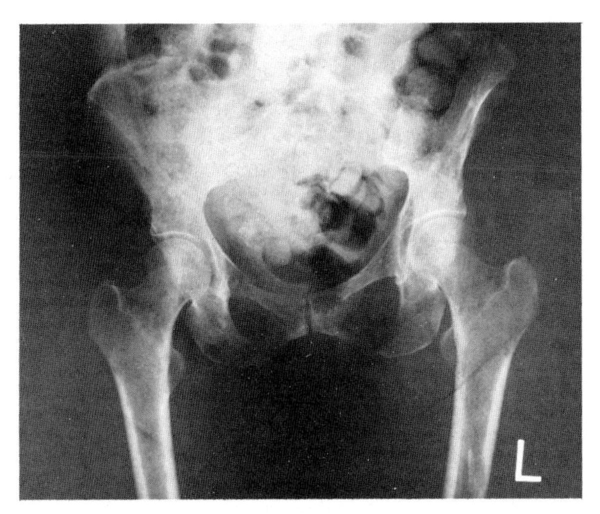

Fig. 6.5. b.

Fig. 6.5. a & b Metastases in the lumbar spine and pelvis from oat cell carcinoma. There is collapse of the right side of the second lumbar vertebra, and a pathological fracture through the right superior pubic ramus.

The Management of Metastatic Disease

In some cancers, for example of the breast, patients commonly survive many months and often years with widespread metastases, especially when these are in bone. In lung cancer the appearance of metastases usually means death within a matter of weeks. Radiotherapy is often useful for palliation, but bearing in mind the short life-expectancy the techniques used must be simple. The minimum radiation dose and the shortest possible time are used that will give symptomatic relief without the production of new symptoms due to the treatment itself.

Metastases in Bone (Fig. 6.5)

These can cause severe pain which may be incapacitating. Lytic lesions may be visible on X-ray, but it must be remembered that at least 50 per cent of the bone substance must be destroyed to produce positive radiographic findings (Edelstyn *et al.*, 1967). Local tenderness and possibly a rise in the serum alkaline phosphatase level give further evidence. Radioisotope scanning using an agent such as $^{87}Sr^{m}$ is sometimes helpful; a relatively high uptake is seen in areas affected by metastases, although osteo-arthritis is also associated with a high uptake. Pathological fracture may occur and is often a pre-terminal event. Paraplegia may result from vertebral collapse. These complications add to the patient's misery and make his terminal nursing much more difficult.

Palliative radiotherapy often relieves the pain of bone metastases and may possibly prevent pathological fracture and paraplegia in some cases. Deposits in the limb bones or in the spine may be treated with single exposures using megavoltage equipment. An incident dose of 1500 rad on a single field often gives pain relief within a few days. When the lumbar spine is so treated transient nausea and vomiting may begin a few hours after the exposure and may persist for a day or so,

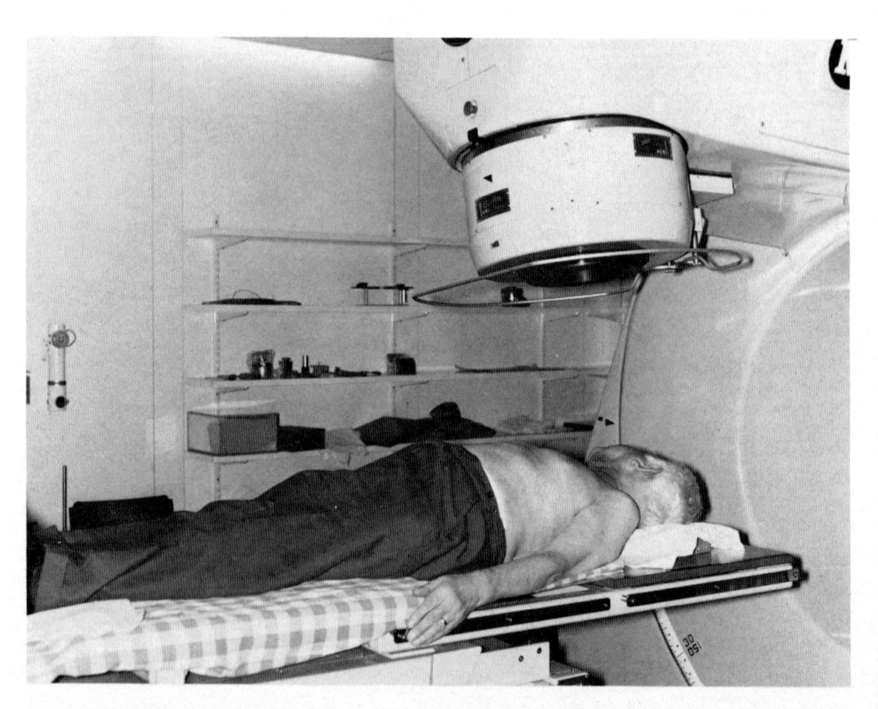

Fig. 6.6. Treatment of a lymph node metastasis in the left supraclavicular fossa, using a linear accelerator. The beam is aimed to avoid the larynx and chest.

but is usually preventable by antiemetics. Skin reactions with megavoltage are negligible although a transient erythema may appear in the treated skin during or immediately after the single exposure.

Sometimes it is necessary to include a large amount of bowel in the treated volume, for example when a hemipelvis is treated using anterior and posterior opposed fields. A single exposure would not be tolerated because of the severe bowel reaction it would produce. A midline dose of 2000–2500 rad in five daily treatments, or 2800 to 3000 rad given in 7 to 10 treatments over two weeks, is therefore used.

Skin nodules may be treated with single exposures of superficial (for example 140 kV) X-rays, giving a dose of 1500 rad.

Lymph node metastases in the supraclavicular fossae or axillae respond well to single exposures of 1500 rad of high-energy radiation. The beam should be directed so that it passes through as little of the patient's body as possible. For example, a mass in the supraclavicular fossa may be treated using a vertical beam, with the patient supine and his head turned to the opposite side. The beam then passes through the mass and the muscles behind it, but avoids the larynx, pharynx and chest, so that no symptoms are caused by the treatment (Fig. 6.6).

The Central Nervous System

Intracranial metastases are common in lung cancer. They may be single or multiple, and their clinical manifestations are those of any space-occupying lesion. Mental deterioration, motor and sensory disturbances, and visual field defects are all common. Raised intracranial pressure may occur, especially when a deposit growing in the posterior fossa interferes with the circulation of the cerebrospinal fluid. The diagnosis is usually made clinically, with help from radioactive brain scanning, electroencephalography and cerebral angiography. Although brain secondaries usually indicate widespread disease, Deeley and Rice Edwards (1968) were unable to find any metastases other than those in the brain in 15 of 63 patients with intracranial deposits from lung cancer who came to autopsy. Although the occasional patient may achieve prolonged survival this does not, in the present author's view, justify the routine treatment of these patients by surgery or irradiation, since of 88 patients treated by Deeley and Rice Edwards with whole brain irradiation, 27 died on treatment and 32 others received no benefit. Only 29 were able to go home and lead a fairly normal life for at least a month, and most of these were dead within three months, although two survived over three years.

Losses of motor and sensory function, once established, are unlikely to be reversed by treatment. Raised intracranial pressure can be often reduced temporarily by a large dose of dexamethasone (4 mg four times a day) with relief of headache and visual disturbance. Irradiation to the whole brain may then be given using opposed lateral fields to a dose of 3000 rad in two weeks. After this it may be possible to reduce the dexamethasone without return of the raised intracranial pressure.

Although two of Deeley and Rice Edwards's patients survived more than three years, it is the present author's opinion that radiotherapy for intracranial metastases from bronchial carcinoma is rarely justified. Possibly intractable headache and threatened blindness are the only strong indications.

Liver Metastases

A common terminal event in lung cancer is involvement of the liver. The patient complains of anorexia, loses weight, and an enlarged, hard, irregular liver is palpable clinically. Occasionally jaundice may occur, but often multiple deposits may exist in the liver with no disturbance of the biochemical liver function. A radioactive liver scan may show filling defects corresponding to masses of growth.

Radiotherapy is of no help here. A temporary improvement in appetite and sense of wellbeing can often be obtained by large doses of steroids, for example 30 to 40 mg of prednisone daily.

The Chemotherapy of Lung Cancer

In a malignancy such as lung cancer, where the disease is so often widespread at the patient's first presentation, it is natural that attempts at systemic treatment should be made. A variety of cytotoxic drugs is now available. These include the alkylating agents such as nitrogen mustard and cyclophosphamide which interfere with cell division, and the antimetabolites such as 5-fluorouracil and methotrexate which block DNA synthesis. There are in addition plant alkaloids such as vincristine and vinblastine, antibiotics including the actinomycins, bleomycin and adriamycin, and many others. None of these agents is a specific 'anti-cancer' drug. Most of them attack any dividing cells, and thus are toxic to the bone marrow and the gut mucosa. Vincristine and bleomycin have relatively little effect upon the bone marrow, but vincristine may produce severe peripheral neuropathy and may impair bowel motility to the point of ileus. Bleomycin produces a peculiar pneumonitis which may be fatal. Other side-effects to be reckoned with are nausea and vomiting, especially with nitrogen mustard, and hair loss, particularly with cyclophosphamide.

Undoubtedly shrinkage of tumour masses can often be produced by chemotherapy, and this effect may sometimes be utilised for palliation. But in an extensive review of the literature Boesen (1973) was able to find little if any evidence of prolongation of life by cytotoxic drug therapy in lung cancer.

A single intravenous injection of 20 mg of nitrogen mustard may produce sufficient tumour regression to relieve superior vena caval obstruction, or tracheal or bronchial compression, particularly in the less-differentiated growths. Nausea and vomiting may occur but may be prevented or ameliorated by antiemetics. Should radiotherapy be given after nitrogen mustard a severe fall in white cell and platelet counts may occur, necessitating curtailment of the radiotherapy.

After the undoubtedly superior results of multiple drug chemotherapy in Hodgkin's disease (see Chapter 7) the technique has been extended to the solid tumours, including bronchial carcinoma. Working upon the principle that a combination of several drugs which act at different points in the cell cycle will be more effective for less toxicity than any single drug, many régimes have been developed. One example is the combination of cyclophosphamide, 5-fluorouracil, vincristine and methotrexate described by Hanham *et al.* (1971), who achieved a short response in six out of fourteen cases of bronchial carcinoma, with a maximum duration of three months.

Since chemotherapy in lung cancer does not as yet hold out the promise of prolongation of life, the degree of palliation it may offer may be considered. Against any relief of the symptoms of the tumour that may be obtained must be weighed the side-effects of the drugs, and the necessity for repeated courses. It seems difficult at present to find any justification for complicated chemotherapeutic techniques for most patients with lung cancer.

The Host Response and Immunotherapy

There is increasing awareness of the fact that resistance to the tumour by its host may occur. This has been held to account for spontaneous regressions of many tumours, including lung cancer (Sutton and Pratt-Johnson, 1970). It is believed the host response is overwhelmed by a large mass of cancer cells, but may be capable of destroying a small residuum when the number of cancer cells has been reduced sufficiently by surgery, radiotherapy or chemotherapy. The main defensive agents of the host are thought to be the 'T' lymphocytes, which attack the malignant cells directly. The 'B' lymphocytes may produce antibodies to the cancer cells, but these antibodies may act as a 'blocking factor', coating them and preventing access by the cytotoxic lymphocytes (Hellstrom *et al.*, 1971).

The object of immunotherapy, once the bulk of the tumour has been reduced as far as possible, is to stimulate the host to produce 'T' lymphocytes lethal to the remaining cells. This response is thought to be mediated through the lymph nodes draining the tumour, but these nodes may be exhausted or even destroyed by metastases. Preparations of cancer cells from the patient's own tumour, heavily irradiated to prevent growth, may be injected at remote sites in the hope of stimulating other lymph nodes to form cytotoxic lymphocytes. Non-specific stimulation of the reticulo-endothelial system, for example by using repeated doses of BCG, is also a possibility, as are attempts at identifying and neutralising a 'blocking factor'.

Immunotherapy is not expected to be a definitive treatment in its own right, but rather an adjuvant to 'mop up' residual cancer cells after the bulk of the tumour has been reduced by other means.

Although present-day methods of treatment may do much to help patients with lung cancer, and may cure some of them, the overall prognosis remains appalling. The outlook seems unlikely to improve until effective means of prevention can be found.

Pleural Mesothelioma

Rare until the second part of the present century, this distressing condition is now seen with increasing frequency. Most cases can be shown to have a history of asbestos exposure, but the latent period is long, usually 20 or more years. Patients come not only from the ranks of asbestos workers, but also from the population living in the vicinity of asbestos factories and mines.

Pathology

Mesothelioma appears on the visceral and parietal layers of pleura, pericardium and peritoneum; there is no evidence, however, that it arises from pre-existing asbestos plaques (Parkes, 1973). Macroscopically it is a waxy whitish or yellow growth, beginning as flat plaques but eventually forming bulky masses compressing the lungs and mediastinal structures and eroding the ribs. Cystic degeneration and effusion formation are common. Microscopically the tumours are very variable, including tubular and papillary forms as well as spindle-cell and anaplastic types. Lymph nodes may be involved, but distant metastases are rare. Diagnosis may be difficult even with biopsy using closed or open techniques. The latter also carries the theoretical risk of fungation of the tumour through the incision.

Clinical Manifestations

Increasing breathlessness and nagging chest pain are prominent symptoms, and may be extremely distressing; pleural effusion is common. Sweating, weight loss and general deterioration occur. Sometimes dysphagia or other obstructive manifestations may be encountered. Chest X-ray shows enlarging opacities protruding into the lung fields from the chest wall and diaphragm, as well as pleural effusion and rib destruction.

The prognosis is poor; most patients are dead by eighteen months or so, although occasionally one survives as long as four or five years.

Treatment

There is no curative treatment for mesothelioma. Radiotherapy and chemotherapy are generally held to be ineffective (Parkes, 1973).

However, temporary pain relief can sometimes be obtained by radiotherapy which may also delay the re-accumulation of pleural effusion. It is usually necessary to irradiate a large volume of the chest, often the whole hemithorax. Anterior and posterior opposing fields are used, giving doses of 3000–3500 rad in two to three weeks. Such doses will probably produce fibrosis of the remaining lung tissue on that side. Intrapleural cytotoxic therapy does not seem to be helpful.

Carcinoma of the Oesophagus

Carcinomas of the thoracic part of the oesophagus may be considered in two main groups; those of the 'middle third', in the region of the arch of the aorta, and those of the 'lower third', near the oesophago-gastric junction. Growths arising in the hypopharyngeal region will not be included in this chapter.

Most of these tumours are squamous cell carcinomas, often of a poorly-differentiated and aggressive type. Sometimes an adenocarcinoma is found in the lower third of the oesophagus; such a growth may in fact be an ectopic focus of gastric carcinoma, although true oesophageal adenocarcinomas probably occur. The oesophagus itself is a thin-walled organ, and the tumour usually spreads readily to invade adjacent structures such as the aorta, the pericardium, the trachea bronchi and pleura as well as extending submucosally well beyond the apparent limits of the growth. Lymph node metastases are common in the supraclavicular and subdiaphragmatic regions as well as in the mediastinum. The peak incidence is in the seventh decade of life, and the dysphagia which is the main symptom may quickly reduce the patient to a condition of starvation and emaciation. All these factors combine to make the management of oesophageal carcinoma a formidable problem.

Nevertheless the oesophagus was first resected for cancer almost 100 years ago in a patient who survived for a year (Czerny, 1877). In 1913 Torek succeeded in removing the oesophagus for carcinoma using a transthoracic approach in a woman who subsequently survived 14 years. In neither of these cases was there any attempt to restore the continuity of the food passage. The patients were fed by permanent gastrostomy, a miserable existence no longer considered acceptable. A thoraco-abdominal approach with oesophago-gastric anastomosis was described by Adams and Phemister (1938), and with the rapid improvements in thoracic surgery, aided by developments in anaesthesia, blood transfusion and antibiotics, surgical treatment of oesophageal cancer became established.

Radiotherapy for this tumour was hampered by technical inadequacy. Treatment with orthovoltage apparatus required multiple fields if an adequate dose was to reach the oesophagus without giving an intolerable dose to the skin, and this meant the irradiation and damage of a large volume of lung. Radium bougies inserted into the oesophagus were of limited value as, although they were able to give a high dose to the surface of the growth, its deeper ramifications were virtually untouched. It was not until the 1950s, when megavoltage apparatus became widely available, that the radiotherapist was able to deliver adequate irradiation to the oesophagus and its surroundings while sparing the skin and the lung.

In order to cure the patient, the surgeon must remove the entire growth, or at least enough of it to allow the body's own defences, if such exist, to overcome the remainder. Because of the nature of the tumour this is difficult, and frequently impossible, and the operation is a major undertaking with a substantial operative mortality. Although patients with distant metastases or very extensive local disease are also incurable by radiotherapy, the criteria of local inoperability do not apply and there is no operative mortality. Radiotherapy must therefore be considered seriously as an alternative to surgery in the curative treatment of carcinoma of the oesophagus.

Preparation of Patients for Treatment

The diagnosis is established by barium-swallow radiographs, with oesophagoscopy and biopsy. Bronchoscopy should be performed at the same time. Evidence of invasion of the trachea or bronchi by the carcinoma may thus be obtained; the risk of a fistula occurring as the tumour regresses is then very great. The patient's general condition should be improved as far as possible before radiotherapy is begun. Anaemia and dehydration should be corrected; if the patient is able to swallow fluids a liquid diet high in calories and vitamins should be given. Some patients may require passage of a nasogastric tube, or even

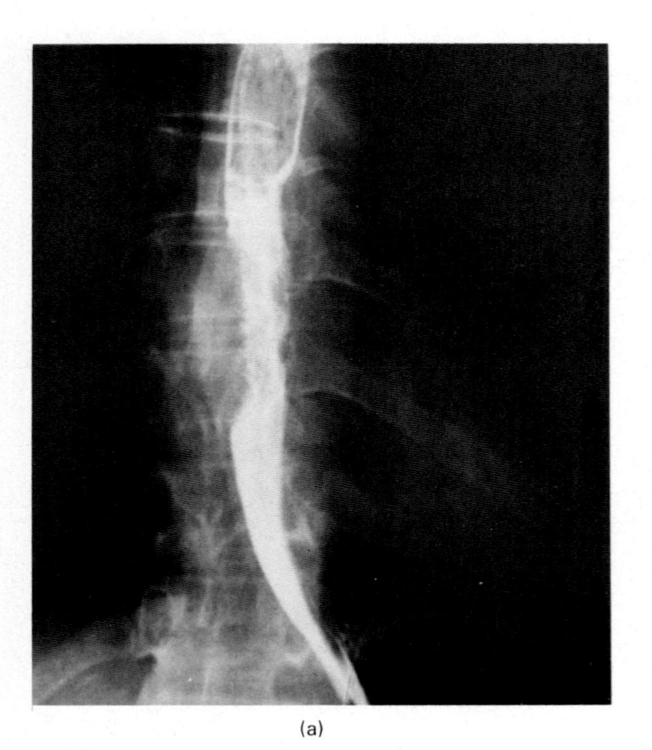

(a)

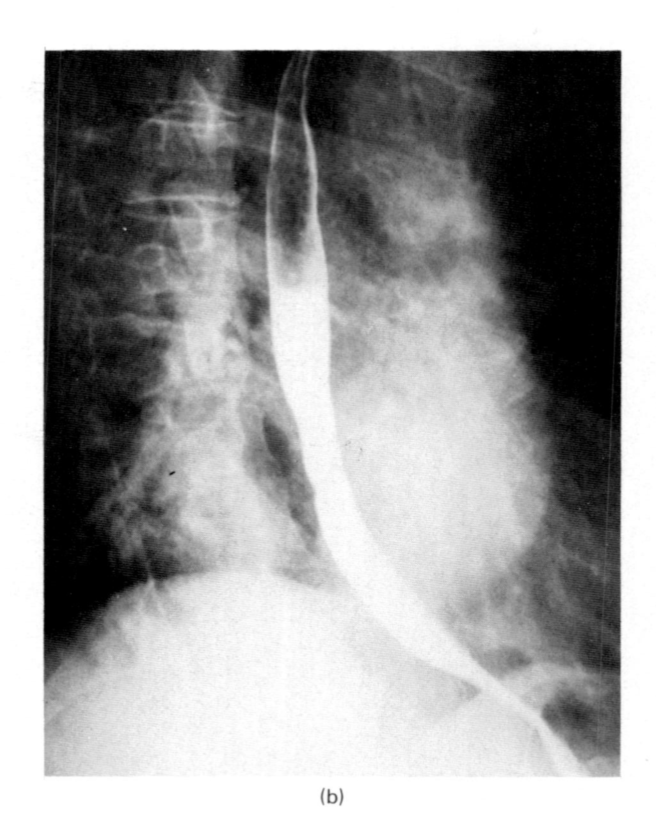

(b)

Fig. 6.7. a Barium swallow showing an oesophageal carcinoma. b The same patient, 4 years after radical radiotherapy.

intravenous fluids to correct dehydration. Distant metastases and bronchial involvement contra-indicate radical radiotherapy.

Technique of Radiotherapy

The object is to irradiate a cylindrical volume enclosing the tumour to a dose which will be adequate to destroy the carcinoma. Since oesophageal growths infiltrate the mucosa microscopically for a considerable distance outside the limits of macroscopic tumour, a margin of about 5 cm at each end of the carcinoma as delimited by barium swallow should be included in the irradiated volume. The technique is further complicated by the fact that the oesophagus is not a straight tube but curves with its concavity anterior, as well as inclining towards the left as it descends. A cylinder of high dose may be required, about 7 cm in diameter and perhaps 14–16 cm long, but meticulous and complicated planning is required to place this cylinder accurately.

The oesophagus and its carcinoma are localised in relation to skin-marks by barium-swallow radiography with the patient in the treatment position. The treatment volume is marked on the films obtained and one or more transverse contours of the patient at the relevant level are drawn. Megavoltage is employed, usually via three fields. The fields are planned so that the amount of radiation reaching the lungs and spinal cord is limited to the tolerance of these tissues; diminished absorption of radiation passing through lung as compared with solid tissue must be taken into account in the calculations. Accurate rotation of the beams about their central axes, and the introduction of specially constructed beam-modifying filters, allow the cylinder of high dosage to be moulded to fit the volume required.

A dose of 5500 rad in twenty fractions over four weeks is suitable. Swallowing often improves during the course of treatment, but may temporarily become slightly painful due to a radiation reaction in the oesophageal mucosa after two or three weeks of treatment. This discomfort is transient and is usually relieved by an aspirin mucilage, or a proprietary preparation such as Mucaine (Wyeth). Skin reactions are negligible. Such treatment, although perhaps complicated and prolonged, is not a severe trial for most patients; there is no mortality and very little morbidity arising from it (Fig. 6.7).

Results of Radiotherapy for Oesophageal Carcinoma

Pearson (1966) reported the results of radiotherapy for oesophageal carcinoma for 1956–64, using a 4 MV linear accelerator. Sixty-one patients had growths involving the middle third of the oesophagus and 40 had growths involving the lower third. The actuarial five-year survival was 23 per cent for middle-third tumours and 17 per cent for lower-third, compared with the corresponding Edinburgh surgical figures of 9 and 11 per cent respectively. McKeown (1974) reported five patients out of seventeen surviving five years after excision of middle-third growths, and eight of 22 living three years after excision of lower-third carcinomas, although his operative mortality was as high as 30·8 per cent in what he described as 'high growths'.

The palliative value of radiotherapy is considerable. In the early days (1957–61) of telecobalt therapy at the London Hospital, 80 patients were treated for oesophageal carcinomas. Only 18 survived one year, but of these 13 were swallowing well at the end of that time. Indeed, if half the patients treated were given a year of normal swallowing this would be a worthwhile achievement in itself.

Management of Recurrent Dysphagia

Dysphagia recurring after radical radiotherapy for oesophageal carcinoma may be due to regrowth of the tumour. This is not invariably the case, as sometimes oesophagoscopy reveals only a fibrous stricture which may be treatable by bouginage.

Where the carcinoma has indeed recurred, the outlook is very poor. Radical surgery seems to meet with little success. Resection was carried out in ten of Pearson's cases, in eight for recurrent tumour and in two for fibrous stricture. Seven patients died post-operatively and the rest within six months. Temporary improvement in swallowing may be obtained by bouginage, or a tube of the Mousseau-Barbin, Celestin, or Souttar type inserted. One of these tubes may enable the patient to swallow for a while but rarely for more than a few weeks. Only about half the patients so treated leave hospital (McKeown, 1974). Ulceration into the mediastinum often occurs as a terminal event; the Souttar tube, made of coiled silver wire, may become dislodged from the oesophagus and may even be passed *per rectum*. Gastrostomy as a means of maintaining nutrition usually results in a state of misery for the patient, who eventually is unable to swallow his saliva.

Pre-operative Radiotherapy in the Treatment of Carcinoma of the Oesophagus

This has been advocated by Nakayama (1967) using a dose of 2000 rad in four fractions. Surgery is carried out in three stages, in the first of which patients with liver or coeliac node involvement are identified and rejected. His results are somewhat difficult to interpret, and are not comparable with those of less highly selective series.

Thymic Tumours

Patients suffering from tumours of the thymus are rarely seen in radiotherapy departments. Only 18 such cases were seen in the London Hospital department over a period of 15 years (Penn and Hope-Stone, 1972).

Clinical Presentation

The age at presentation varies greatly, 19 and 69 being the extremes in the London Hospital series, and the sexes are evenly represented. About half the patients are asymptomatic, the lesion being discovered on radiography. Others complain of a variety of symptoms, including pain in the chest, neck and arm, chest wall swelling, hoarseness, tiredness, or anorexia. Myasthenia gravis may occur in perhaps a third of all patients with thymic tumours (and rather less than one-third of patients with myasthenia gravis have a thymoma). Disorders of the blood cells may occur, notably red cell aplasia (Havard and Scott, 1960). Thymomas may be benign or malignant, but distant metastases are unusual: Rachmaninoff and Fentress (1964) found only ten cases of metastases from thymomas in the world literature, including one of their own.

Histological Classification

Thomson and Thackray (1957) classified thymomas into three groups: *epithelial*, *lymphocytic* and *teratomatous*. The epithelial group includes growths of epidermoid appearance and the lymphoepitheliomas, as well as oval or spindle-cell and undifferentiated tumours and the granulomatous thymomas which histologically may be indistinguishable from Hodgkin's disease. The lymphocytic thymomas consist of masses of lymphocytes, the malignant forms being lymphosarcomas, while the lymphoepitheliomas form an important group. The teratomas consisting of cells from all three germ layers, include benign dermoids but also some frankly malignant growths. For clinical purposes, Penn and Hope-Stone suggested the following classification:

1. *Benign lymphoepitheliomas* (the group most frequently associated with myasthenia gravis)
2. *Invasive thymomas* of epithelial, lymphocytic, or mixed type
3. *Granulomatous thymomas*
4. *Teratomas*

Investigation

An anterior mediastinal mass is demonstrated by radiography and tomography may be helpful. A technique of selective thymic venography has been described by Kreel (1967). Surgical exploration is necessary; if possible the thymoma should be removed, and if inoperable a biopsy should be taken to establish the diagnosis.

Radiotherapy in the Management of Thymoma

Pre-operative radiotherapy was advocated by Keynes (1949) when myasthenia gravis was present, but this is no longer current practice. A thymoma may be completely excised and no invasive property demonstrated, in which case no radiotherapy is indicated. Penn and Hope-Stone advocate post-operative radiotherapy in all cases of invasive thymoma, whether excision seems complete or not. For the inoperable or incompletely excised invasive growth, radiotherapy offers the possibility of tumour regression and prolonged survival (Fig. 6.8); indeed, for the macroscopically invasive tumour, limitation of surgery to biopsy, with complete reliance on radiotherapy for treatment, may well be the best approach (Sturridge, 1974).

Technique of Radiotherapy

A dose of 4000 rad in twenty treatments over 28 days is feasible using megavoltage apparatus. A small thymoma may be adequately

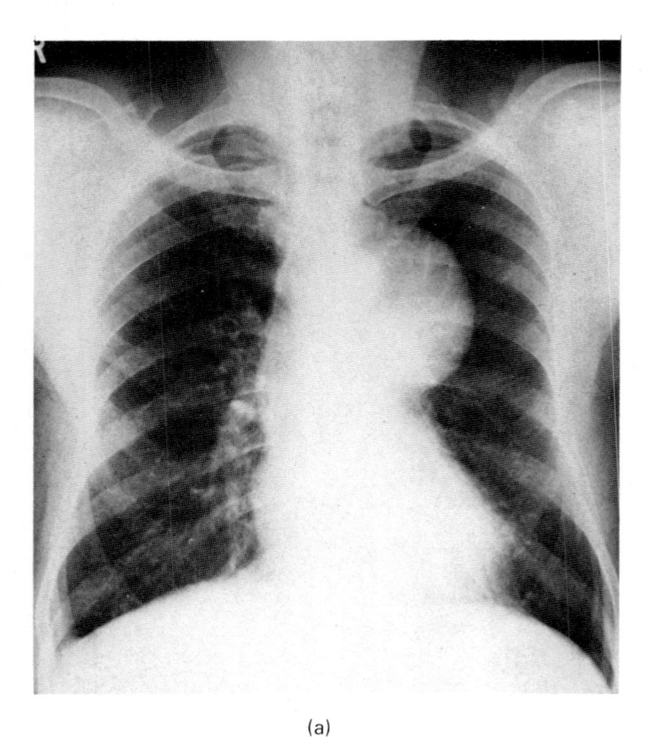

(a)

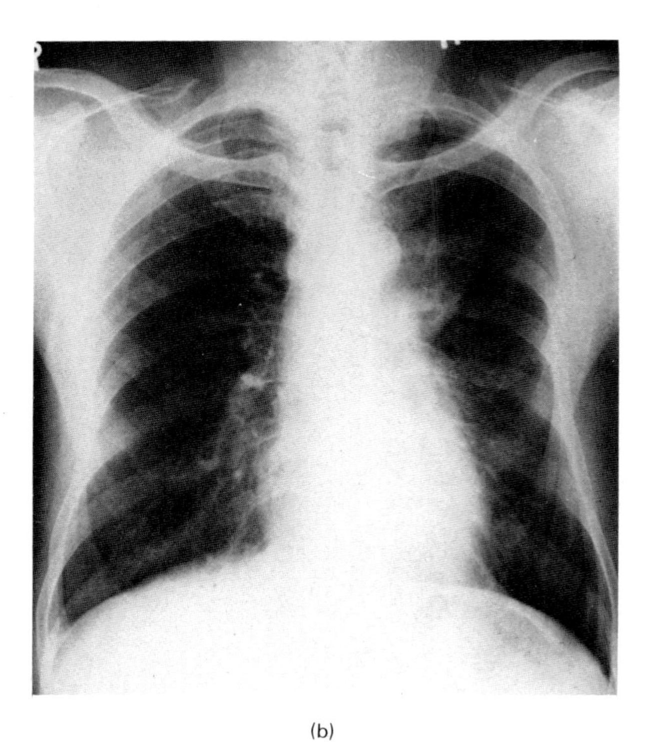

(b)

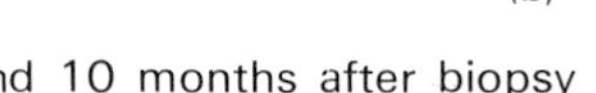

Fig. 6.8. Radiographs of a case of malignant thymoma before and 10 months after biopsy and radical radiotherapy (courtesy Drs C. R. H. Penn and H. F. Hope-Stone and the Editor, *British Journal of Surgery*).

irradiated by a pair of anterior oblique wedged fields, but larger tumours may require anterior and posterior parallel opposed beams. A certain amount of lung tissue is necessarily included in the irradiated volume; pneumonitis may occur and fibrosis can follow. Careful planning of treatment will diminish the likelihood of serious symptoms arising from this source. More serious side-effects, including mediastinitis and pericarditis, have been described (Skeggs, 1968) but only in patients treated to a much higher dose than that suggested. Similarly, permanent spinal-cord damage has not been recorded in the London Hospital series.

Results of Radiotherapy for Thymoma

Thymoma is a rare tumour, and individual experience is of necessity limited. In the London Hospital series only seven patients were selected for a full radical dose of 4000 rad; of these, three had macroscopically complete excision of the tumour. All seven patients survived for three years, and all four who were followed for five years survived for that time. Three of four lived ten years, all of these having growths of mixed histological type; one of them had macroscopic tumour left behind at thoracotomy.

While sound statistical evidence is difficult to obtain, it seems justifiable to regard adequate radiotherapy as the main treatment for invasive thymoma, and to employ it after surgery whether excision appears complete or whether biopsy only has been performed.

Primary Lymphoma of the Lung

Invasion of the lung by a lymphosarcoma or other reticulosis arising in the lymph nodes is well known. Lymphoma may also appear *de novo* in the lung. It is extremely rare, only seven cases occurring in 20 years at the Brompton Hospital (Rees, 1973). It may present as an opacity in the chest X-ray of an asymptomatic patient, or may be associated with chest pain, dyspnoea, pleural effusion, or even vocal-cord palsy. There is no evidence of generalised disease in the early stages, but dissemination may eventually occur. Thoracotomy is required to allow a good biopsy to be taken, and sometimes the lesion can be resected.

The value of radiotherapy and chemotherapy is uncertain, and in a condition of such variety, difficult to determine. It might be expected that irradiation of the tumour mass with a margin of 3 cm or so to a dose of 3000 to 4000 rad in three to four weeks might sterilise a primary lymphosarcoma. Papaioannou and Watson (1965) found similar five-year survival rates of 40 to 44 per cent, whether radiotherapy, surgery or both were used. Prolonged survival has been reported using simple chemotherapy with oral chlorambucil (Rees, 1973) or even after no treatment at all (Jenkins and Salm 1971), but many patients die with generalised disease in spite of the above treatments.

Total Thoracic Irradiation for Multiple Pulmonary Metastases

For most patients with malignant disease the appearance of multiple pulmonary metastases is a grave prognostic pointer. The metastases themselves may cause cough, dyspnoea and sometimes pain. Chemotherapy may sometimes afford some palliation, but radiotherapy has been little used in these circumstances. The dose of radiation that can be delivered to the whole chest is necessarily limited not only by the bone-marrow depression resulting from the irradiation of so large a portion of the body, but also by the risk of radiation pneumonitis. Nevertheless Newton and Spittle (1969) have shown that a dose of 2000 to 2500 rad may be delivered to the whole chest over a period of three to four weeks without ill effect. Regression of metastases with relief of symptoms and sometimes prolonged survival has been obtained.

Megavoltage is used, with large anterior and posterior opposed fields each subtending the whole chest, shaped with lead blocks to limit the radiation to the mediastinum and lung fields. The dose is calculated at the centre of the chest and 150 rad given daily at this point, treating on five days a week. The blood count is checked weekly.

In Newton and Spittle's series complete radiological regression of metastases was observed in 15 out of 60 cases, with lesser degrees of regression in another fifteen. Of 18 patients complaining of chest symptoms, two-thirds obtained complete relief. The most favourable groups were Ewing's sarcomas, Wilms's tumours and testicular tumours, teratomas as well as seminomas. The present author has seen complete regression with prolonged survival in a case of the highly malignant MTIB testicular teratoma. The long survivors in Newton and Spittle's group include two cases of seminoma alive at four years after treatment, and a patient with Wilms's tumour alive at nearly five years after treatment; there is no mention of concomitant chemotherapy. In no case treated as above were there early or late complications attributable to radiotherapy.

Clearly total thoracic irradiation is a safe procedure which may be of considerable help to patients in a desperate situation.

References

ADAMS, W. E. and PHEMISTER, D. B. (1938) *Journal of Thoracic Surgery*, **7**, 621.

ALEXANDER, P. (1965) *Atomic Radiation and Life*, Penguin, Harmondsworth, 81.

BATES, M., HURT, R. L., LEVISON, V. B. and SUTTON, M. (1974) *Lancet*, **1**, 1134–1135.

BELCHER, J. R. (1974) Personal communication.

BLANSHARD, G. (1955) *Lancet*, **2**, 897–901.

BOESEN, E. (1973) *BTTA Review*, **3**, 17–25.

CAMERON, S. J., GRANT, I. W. B., LUTZ, W. and PEARSON, J. G. (1969) *Clinical Radiology*, **20**, 12–18.

CAMERON, S. J., GRANT, I. W. B., PEARSON, J. G. and MARQUIS, C. (1972) *British Medical Journal*, **1**, 535–537.

CHAJEK, T. and FAINARU, M. (1973) *British Medical Journal*, **1**, 782–783.

CZERNY, V. (1877) *Zentralblatt für Chirurgie*, **4**, 433.

DEELEY, T. J. (1966) *Clinical Radiology*, **17**, 299–301.

DEELEY, T. J. and RICE EDWARDS, J. M. (1968) *Lancet*, **1**, 1209–1212.

DURRANT, K. R., BERRY, R. S., ELLIS, F., RIDEHALGH, F. R., BLACK, J. M. and HAMILTON, W. S. (1971) *Lancet*, **1**, 715–719.

EDELSTYN, G. A., GILLESPIE, P. J. and GREBBELL, F. S. (1967) *Clinical Radiology*, **18**, 158–162.

FOX, W. and SCADDING, J. G. (1973), *Lancet*, **2**, 63–65.

GUTTMAN, R. J. G. (1965) *American Journal of Roentgenology*, **93**, 99–103.

HANHAM, I. W. F., NEWTON, K. A. and WESTBURY, G. (1971) *British Journal of Cancer*, **25**, 462–478.

HARE, E. S. (1838) *London Medical Gazette*, **23**, 16–18.

HAVARD, C. W. H. and SCOTT, R. B. (1960) *British Journal of Haematology*, **6**, 178–190.

HELLSTROM, I., HELLSTROM, K. E., SJOGREN, H. O. and WARNER, G. A. (1971) *International Journal of Cancer*, **7**, 1.

HICKMAN, J. A. and JONES, M. C. (1970) *Thorax*, **25**, 226–229.

HOPE-STONE, H. F. (1967) *British Journal of Diseases of the Chest*, **61**, 57–69.

HOPE-STONE, H. F. and KEY, J. J. (1961) *British Medical Journal*, **2**, 1126–1128.

JENKINS, B. A. G. and SALM, R. (1971) *British Journal of Diseases of the Chest*, **65**, 225.

JOHNSON, R. J. R., WALTON, R. J., LIM, M. L., ZYLAK, C. J. and PAIN-CHAUD, L. A. (1973) *Clinical Radiology*, **24**, 494–497.

KEYNES, G. (1949) *British Medical Journal*, **2**, 611–616.

KREEL, L. (1967) *British Medical Journal*, **1**, 406–407.

LENNOX, S. C., FLAVELL, S. G., POLLOCK, D. J., THOMPSON, V. C. and WILKINS, J. L. (1968) *Lancet*, **2**, 925–927.

LEVISON, V. B. (1961) *British Medical Journal*, **1**, 1143–1145.

MANTELL, B. S. (1973) *British Journal of Diseases of the Chest*, **67**, 315–317.

MCKEOWN, K. C. (1974) *Proceedings of the Royal Society of Medicine*, **67**, 389–395.

MORRISON, R., DEELEY, T. J. and CLELAND, W. P. (1963) *Lancet*, **1**, 683–684.

NAKAYAMA, K., ORIHATA, H. and YAMAGUCHI, K. (1967) *Cancer*, **20**, 778–788.

NEWTON, K. A. and SPITTLE, M. F. (1969) *Clinical Radiology*, **20**, 19–22.

PANCOAST, H. K. (1932) *Journal of the American Medical Association*, **99**, 1391.

PAPAIOANNOU, A. N. and WATSON, W. L. (1965) *Journal of Thoracic and Cardiovascular Surgery*, **49**, 373–387.

PARKES, W. R. (1973) *British Journal of Diseases of the Chest*, **67**, 261–300.

PATERSON, R. and RUSSELL, M. H. (1962) *Clinical Radiology*, **13**, 141.

PEARSON, J. G. (1966) *Clinical Radiology*, **17**, 242–257.

PENN, C. R. H. and HOPE-STONE, H. F. (1972) *British Journal of Surgery*, **59**, 533–539.

RACHMANINOFF, N. and FENTRESS, V. (1964) *American Journal of Clinical Pathology*, **41**, 618–625.

REES, G. M. (1973) *Thorax*, **28**, 429–432.

SHIELDS, T. W., HIGGINS, G. A., LAWTON, R., HEILBRUNN, A. and KEEHN, R. J. (1970) *Journal of Thoracic and Cardiovascular Surgery*, **59**, 49–61.

SKEGGS, D. B. C. (1968) *Proceedings of the Royal Society of Medicine*, **61**, 760–762.

SMART, J. (1966) *Journal of the American Medical Association*, **195**, 1034.

SMART, J. and HILTON, G. (1956) *Lancet*, **1**, 880–881.

SMITHERS, D. W. (1955) *Journal of the Faculty of Radiologists*, **6**, 174.

STEEL, S. J. (1971) in *Modern Radiotherapy, Carcinoma of the Bronchus*, ed. Deeley, T. J., Butterworth, London.

STURRIDGE, M. F. (1974) Personal communication.

SUTTON, M. and PRATT-JOHNSON, J. H. (1970) *Clinical Radiology*, **21**, 256–258.

SZUR, L. and BROMLEY, L. L. (1956) *British Medical Journal*, **2**, 1273–1276.

THOMSON, A. D. and THACKRAY, A. C. (1957) *British Journal of Cancer*, **11**, 348.

TOREK, F. (1913) *Journal of the American Medical Association*, **60**, 1533.

CHAPTER SEVEN

The Reticuloses and Allied Disorders

H. F. Hope-Stone

The reticuloses is a generic name given to a group of allied diseases which may be considered under the following headings: Hodgkin's disease, lymphosarcoma, reticulum cell sarcoma, lymphoid follicular reticulosis and Burkitt's lymphoma. One might wish to include the leukaemias and myelo-proliferative diseases, but this is probably too wide a definition. Since irradiation is now being used more frequently in these latter conditions, references will be made to them later.

Epidemiology

The incidence of the reticuloses varies according to type, sex, and race. Hodgkin's disease is the most frequent (30–50 per cent), then lymphosarcoma (30–40 per cent), reticulum cell sarcoma (10–20 per cent), and lymphoid follicular reticulosis (2–10 per cent) (Moss, 1969). There is a preponderance of males over females in Hodgkin's disease, of the order of 2 to 1 (Easson and Russell, 1963). In lymphosarcoma this is less marked, being 1·3 to 1 in the author's series, while reticulum cell sarcoma shows no difference in the sex ratio (Hope-Stone, 1969).

The average age in all groups is 40, but ranges from 2 to 80 years. The majority of cases of Burkitt's lymphoma occur in children.

There is a variable incidence throughout the world of Hodgkin's disease, ranging from 80 per million per year of the population in the United Kingdom to 4 per million per year in Japan. MacMahon (1957) suggested that the low incidence in Japan might be related to its virtual absence below the age of 40. He was also the first to point out the bimodal behaviour of Hodgkin's disease, as shown by an additional peak between the ages of 15 and 40 years. The other reticuloses, when plotted semi-logarithmically, exhibit roughly linear increases from childhood to 75 years.

Burkitt's lymphoma, first described in the central African area below 5000 ft (Burkitt, 1958), has also been found endemically in New Guinea, and sporadically in North and South America and Europe, occurring in both nationals and immigrants of these regions.

An increased incidence of Hodgkin's disease in local communities has been described in an American group of High School students and their female relatives (Vianna *et al.*, 1972). It has been suggested that the disease spreads like an infection in a community, showing variable susceptibility.

Aetiology

Little is known of the actual causation. Smithers (1973) suggested that the disease may be induced in susceptible subjects by a virus, and could therefore be transmitted from person to person like an infection, although development of the disease would be unlikely in the absence of a reduced immune response in any individual. In Burkitt's lymphoma the Epstein–Barr virus has been indirectly implicated as an oncogenic agent, but definite proof is still lacking (*The Lancet*, 1974).

The unifocal theory of origin (Thompson, 1955), although incorrect in suggesting the thymus as the only primary site, nevertheless receives much support, and suggests that the reticuloses are potentially curable. Metastases can be accounted for by the fact that lymphocytes can circulate between the lymph and blood streams (Yoffey, 1960). Certainly, if one studies the first signs of spread of the disease after radical treatment of a localised primary reticulosis, the adjacent lymph nodes are found to be most commonly first involved, being 60 per cent in

Sheer's series (1955). If the tumour were multifocal in origin, new deposits would not be likely to present in this way.

Immunology

Although after intense irradiation or chemotherapy the immune response would be expected to be reduced, no definite evidence exists of such a deficiency in the untreated early cases, although it may present when the disease is advanced. It is well to remember that when there is a possibility of immune deficiency, certain procedures that are potentially hazardous should be avoided: e.g. smallpox vaccination should not be carried out.

Histology

Hodgkin's Disease

The old classification of para-granuloma, Hodgkin's disease, and Hodgkin's sarcoma has been abandoned in favour of Lukes and Butler (1966), and the Rye Classification (*Cancer Research*, 1966):

Rye Classification and Frequency (Kaplan, 1972)

	Relative frequency (%)
Lymphocyte predominant	10–15
Nodular sclerotic	20–50
Mixed cellularity	30–40
Lymphocyte depleted	5–15

This histological classification is important, since the prognosis for the first two groups is better than the last.

Reticulum Cell Sarcoma

This appears to be a fairly easily identifiable entity, but difficulty can be encountered with some very anaplastic carcinomas, which are often indistinguishable from a reticulum cell sarcoma.

Lymphosarcoma

This presents more difficulties, as it is often impossible to differentiate from lymphatic leukaemia. Detailed classification of this group has been described by Millet *et al.* (1969):

	Frequency (%)
Lymphoblastic	27
Diffuse	34
Follicular lymphoma	37
Nodular sclerotic	65

These authors show that the nodular sclerotic group have a better prognosis than the others.

Lymphoid Follicular Reticulosis (Brill-Symmers disease, follicular lymphoma)

This group, included as a form of lymphosarcoma in Millet's classification, is believed to be a separate entity by other authors (Hilton and Sutton, 1962).

All the non-Hodgkin's lymphoma have now been reclassified histologically by Rappaport *et al.* (1956) and Farrer-Brown *et al.* (1974) (Table 7.1, opposite).

Burkitt's Lymphoma

Histologically this can be distinguished from the other reticuloses by the closely-packed lymphoblasts with a scattering of pale macrophages, giving the characteristic 'starry sky' appearance. However, morphologically there are many points of resemblance.

Presentation

In early cases the commonest symptom and sign is an enlarging lymph node, usually in the neck. Although it is unusual to find Hodgkin's

Table 7.1. Classification of Non-Hodgkin's Lymphomas

Grade	*TRADITIONAL*	*BENNETT, FARRER-BROWN, HENRY*			*RAPPAPORT*
		Follicular lymphoma		(FL)	*Nodular lymphomas*
GRADE I	Follicular lymphoma	Follicle centre cell	Predominantly small		Lymphocytic poorly-differentiated
		Follicle centre cell	Mixed small and large		Mixed lymphocytic and 'histiocytic'
		Follicle centre cell	Predominantly large		'Histiocytic'
		Diffuse lymphomas			*Diffuse lymphomas*
	Lymphosarcoma Well-differentiated	Lymphocytic	Well-differentiated small cell	(DLWD)	Lymphocytic well-differentiated
		Lymphocytic	Intermediate differentiation Small follicle cell	(DLI)	Lymphocytic poorly-differentiated
GRADE II	Lymphoblastic Lymphosarcoma	Lymphocytic	Poorly-differentiated	(DLPD)	Lymphocytic poorly-differentiated; Undifferentiated
	Reticulum cell sarcoma	Mixed large, undifferentiated and small lymphoid cells		(D Mixed)	Mixed lymphocytic and 'histiocytic'
		Undifferentiated large cells		(DUL)	'Histiocytic'

disease presenting at sites other than lymph nodes, the other reticuloses may first be seen in the stomach, small bowel, tonsils, thyroid, nasopharynx, antrum, testis or even lung parenchyma. Pericardial involvement rarely occurs at an early stage, but it may be seen when the disease is more advanced (Fig. 7.1). Pleural effusion and ascites may be seen early, particularly in lymphoid follicular reticulosis.

Other sites which may be involved include the breast and orbit, the

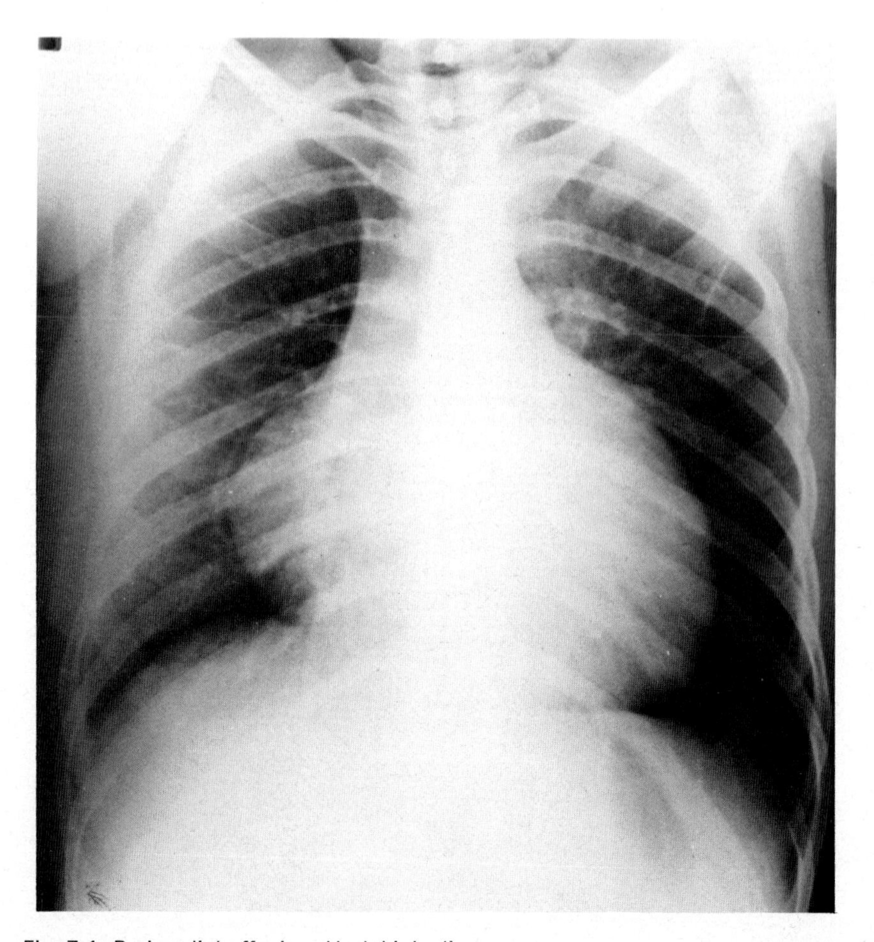

Fig. 7.1. Pericardial effusion: Hodgkin's disease.

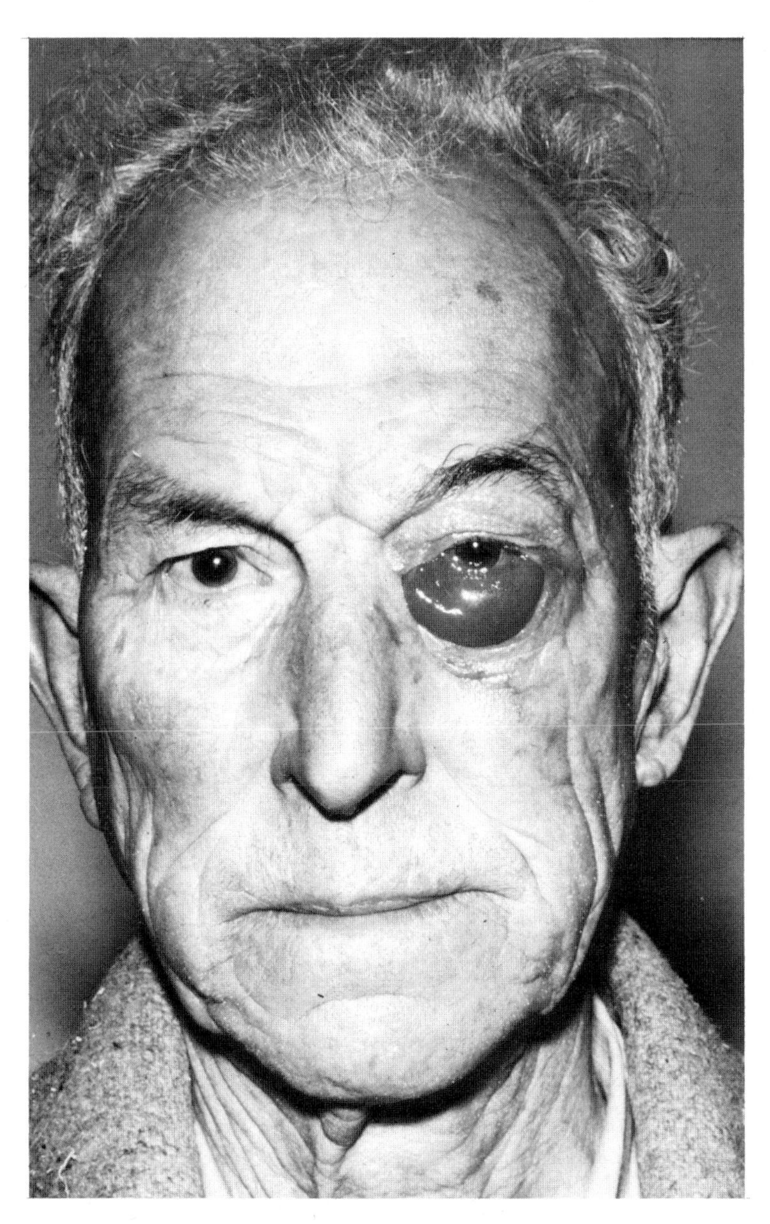

Fig. 7.2. Orbital involvement: lymphosarcoma.

latter site being most commonly seen in lymphosarcoma (Fig. 7.2). The spleen can be involved relatively early in the disease, but liver involvement occurs at a late stage and is usually associated with splenic disease.

Primary cutaneous Hodgkin's disease would appear to be a recognised entity, and to have a better prognosis than when this is a secondary manifestation. Reticulum cell sarcoma may present with direct

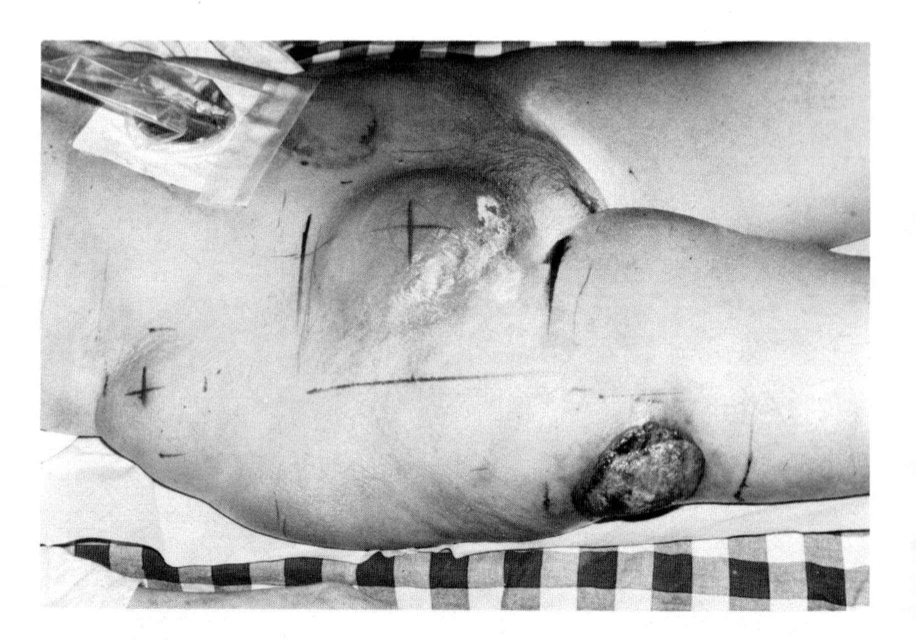

Fig. 7.3. Skin ulceration: reticulum cell sarcoma.

skin involvement (Fig. 7.3). Lymphosarcoma cutis is also rare, which is fortunate as it is usually succeeded by rapid dissemination of the disease. Mycosis fungoides (Fig. 7.4), which is histologically similar, develops in three stages: initially erythematous, it then shows a series of discrete irregular plaques, and finally the typically ulcerated and tomato-like plaques appear. It may subsequently develop into a generalised reticulosis.

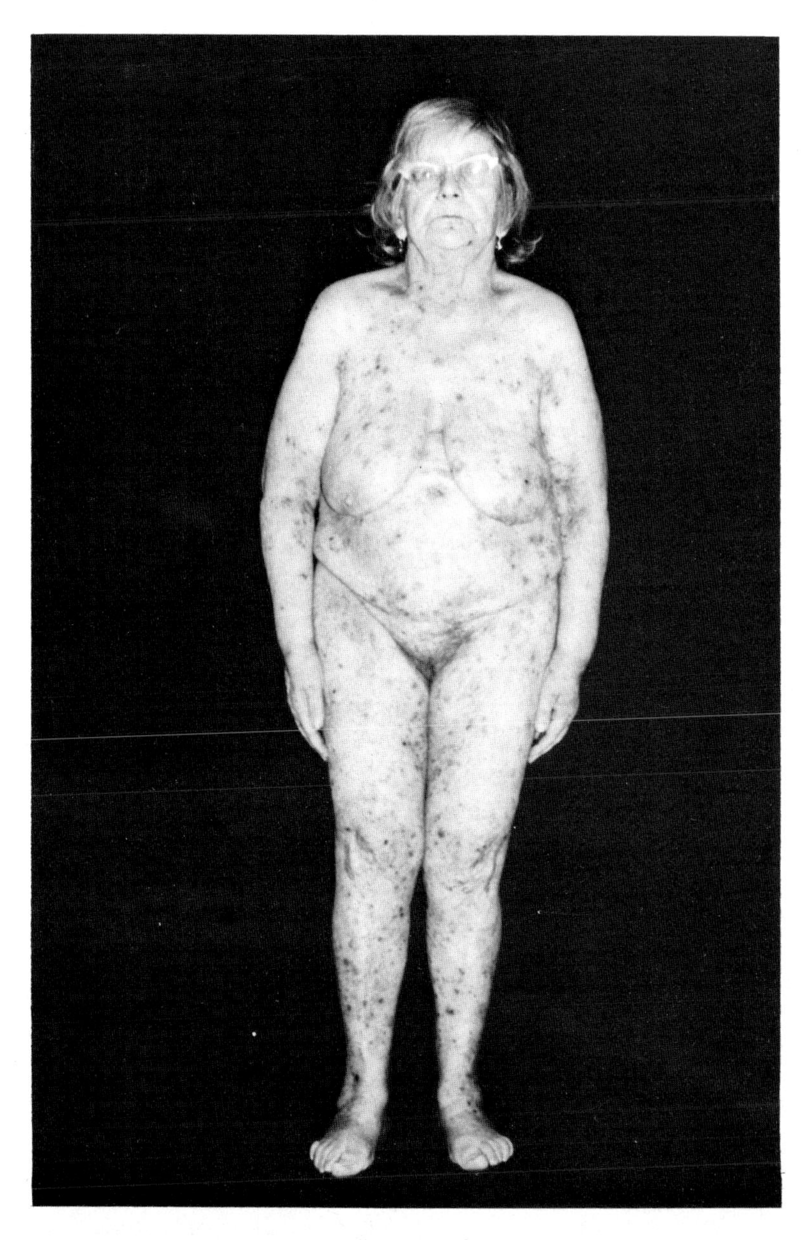

Fig. 7.4. Mycosis fungoides.

Herpes simplex is found in the reticuloses (Jensen, 1973), but more common is herpes zoster, with an incidence of 15–25 per cent in Hodgkin's disease and 7–8 per cent in the other lymphomata. Impairment of the patient's immunological response is probably an important factor, and this will be made worse by irradiation, cytotoxic drugs and cortico-steroid therapy. The use of the latter drugs is particularly worrying, as generalised varicella may follow, and can be fatal (Dayan *et al.*, 1964). If at all possible, the cortico-steroid therapy should be stopped or reduced.

Bone involvement can occur primarily, as in reticulum cell sarcoma, but it is not uncommon as a secondary manifestation, particularly in Hodgkin's disease, producing the so-called 'vertebra nigrans'.

Neurological involvement is usually secondary, and may show as meningeal deposits, which are rare, and can present with epilepsy (Currie and Jardine, 1969). Spinal cord involvement is usually due to extra-dural deposits, originating from paravertebral lymphadenopathy, and from direct pressure by collapsed vertebrae. Direct brain involvement is rare, but can occur as a diffuse lesion in microgliomatosis. This is considered to be a primary reticulosis, histologically identical with reticulum cell sarcoma (Fisher *et al.*, 1969).

Marrow infiltration occurs late in the disease. This may present as hypochromic anaemia, haemolytic anaemia or pancytopenia. It is only in the last group that direct infiltration by neoplastic cells is likely to be seen.

Burkitt's lymphoma, first described as occurring in the jaws of young African children, may be seen presenting in any part of the reticulo-endothelial system, as well as many other organs including the ovaries and kidneys. Massive abdominal lymphadenopathy may occur, with other nodes only moderately enlarged.

Natural History

Many cases of the reticuloses, if treated correctly, can be cured. If left alone they are usually rapidly fatal. During the course of the treated disease, leukaemia may occur, particularly in the lymphosarcoma and follicular lymphoma group. Lymphoid follicular reticulosis has the unusual propensity of spontaneous resolution, and one should not be too pessimistic with regard to the outcome of the disease, even in the more advanced case. There is no evidence that pregnancy alters the prognosis in any way, at least in Hodgkin's disease, and this appears to be true whether the pregnancy develops in remission or relapse (Hartvigsen, 1955).

Diagnosis

The only certain way to confirm the diagnosis is by obtaining adequate biopsy material. If there is an easily accessible lymph node this should be removed *in toto*. The drill biopsy technique, useful as it is for confirming advanced malignancy, is second best in the reticuloses, where as much undisturbed histological material as possible should be obtained. The same applies to both gut and bone involvement. Radiotherapy should not be given prior to obtaining histological material, as such treatment will only make diagnosis more difficult.

Relationship of the Four Main Groups of Reticuloses

Although four main groups are described as separate entities with different morphological and clinical characteristics, there are many similarities between them, particularly in relation to their response to treatment and prognosis. Histologically there is well-documented evidence of the presence of two or more types of reticuloses occurring in one patient: e.g. lymphosarcoma and Hodgkin's disease, or even lymphosarcoma, reticulum cell sarcoma and Hodgkin's disease (Herbert and Miller, 1945). It may well be that subdivision of the reticuloses is mainly arbitrary, and based on morphological grounds rather than on the natural history of the disease (Hope-Stone, 1969).

Staging

The simple classification of early localised and late generalised disease, as described by Boden (1951), has been modified a number of times. Recently the Rye Classification has been widely adopted (*Cancer Research*, 1966):

Stage I	Disease limited to one group of lymph nodes, or two groups if they are contiguous.
Stage II	Disease of more than two contiguous lymph node groups or two non-contiguous groups provided they are all on the same side of the diaphragm.
Stage III	Disease on both sides of the diaphragm, limited to the nodes and spleen thymus and/or Waldeyer's ring.
Stage IV	Involvement of the bone marrow, lung parenchyma, pleura, liver, bone, skin, kidneys, gastrointestinal tract, or any tissue or organ in addition to the lymphoid tissue.

The four stages are divided into A and B: A denotes no constitutional symptoms; B denotes constitutional symptoms as defined by *pyrexia*, 38°C or higher on three occasions in two weeks; *night sweats*, considered significant when the patient is woken by them; *weight loss*, over 10 per cent in three to six months.

The chief problem of staging is the desirability of pursuing relentlessly every conceivable investigation to its maximum degree, and this may include laparotomy, splenectomy and liver biopsy. The more thorough the investigation, the more likely are the patients with advanced disease to be recognised.

There are certain essential investigations, and these should include a full blood count with haemoglobin, ESR, WBCs and a differential and platelet count. The neutrophil alkaline phosphatase score (NAP) is said to indicate active Hodgkin's disease when raised (80–140), and is also useful in polycythaemia rubra vera where it can be very high (more than 150), and myeloid leukaemia, when it is very depressed (less than 10) (Bennet *et al.*, 1968). The test can also be used to monitor the activity of the disease after therapy.

Bone marrow investigation is essential in lymphosarcoma when there is any doubt about the possibility of lymphatic leukaemia being present. In the other reticuloses it may be helpful in advanced cases to elucidate the haemolytic anaemias and pancytopenias. Tumour cells are rarely seen even in generalised disease, unless an open bone biopsy is carried out (Jelliffe *et al.*, 1970). If previous irradiation has been given, the marrow specimen should be obtained if possible from a non-irradiated area. A Coombs test and a reticulocyte count may be useful in the diagnosis of the haemolytic anaemias. Biochemical investigations should include the serum uric acid and liver function tests, but the latter are only really useful if positive.

Radiology plays a very important role – a straight X-ray and lateral of the chest are not sufficient to exclude early mediastinal involvement, and tomography should always be considered. Straight X-rays of the abdomen often show enlargement of the liver and spleen. Lymphangiography has proven to be of tremendous value in providing evidence of intra-abdominal and pelvic node involvement, although if negative this does not rule out the presence of occult disease; this investigation will not demonstrate involved glands in the mesentery, porta hepatis, coeliac axis or hilum of the spleen.

The classical floccular pattern of Hodgkin's disease (Fig. 7.5) is easy to recognise, but the other reticuloses are not so easily distinguished, and may show only by a filling defect of a node or complete failure of the nodes to fill. The investigation is always carried out with an IVP, as displacement of the ureters may be the only sign of involved nodes when the lymphogram is negative. Lymphangiography is not without side-effects; these include sepsis at the site of the injections, allergic skin reaction to the dye used to outline the lymphatics, and local thromboembolism. Worse still, multiple pulmonary emboli can cause acute respiratory embarrassments which in the chronic bronchitic or asthmatic may be potentially fatal. For the same reason, lymphangiography should not be carried out if the whole lung has recently been irradiated. In about one per cent of patients the investigation itself is technically impossible, due to failure to cannulate the lymphatics (McDonald, 1969).

If the above investigations are negative, inferior vena cavography may prove helpful, particularly in the presence of spinal cord involvement. Myelography may be required, however, to show the precise site of obstruction even when the lymphangiogram is positive (Fig. 7.6).

Radioactive isotope scans of the liver and spleen may give positive evidence of disease, but false negative results can be misleading. Bone metastases can often be shown up by ^{85}Sr or ^{18}F before they are evident radiologically. Whole lung scanning with ^{67}Ga is less likely to show up early metastases than is whole lung tomography (Kay and McCready, 1972). The former method can be used to detect early lymph node involvement, particularly in the mediastinum (Edward and Hays, 1970).

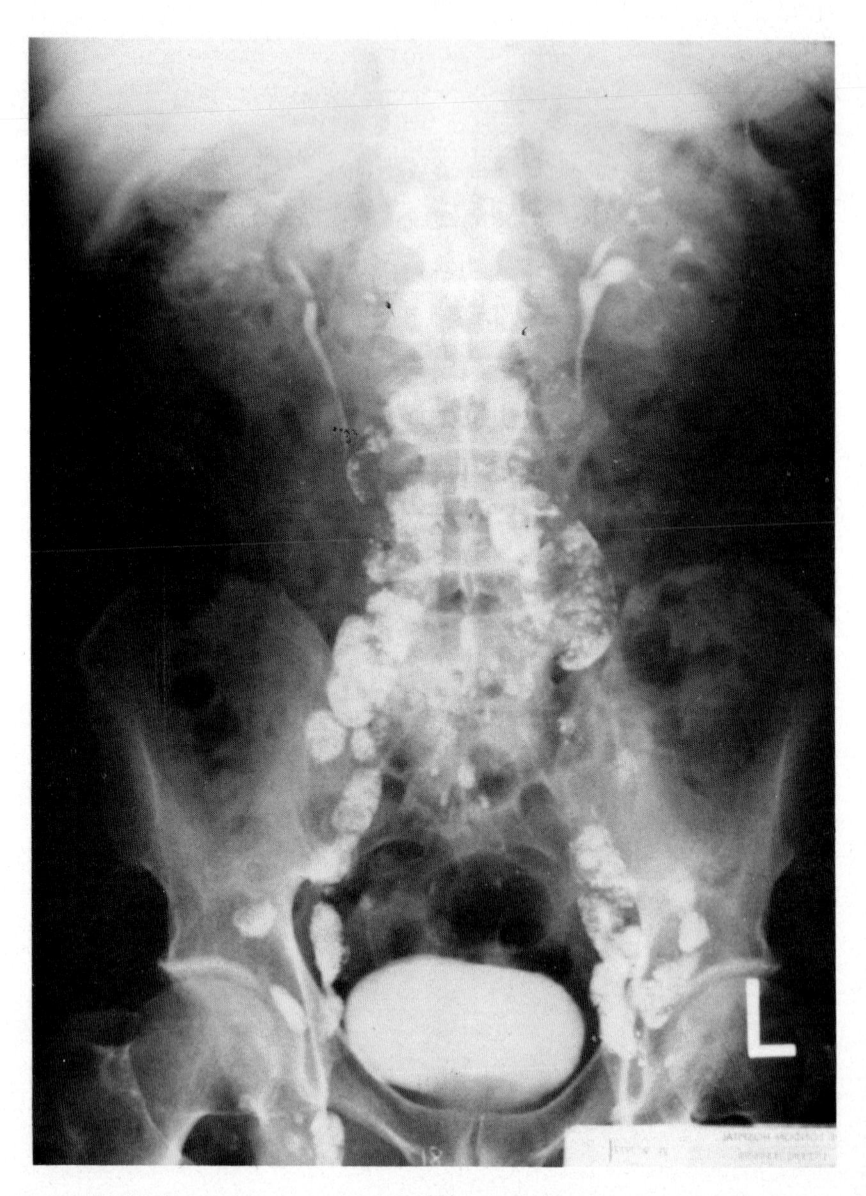

Fig. 7.5. Lymphangiogram showing floccular pattern: Hodgkin's disease.

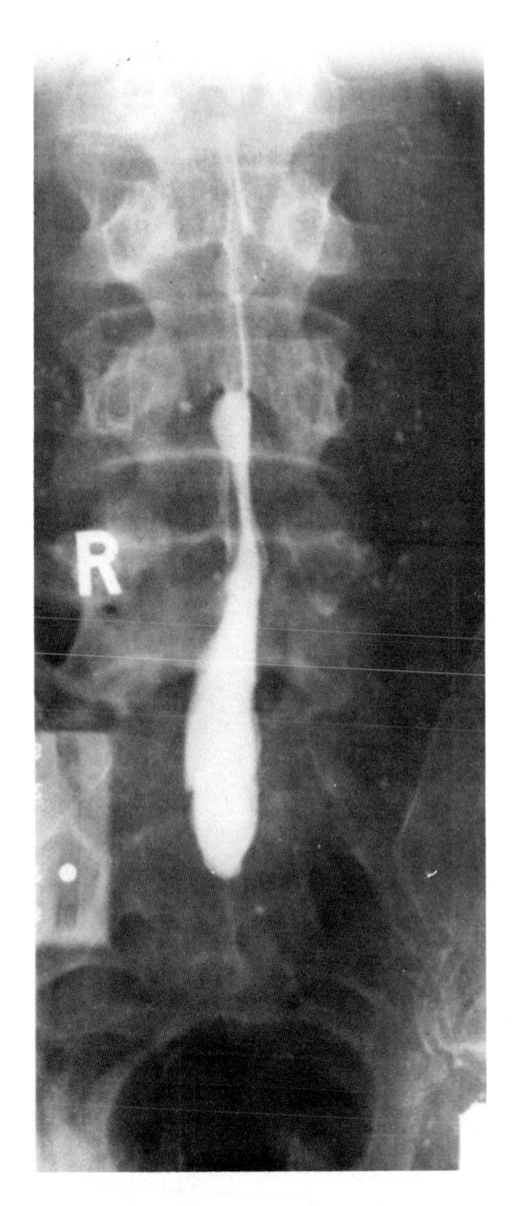

Fig. 7.6. Myelogram: Hodgkin's disease with paraplegia.

Brain scanning with ^{99}Tc is relatively easy to perform, and is without side-effects. It may well give unequivocal evidence of intracerebral involvement (Currie and Jardine, 1969).

The most pleasant test of all is always worth considering and is based on the fact that injection of alcohol may produce a very painful response in an involved bone long before there is any radiological evidence of disease.

Laparotomy and Splenectomy

In the presence of active disease, and since all the previous investigations may prove negative, it has been suggested that every patient with Hodgkin's disease should have a laparotomy (Glastein *et al.*, 1969). The same suggestion has been made for the other lymphomata.

Goffinet *et al.* (1973) described 67 cases where splenectomy was positive in 27 (the spleen being impalpable in 26 and the lymphangiogram negative in 16). Jelliffe *et al.* (1970) describe 21 patients with Hodgkin's disease, in whom splenectomy was performed; in 12 this helped to evaluate the extent of the disease. Liver involvement may be diagnosed at laparotomy by inspection, deep-needle biopsy, or by wedge excision. It should be remembered that serial section of every suspected organ – liver, spleen and lymph node – is the only way of being certain that no focus of disease is present; but this is not a practical proposition. Fortunately it would appear that liver involvement is uncommon unless the spleen is affected.

Splenectomy is not without danger (Host *et al.*, 1973). An anaesthetic is required, which in itself has its own morbidity and mortality rate. Pulmonary emboli occur, and it would seem that further thromboembolic episodes are more likely in splenectomised patients, due possibly to the subsequent thrombocythemia. Because of this latter complication, this operation should not be undertaken in patients taking an oestrogen contraceptive drug. Sub-diaphragmatic abscesses and atelectasis of the left lung have also been described. Thus, if splenectomy is to be carried out routinely the greatest care must be taken, as the procedure is being used for diagnostic and not therapeutic purpose.

The present author is not impressed by the arguments advanced in favour of this form of surgery. A very small percentage of unsuspected cases will certainly be found to have more advanced disease, but if these cases were observed both clinically and by the more simple investigations it is quite possible that further spread of the disease would manifest itself fairly rapidly. Furthermore, there is as yet no definite evidence that early aggressive treatment of every possibly involved site will produce better long-term results than a careful watching policy, followed by treatment when further active disease occurs. Only a randomly selected prospective trial to compare the two methods could solve this problem, and this should be undertaken before such radical investigation procedures are carried out as a routine.

Treatment

In the textbooks of medicine as late as the mid-1960s, the reticuloses were considered to be incurable, treatment by irradiation being purely palliative (Davidson, 1966). Today it is accepted that the situation is different, and one can now offer the prospect of 'cure' if the disease is treated in its early stages by irradiation alone (Easson and Russell, 1963). Combination with surgery does not offer any better results, the latter being confined to that of diagnosis, and occasionally the relief of obstructive conditions arising in the gastrointestinal tract or, more rarely, in the vertebral canal. Chemotherapy should be reserved for the more advanced conditions – namely Stages IVA and B, IIIB, and possibly IIIA. Irradiation and chemotherapy have been advocated in the last group.

Immunotherapy is very much in its infancy, and has no definite role to play in the management of the early case. It may well be that after eradication of the primary disease by radiotherapy it will be of value in controlling any residual malignant cells that may be left behind (Halnan, 1973).

Radiotherapy can be used radically to cure the disease, or palliatively to relieve symptoms and prolong survival. Since the reticuloses are radiosensitive tumours, the very high doses used to cure squamous carcinomas, for example, are not required, and thus side-effects are reduced, allowing the treatment of relatively large volumes of tissue at any one time.

Curative radiotherapy is aimed at eradicating all known tumour without permanently damaging the normal surrounding tissue. This method of treating Hodgkin's disease was first tried successfully by René Gilbert in the years 1920–39 (Gilbert, 1939); treatment was with conventional deep X-rays (180–240 kV). Even in the late 1940s and early 1950s similar apparatus with a maximum of 300 kV was used with remarkably good results (Boden, 1951). The disadvantage of such apparatus was the long time taken to treat each patient, owing to the low output of these machines, and also the skin reaction produced by kilovoltage therapy. Differential bone absorption led to high and low doses, which caused either bone necrosis or shielding of the tumour itself. Megavoltage therapy has reduced these problems, and although it may well not increase the chances of cure it will certainly reduce the discomfort to the patient and increase the ease of treatment (Jelliffe *et al.*, 1970). Such apparatus in the 2–10 MV range, using either ^{60}Co teletherapy units or linear accelerators, is now readily available in most radiotherapy centres throughout the world. In the majority of cases an ambulant and relatively fit subject can be treated as an outpatient.

Technique

Stage I

An adequate dose of irradiation should be given to the known lymph nodes or organs involved. A wider margin than the conventional 1 cm used in the treatment of squamous carcinomas of the skin should be used, as it is likely that undetectable microscopic spread of the disease to adjacent lymph nodes has already occurred. It is customary to use at least a 5 cm margin around the known tumour area; in the neck, field-sizes of the order of 15–20 × 12 cm are most commonly used. For a reticulosis limited to a unilateral organ, such as the tonsil, antrum or thyroid, the wedge technique first described at the London Hospital by Ellis and Miller (1944), using 220 kV, and subsequently modified for megavoltage therapy at the same hospital by Cohen *et al.* (1960), can be used. The advantage of this latter method is that it can produce a very homogeneous dose of irradiation to a relatively small area, and spare the rest of the region from unnecessary irradiation. This is particularly useful in the head and neck region, where vital structures such as the spinal cord and salivary glands can be avoided.

Stage II

Here large volumes of tissue need to be irradiated, and a pair of parallel and opposed fields will be required. If it is necessary to treat the neck, mediastinal and axillary nodes, this can easily be achieved, but lung shielding is required. At the London Hospital since 1948 The 'Gothic cut-out' technique has been used with great success (Fig. 7.7). This is similar to the more recently described 'mantle' technique (Peters, 1968). Lead blocks mounted on a suitable tray, or attached to the therapy machine itself, can delineate the fields. Further shielding can be introduced if it is intended to treat only one side of the neck and mediastinum concurrently.

In the abdomen, similar techniques can be used in treating the pelvic and para-aortic lymph nodes. Here the vital structures requiring protection are the kidneys; an IVP marker-film technique can be used (Fig. 7.8).

Stage IIIA

If irradiation is to be used, all the known lymph node areas will need to be irradiated. In order to minimise marrow depression and irradiation sickness, the groups of nodes above and below the diaphragm are treated separately. It is customary to treat first that group of nodes which is producing the most symptoms; a month's gap is given before treating the next area, in order to allow the marrow to recover and to give the patient a rest from treatment.

Post-operative Irradiation

This is almost entirely confined to irradiation of the abdominal lymphatic drainage areas after surgical resection of involved gut. This is most commonly seen in lymphosarcoma of the small bowel or stomach.

Prophylactic Irradiation

In very early Hodgkin's disease, Peters and Middlemiss (1958) suggested that, since the tumour spreads from one lymph node to an adjacent one, it would be wise to irradiate not only the known lymphatic involvement but all the adjoining groups of lymph nodes as well.

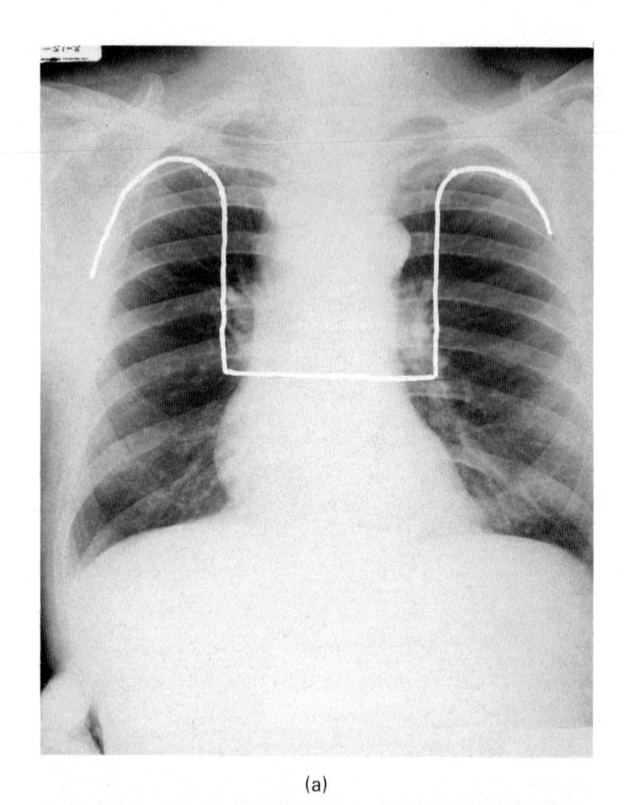

(a)

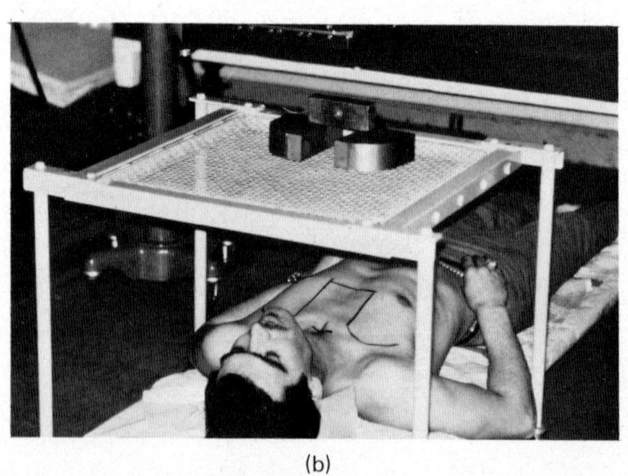

(b)

Fig. 7.7. a Gothic cut-out: Hodgkin's disease.
b Set-up for Gothic cut-out.

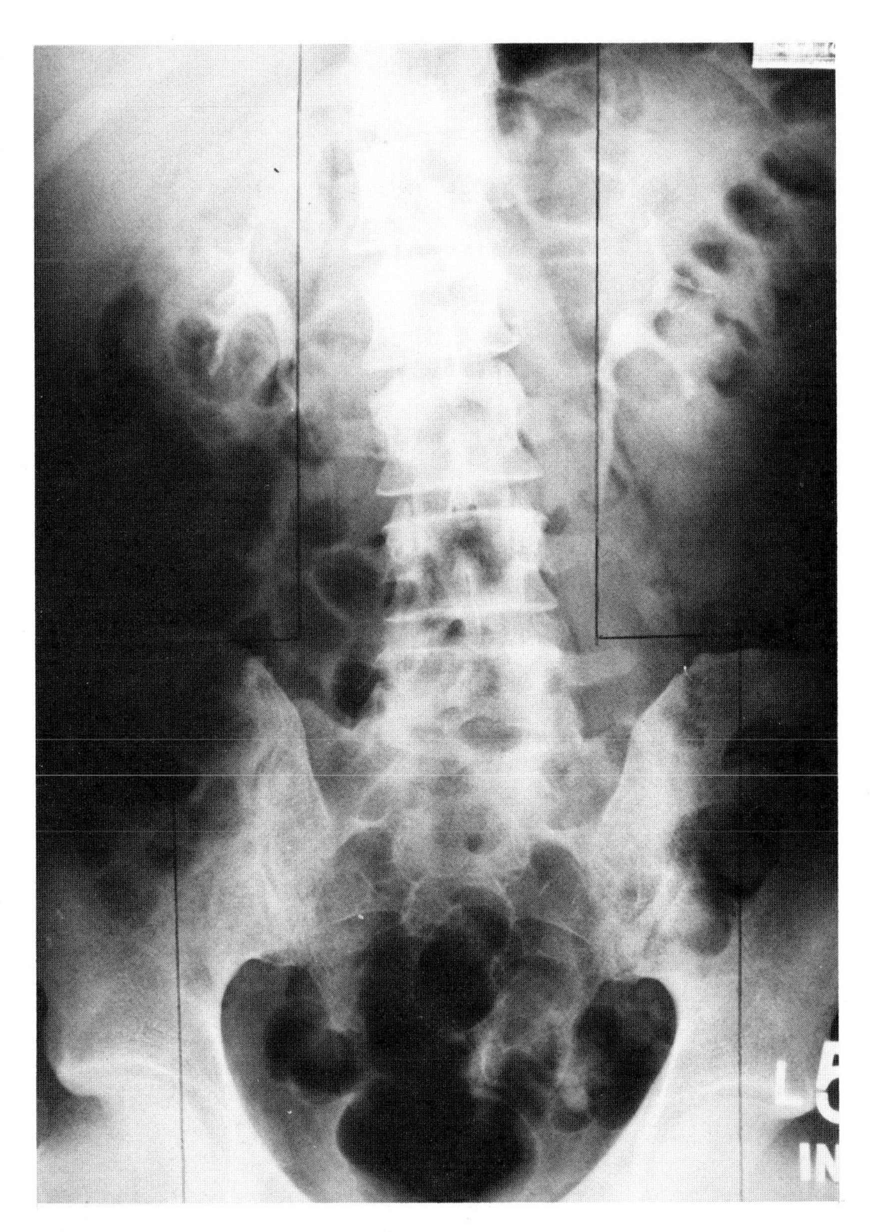

Fig. 7.8. IVP marker film.

If nodes on one side of the neck are involved, then the nodes on the opposite side, both axillae, and the mediastinum should all be treated. Similarly, in the abdomen, even if only one side of the pelvis is involved, all the other lymphatic tissue below the diaphragm should be treated. Relatively low doses (1500–2000 R) were used for the prophylactic sites, and normal doses for the involved nodes (3000–4000 R). Kaplan (1962) advocated an even more aggressive approach – he suggested that much higher doses of irradiation (4000–4500 R) should be given to all the prophylactic areas; subsequently he advocated irradiation of every lymph node area in the body, even in Stages I and II.

The present author strongly disagrees with the idea of prophylactic irradiation, on the grounds that, in 1969 at least, there was no concrete evidence that such treatment had improved the results, although the complication rate from such wide-field irradiation must inevitably be higher. The published five- and ten-year survival figures were no better for those treated with localised irradiation than those treated prophylactically (Hope-Stone, 1969). He therefore concluded that 'the only way to establish the truth would be to carry out a random selective prospective survey'. Such a trial is now in progress (Co-operative Clinical Cancertherapy Group: Jeliffe, 1973).

In the other reticuloses some attempt has been made to establish the value of prophylactic treatment; thus Jones *et al.* (1973), reporting on a large series of non-Hodgkin's lymphoma, have not been able to show any advantages in the diffuse histiocytic lymphosarcoma group, and probably no advantages in the other groups either.

Irradiation Dosage and Fractionation

Patients treated radically require a fractionated tumour-dose to be given, either daily or three times weekly, from Monday to Friday, over a period of three to five weeks.

Total dosage has ranged from 2400 R (orthovoltage, 240 kV (Hilton and Sutton, 1962)) to 4400 rad (megavoltage (Kaplan, 1972)). In Hodgkin's disease, a tumour-dose of 2850 rad produces as good results in terms of survival rate, resolution of the primary neoplasm and local recurrence rate as any other dose-level (Hope-Stone, 1969).

This dose can be given over a period of two weeks for small volumes and 3–4 weeks for large volumes. The advantages of giving the smallest dose compatible with the best survival is that the side-effects and late complications will be reduced. Kaplan (1972) claims that his overall better results are due to the higher doses used, although Jelliffe and Thompson (1955), using very nearly the radiobiologically equivalent dose (3500 R: 4250 rad) could not obtain such a good survival rate. In lymphosarcoma and lymphoid follicular reticulosis, which are more radiosensitive, a lower dose of 2500 rad is compatible with an excellent survival rate. By contrast, reticulum cell sarcoma appears to be more radioresistant, and a minimum of 3500 rad has been suggested (Hope-Stone, 1969).

Side-effects

Side-effects occur most often when the total dose is very high, and when large volumes of tissue are irradiated. They can be kept to a minimum by careful attention to treatment planning. The general effects of tiredness and depression are inevitable when large volumes of tissue need to be irradiated, but keeping up a good haemoglobin level will reduce the former, and a helpful attitude to the patient's morale will aid the latter.

Radiation sickness should not be a problem unless large volumes are treated, and this usually applies only to abdominal irradiation. Thus, if the neck alone is being treated, nausea should not occur, and indeed if it does it is probably psychological and can often be relieved by a placebo. If the nausea occurs with a large field treatment, anti-emetics may be helpful – e.g. Pyridoxine 50 mg q.d.s., Torecan 10 mg t.d.s., Maxalon 10 mg t.d.s., and Ancoloxin 2 tabs t.d.s. Pyridoxine produces no side-effects; the others can cause tiredness and lightheadedness. If severe vomiting occurs and continues, other causes should be ruled out before assuming that the irradiation is at fault. Serious conditions such as intestinal obstruction have been missed by not following this rule.

Radiotherapy or chemotherapy may cause the production of large quantities of uric acid by the destruction of masses of lymphomatous tissue; excretion of this uric acid through the kidneys gives rise to crystaluria. Vomiting may be associated with renal colic due to this uric acid crystaluria, and can be fatal (Greenbaum and Hope-Stone, 1959). This complication can be avoided by estimation of the serum uric acid before starting treatment, and at weekly intervals throughout the course of treatment. If the uric acid level is elevated, Allopurinol should be given in a dosage of 100 mg t.d.s.; if crystaluria occurs the danger can be reduced by alkalinisation of the urine, combined with a high fluid diet and Allopurinol.

Intestinal upsets occur mainly in the form of diarrhoea, and can usually be controlled with Kaolin et Morphine or Lomotil 2 tabs t.d.s. It rarely occurs before a dose of 2000 rad is given to the abdomen or pelvis. However, in a patient with pre-existing bowel disease, such as diverticulitis, diarrhoea may occur at a lower dose-level, and is potentially dangerous; it may be necessary to stop treatment until the symptoms subside. The oesophagus can tolerate doses up to 3000–3500 rad without effect; above this level, oesophagitis may occur, but will usually respond to aspirin or Mucaine emulsions.

Skin reactions are minimal, unless orthovoltage is used, but some erythema and dry desquamation may occur, particularly at the sites of friction and in naturally moist areas, such as the groins, axillae and vulva. The latter site can often be protected by lead shielding. Water on the skin will make the reaction worse, so washing is discouraged (this, incidentally, also prevents the skin-marks, used to outline the treatment field, from being washed off inadvertently).

When the head and neck region is treated, the biggest upset is caused by drying up of the salivary secretions, so that the patient complains of a dry mouth, loss of taste, or a salty taste. The last two symptoms will clear up within a month of finishing treatment, but the former may take up to six months before returning to normal. Epilation will occur when the base line of the skull is included in the treatment fields, but with megavoltage therapy the hair will regrow normally in 6–9 months.

Lung complications should not occur with good shielding, but some patients are unusually sensitive, and if the mediastinal fields are very wide some lung tissue may have to be irradiated. Pneumonitis is the first sequela, presenting with a dry hacking cough, chest pain and dyspnoea, but no fever. Radiologically there is a typical hilar flare with a ground-glass appearance; fibrosis may follow. Antibiotics and steroids have been recommended as treatment, although whether they actually improve the outcome is not certain (Hope-Stone, 1967). Good resolution can occur within a few months. The incidence of these complications is related to dosage, so it is not surprising that Kaplan (1972) quotes an incidence of 6·4 per cent.

The gonads are, of course, susceptible to irradiation. The testes can be shielded, but indirect irradiation will cause some dosage to be received. Gonadal dose measurements in patients receiving pelvic irradiation give a figure of 50–150 rad; this will certainly not produce sterility, but may cause temporary infertility and genetic damage (Blandy *et al.*, 1970).

The ovaries present a more difficult problem for, unless they are surgically removed out of the irradiation field, permanent sterility will ensue. Oophoropexy has been tried, moving the ovaries to the midline anteriorly, just above the pubic symphysis; this would allow appropriate lead protection to be used without shielding the involved lymph nodes.

Late Complications

If a long section of the spinal cord receives a dose of about 3500 R in 17 days, radiation myelitis may occur, and can be fatal (Boden, 1950). Fortunately, such a high dose-level, equivalent to 4500 rad in 28 days (megavoltage) is not required in the treatment of the reticuloses. Transient radiation myelopathy can be seen at lower doses, and presents with paraesthesia in the limbs, exacerbated by neck flexion (Jones, 1964). These neurological complications commonly occur within one to eighteen months after treatment. The kidneys are much more susceptible; if the whole of one kidney receives a dose of more than 2500 rad, radiation nephritis may follow within nine to eighteen months, and may be fatal (Luxton, 1953).

The teeth may be affected if at the time of treatment dental caries is present. Prophylactic removal of severely carious teeth is to be recommended, in order to reduce the risk of bone necrosis. If teeth have to be extracted at a later date, this is much less likely to occur following megavoltage therapy than when orthovoltage has been used.

The lens is very radiosensitive, and a cataract may result from a dose in excess of 1200 rad. Lead shielding will prevent this complication, but such shielding should not be used if it would mean that the tumour itself were not to receive the full dose. Thus, if an antral tumour invades the orbit, the risk must be accepted, as a mature cataract can be removed at a later date (Fig. 7.9). Glaucoma and sympathetic ophthalmia are rarely seen, even if the whole eye is irradiated.

In children, both the thyroid and bone are susceptible. In the former, thyroid carcinoma can follow many years later. In growing bone, epiphyseal damage can occur with doses as low as 400 rad; unequal bone-growth may lead to stunting or kyphoscoliosis.

Cardiovascular damage is rare at moderate dose-levels, but at 4400 rad to the whole mediastinum Stewart *et al.* (1967) reported an incidence of 54 per cent of ECG changes, although only 9 out of 25 cases had symptoms, and complete recovery occurred in the whole group.

Leukaemia may be induced by irradiation; it would be difficult to attribute this to treatment alone, as all the reticuloses can develop leukaemia as part of the natural history of the diseases.

Palliative Irradiation

In the more advanced cases (Stages IIIB and IV), chemotherapy will be used first; local control of the tumour masses will not always be achieved, however, and their presence will be upsetting to the patient. Moderate doses of irradiation can easily produce a regression, and will certainly prevent fungation.

Bone involvement can be very painful, and potentially dangerous if the lesions are osteolytic rather than sclerotic. Local irradiation is almost always effective in relieving symptoms and preventing fracture.

Oesophageal and mediastinal obstruction are unusual; if they do occur, more rapid relief of symptoms can be produced by irradiation than by chemotherapy.

Spinal cord compression by direct infiltration or vertebral collapse may be prevented by palliative irradiation. Paraplegia can be treated in this way, although laminectomy with post-operative radiotherapy is to be preferred, since the compression is relieved more rapidly. The danger of producing oedema by irradiating the spinal cord is probably

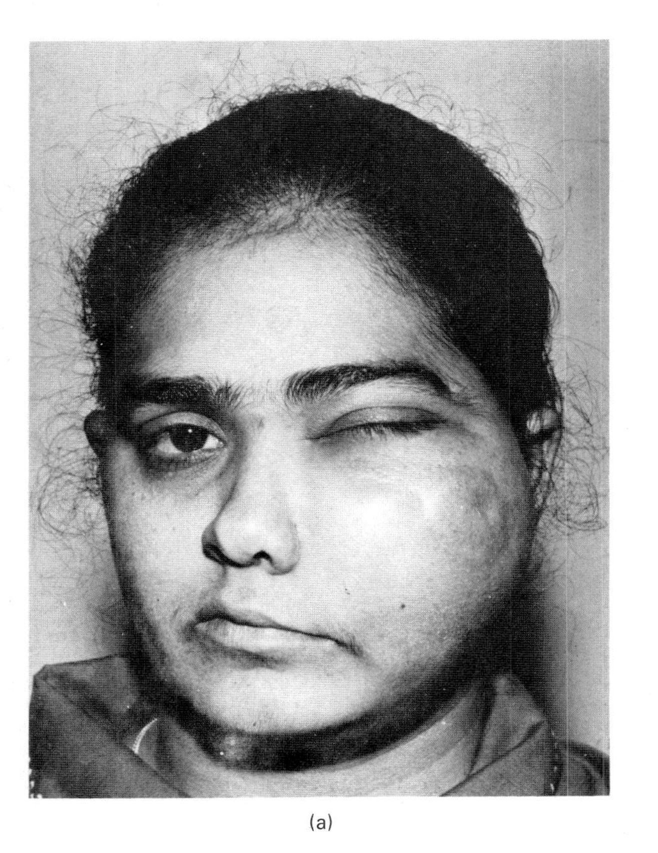

(a)

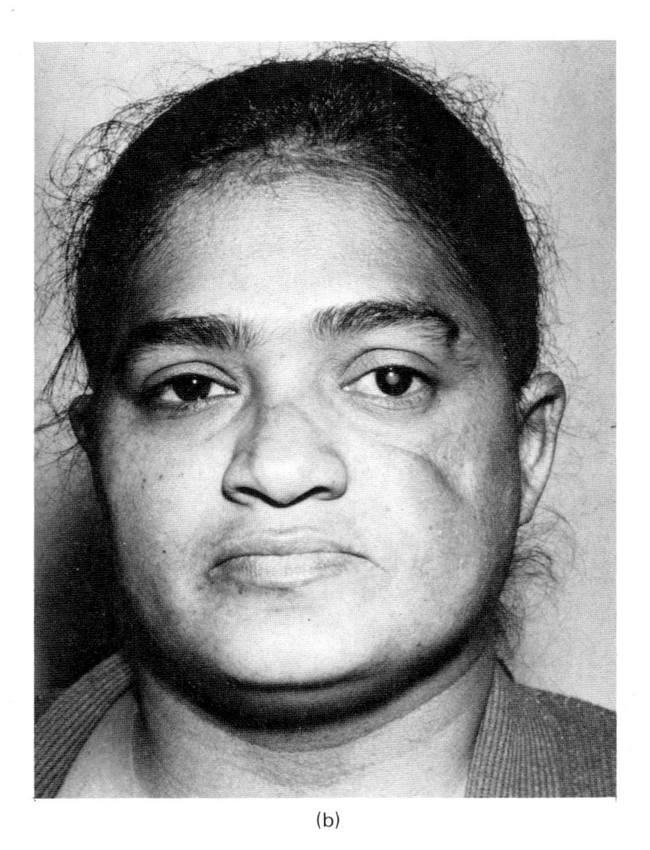

(b)

Fig. 7.9. a Reticulum cell sarcoma of antrum, before radiotherapy. b Seven years later, with cataract left eye.

over-exaggerated, but steroid therapy using dexamethasone, 4 mg t.d.s., will help prevent this complication.

Irradiation of Allied Diseases

Burkitt's Lymphoma

Although all the original cases were treated with chemotherapy, with some degree of success, one would expect irradiation to be very effective in managing the local manifestation of the disease. To overcome the rapid proliferation of cells, superfractionation is used; this has now been tried in Kenya, using three fractions daily, giving a tumour dose of 3000 rad in ten treatments, and this may be combined with chemotherapy (Zeigler, 1974).

Mycosis Fungoides

Since this is a very slow-growing lesion, yet extremely depressing to the patient by its disfigurement of the skin, some form of therapy to control the local lesion is desirable. Chemotherapy and radioactive phosphorus have been tried, but usually fail to control the lesions. Treatment with superficial X-rays (100–140 kV) can eradicate the local lesion, but since the area covered by one applicator is never greater than 15–25 cm, numerous areas have to be treated, which is both time-consuming and tedious for the patient. As there is a danger of overlapping the fields, lead shielding is required, and this in turn may lead to failure to control the lesion at the junctional points. Deep X-rays (240 kV) can cover a much wider area of the body, but bone marrow depression will certainly follow such deeply-penetrating X-rays.

Electrons penetrate the skin only to a limited depth, and will destroy the lesion without affecting the marrow. Electron beam therapy, using a linear accelerator, would seem ideal for this purpose (Szur *et al.*, 1962), but it is very time-consuming. ^{90}Sr, a pure beta emitter, is an excellent source of electrons, and if a large source of this isotope is incorporated in a moving head the whole body surface can be quickly and easily treated. A very elegant technique has been described by Bratherton (1972), who suggests using a skin-dose of 2000 rad, giving ten fractions daily in two weeks.

Chronic Myeloid Leukaemia

Myeleran would appear to have superseded irradiation of the spleen in this condition (MRC Working Party, 1968). However, some cases are resistant to drug therapy, and local irradiation to the spleen is well worth trying. Doses of the order of 20–50 rad can be given daily, until the white cell count drops to about 5000 per mm^3 or the haemoglobin rises to a reasonable level.

Myelosclerosis

Cytotoxic drug treatment may be hazardous, and splenectomy is an irreversible procedure. Splenic pain is often the only symptom and this, together with severe thrombocytopenia, can often be controlled by very careful irradiation to the spleen. Ten to 20 rad daily can be given; if thrombocytopenia is present, prednisone, 5 mg q.d.s., may be given concurrently. Treatment is continued until the spleen becomes much reduced in size, or until the platelet count returns to normal. Undue depressions of the white cell count should not be allowed to occur.

Chronic Lymphatic Leukaemia

While chemotherapy may be preferred for the generalised disease, local lymph node masses and infiltration of organs such as the orbit, eye, bone and testis are better treated by local irradiation, which has the advantage of producing a more rapid response without producing bone marrow depression.

Acute Lymphoblastic Leukaemia

Irradiation was used many years ago in the initial treatment of this disease, but it appeared to do more harm than good. Chemotherapy has been used with increasing success over the past few years.

It is now being realised that undetectable disease may remain in the central nervous system when the rest of the leukaemia cells appear to have been eradicated. These residual cells can repopulate the marrow and cause relapse of the whole disease. Presumably the blood–brain barrier does not allow the passage of the cytotoxic drugs into the CSF. Such drugs can, of course, be given intrathecally, but may not reach the brain either. Leukaemic cells are very radiosensitive, and Pinkel (1972) advocated that the whole of the brain and spinal cord should receive prophylactic irradiation, when the rest of the disease was in remission. A tumour-dose of 2400 rad can safely be given in ten daily treatments over two weeks. Alternatively, only the brain need be irradiated, and intrathecal methotrexate used to deal with the potential spinal cord involvement. Either method seems to be effective both in preventing CNS relapse and prolonging survival (MRC Working Party, 1973).

The technique of irradiation may be achieved simply with a series of direct or matching fields, or more homogeneously and scientifically with the somewhat more difficult technique used successfully in the treatment of medulloblastoma (Hope-Stone, 1970). The chief side-effect is epilation, but the hair will regrow within 6–9 months. One should not expect to see any more long-term complications than we are already prepared to accept with the cured medulloblastoma patients (Hope-Stone, 1970) – i.e. the possibility of a slight chance of growth stunting and the occasional case of thyroid carcinoma 20 years later.

Chemotherapy

Since this book is concerned with irradiation methods, a detailed description of drug therapy would be out of place. Suffice to say that in Hodgkin's disease (Stages IIIB and IV) chemotherapy would appear to be the treatment of choice. In Stage IIIA the choice lies between total nodal irradiation, as so persistently and ably advocated by Kaplan (1972), and quadruple chemotherapy. The latter was shown to be successful in producing a high remission rate by Nicholson *et al.* (1970).

The régime consists of four main drugs – vincristine or vinblastine, mustine, procarbazine, and prednisone (MOPP). These are given in two-weekly courses for a total of six cycles, with a gap of 3–6 weeks between each course. Since we do not know whether irradiation or chemotherapy is more likely to produce cure as opposed to good palliation, a random controlled trial would be the best method of finding the answer. Such a trial, in Stage IIIA Hodgkin's disease, is in progress now (Co-operative Clinical Cancertherapy Group: see page 211).

For the other advanced reticuloses, different forms of quadruple therapy are advocated. Again, we do not yet know whether this is better than total nodal irradiation, and a trial would be needed to give the answer. Such a trial is now being organised by the above-named Co-operative Group.

Results: The Cure of the Reticuloses

Untreated Hodgkin's disease has an overall five-year survival figure of about 2 per cent (Croft, 1940). Using kilovoltage irradiation only, by 1955 Jelliffe and Thompson reported a 29 per cent overall five-year survival rate. In 1972 Kaplan reported a 58 per cent five-year figure.

However, five-year survivors are not necessarily cured. Easson and

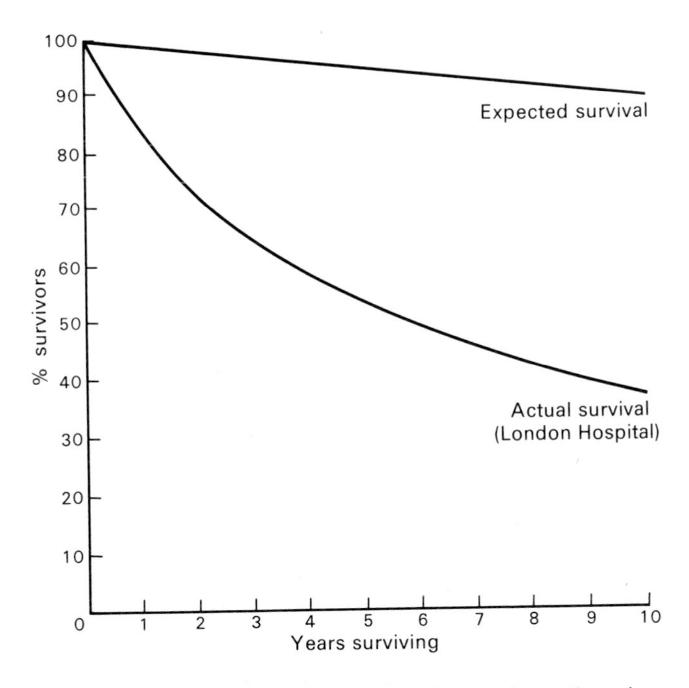

Fig. 7.10. Hodgkin's disease: localised cases. Comparison of crude survival rate with the expected survival rate in the normal population (courtesy the Editors, *British Journal of Radiology*).

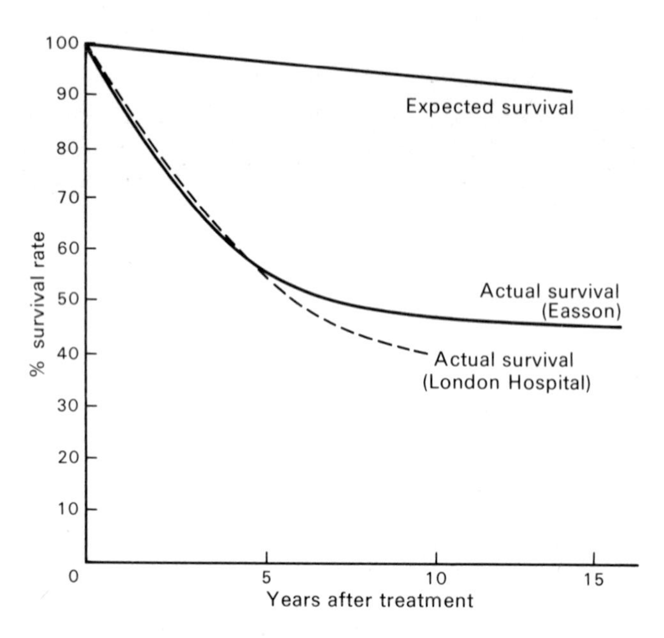

Fig. 7.11. Localised reticuloses. Comparison of crude survival rate with the expected survival rate in the normal population (courtesy the Editors, *British Journal of Radiology*).

Russell (1963) were the first to define cure in a rational way, and stated that 'if a group of patients was followed over a period of 10–15 years and the survival curves were compared with those of a control group matched for age and sex, then cure could be said to have occurred when the two curves ran parallel to each other'.

In the author's series (Hope-Stone, 1969), these curves are shown for both early Hodgkin's disease (Fig. 7.10) and all the other reticuloses (Fig. 7.11). Easson and Russell's ten-year survival figure for early Hodgkin's disease was 42 per cent, and Hope-Stone's 44·5 per cent. These figures are nowhere near as good as those claimed by Kaplan. However, it should be remembered that staging of these cases was by very simple investigations, usually limited to chest X-rays, haematological and clinical examinations; tomography of the mediastinum, lymphangiography and liver and spleen scanning, exploratory laparotomy and splenectomy were not used to stage these cases. Thus it is very probable that a proportion of the so-called Stage I and II cases were in fact Stage III or even IV. Constitutional symptoms were not used in the staging, so some of the early cases were probably in the B group and would be expected to do worse.

One would therefore expect better survival rates in 1972 without suggesting that these were entirely due to the use of megavoltage irradiation. Nevertheless, more thorough investigation may lead to a higher cure-rate, as all known areas of involvement would be treated to a radical dose. Thus Peters's five-year results in 1968 were 60–90 per cent in Stage I and II Hodgkin's disease. Kaplan (1972), in 121 cases, has an overall actuarial five-year survival rate of 78·6 per cent, rising to 86·8 per cent in Stage IA, and only falling to 43 per cent in IIIB. Although the numbers are relatively small, they do seem to show the advantages of the more radical techniques of irradiation which he so strongly advocates.

These last two series appear to show the extra value of prophylactic irradiation. In the Co-operative Clinical Cancertherapy Group, a random trial to assess the value of prophylactic versus local irradiation in Hodgkin's disease Stages I and II, above the diaphragm, shows the following results (Jelliffe, 1973):

	Number of cases	Alive and well 6–48/12 (crude survival)
Local radiotherapy	85	60 (71%)
Prophylactic radiotherapy	89	67 (75%)

These results can be compared with those both of Kaplan and Peters, since the dose-levels are nearly as high – i.e. 3500–4000 rad in daily fractions over 3–4 weeks – and these latter authors use an actuarial survival rate which is always higher than the crude rate. It does not appear, however, from these trial figures that Kaplan and Peters's more aggressive approach is really necessary.

The Group's assessment, by the same method, of the value of chemotherapy in Stage IIIA Hodgkin's disease, gives the following:

	Number of cases	Complete remission 6–48/12
Total nodal irradiation	31	26 (83%)
Chemotherapy (MOPP)	32	24 (75%)

It is interesting to see that irradiation may be of the greater value.

Results in Relation to Histology in Hodgkin's Disease

The lymphocyte-predominant and nodular sclerotic groups have the most favourable prognosis. The mixed cellularity group is intermediate, and the lymphocyte-depleted the worst. This correlation is shown even if the analysis is restricted to Stages I and II (Keller *et al.*, 1968).

Children

Hodgkin's disease is always thought to run a more rapid and fatal course in children. However, Jenkins *et al.* (1967), in a series of 75 children, reported a 33 per cent overall five-year survival rate, with 62 per cent in Stages I and II. More recently, Fuller (1973) showed an 80 per cent five-year survival rate in 47 children in Stages I and II. Thus the prognosis in children is improving in a similar measure to that in adults.

Results in the Other Reticuloses

Lymphosarcoma

In the author's series (Hope-Stone, 1969) a five-year survival figure of 61 per cent was shown in the localised cases. Cure, as previously defined, was obtained in 40 per cent (Fig. 7.12). The overall five-year survival rate was 36 per cent. Histological grading is certainly helpful with regard to prognosis. Millet *et al.* (1969) reported for localised cases a 51–68 per cent five-year survival rate in the nodular sclerotic, follicular lymphoma and diffuse lymphosarcoma group, but only 37 per cent in the lymphoblastic lymphosarcoma.

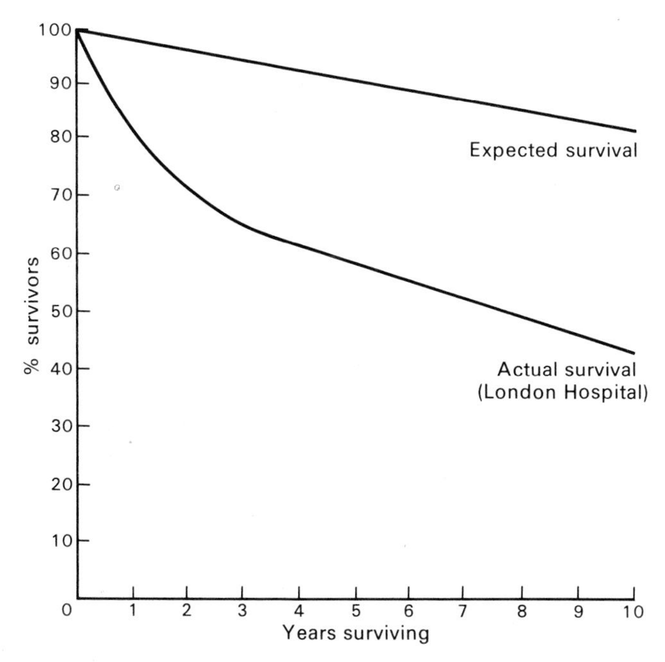

Fig. 7.12. Lymphosarcoma: localised cases. Comparison of crude survival rate with the expected survival rate in the normal population (courtesy the Editors, *British Journal of Radiology*).

Follicular Lymphoma

This was included in Millet's series of lymphosarcoma, with a 70 per cent five-year survival in 16 cases that were localised, and 30 per cent in 27 generalised cases – i.e. an overall 40 per cent five-year survival rate.

Reticulum Cell Sarcoma

Cure can be obtained in localised disease in some 40 per cent of cases (Fig. 7.13). Staging of this disease certainly is useful from a prognostic point of view. Some 66 per cent of Stage I cases survive five years, compared with 27·5 per cent in Stage II and 2·2 per cent in Stage III (Hope-Stone, 1969).

In these last three groups more careful investigation and more radical treatment might further improve the results.

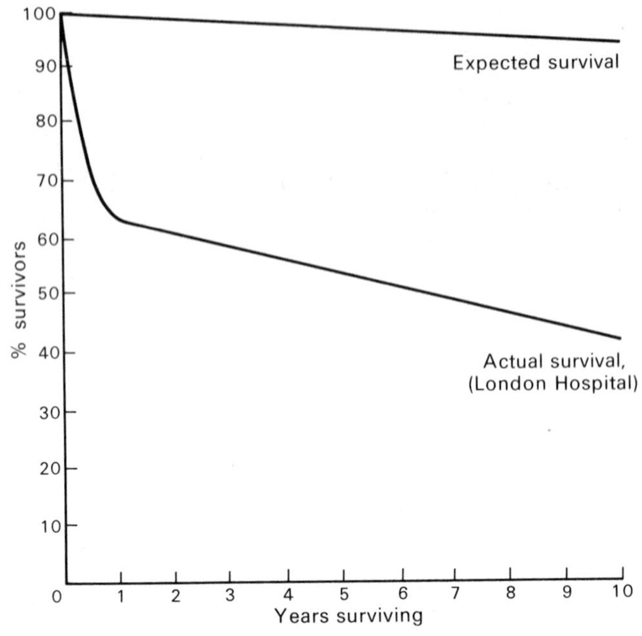

Fig. 7.13. Reticulum cell sarcoma: localised cases. Comparison of crude survival rate with the expected survival rate in the normal population (courtesy the Editors, *British Journal of Radiology*).

Future Methods of Treating Advanced Cases

Combination of chemotherapy and irradiation in the management of advanced Hodgkin's disease has been advocated by Bull *et al.* (1970). They used total nodal irradiation to a dose of 4400 rad; this was followed by six courses of MOPP after a 6–8 week rest. Surprisingly, the marrow tolerated this dosage, and the results are so far encouraging.

For the very aggressive generalised lymphosarcoma, another method that is now being tried is to use whole body irradiation, giving doses to the order of 150 rad in 3–4 weeks; early results are promising.

Future Developments in the Management of the Reticuloses

Irradiation techniques, histological grading and clinical staging have probably reached their zenith, and it is unlikely that further improvement will be obtained in this way. Chemotherapy will certainly play an important role in the more advanced cases.

The only possibility that has not been fully explored is the role of immunotherapy in the management of the early cases, and the possibility of enhancing the natural immune response of the host needs to be considered. If after apparent eradication of the tumour from the lymph nodes immunotherapy were to be given, then unsuspected minute foci of disease, either outside the treated zone or those not dealt with in the treated area, might well be subsequently destroyed. The present crude methods of BCG vaccination or re-injection of irradiated tumour cells would need to be replaced by more sophisticated techniques.

Conclusion

Over the past twenty years there has been a marked change in the approach to treatment of the reticuloses. Physicians and surgeons alike have come to realise that these are not all incurable conditions, with the occasional unexpected lucky response after irradiation; radiologists have improved our investigating ability; and pathologists, too, have done their part in reclassification of the diseases so that we can pick out the more favourable prognostic groups.

Radiotherapists will now have a chance to see and treat all the early cases, and then the chances of curing the disease become very much higher. Even in the more advanced cases, enthusiastic co-operation between clinician, radiotherapist and haematologist can decide which is the best form of treatment – radiotherapy, chemotherapy, or a combination of both – and apply these modalities in the best interests of their patients.

References

BENNETT, J. M., RUBENBERG, A. M. and NATHANSON, L. (1968) *Archives of International Medicine*, **121**, 338–341.

BLANDY, J. P., HOPE-STONE, H. F. and DAYAN, D. (1970) *Tumours of the Testicle.* Heinemann, London.

BODEN, G. (1950) *Journal of Faculty of Radiologists*, **2**, 79–94.

BODEN, G. (1951) *British Journal of Radiology*, **24**, 285, 494–498.

BRATHERTON, D. G. (1972) *Modern Trends in Radiotherapy–2*, ed. Deeley, T., Butterworth, London, 176–187.

BULL, J. M., DE KIEWIT, J. W., ROSENBERG, S. A. and KAPLAN, H. S. (1970) *Clinical Research*, **18**, 189.

BURKITT, D. P. (1958) *British Journal of Surgery*, **41**, 218–223.

Cancer Research (1966) **26** Part 1, 1090–1094. Report on Conference of the National Cancer Institute and American Cancer Society, Rye, NY, 1965.

COHEN, M., BURNS, J. E. and SEAR, R. (1960) *Acta radiologica*, **58**, 401–486.

CROFT, C. B. (1940) *Bulletin of Staff Hospital, University of Minnesota*, **11**, 391–409.

CURRIE, S. and JARDINE, G. W. H. (1969) *Journal of Neurology and Neurosurgery and Psychiatry*, **32**, 31–33.

DAVIDSON, S. D. (1966) *Principles and Practice of Medicine.* Livingstone, London.

DAYAN, A. D., MORGAN, H. G., HOPE-STONE, H. F. and BOUCHER, B. J. (1964) *American Journal of Roentgenology*, **xcii**, 1, 116–123.

EASSON, E. C. and RUSSELL, M. H. (1963) *British Medical Journal*, **2**, 1704–1707.

EDWARD, C. H. and HAYES, R. C. (1970) *Journal of American Medical Association*, **212**, 1182.

ELLIS, F. and MILLER, H. (1944) *British Journal of Radiology*, **17**, 904–915.

FARRER-BROWN, G., BENNETT, M. H. and HENRY, K. (1974) *Lancet*, **ii**, 405–406.

FISHER, D., MANTELL, B. S. and URICH, H. (1969) *Journal of Neurology, Neurosurgery and Psychiatry*, **32**, 474–477.

FULLER, L. M., SULLIVAN, M. P. and BUTLER, J. J. (1973) *Cancer*, **32**, 640–645.

GILBERT, R. (1939) *American Journal of Roentgenology*, **41**, 198–241.

GLASTEIN, E., GUERNSEY, J. M., ROSENBERG, S. A. and KAPLAN, H. S. (1969) *Cancer*, **24**, 709–718.

GOFFINET, R. W., CASTELLINO, R. A., KIM, H., DORFMAN, R. F., FUKS, Z., ROSENBERG, S., NELSEN, T. and KAPLAN, H. S. (1973) *Cancer*, **32**, 672–681.

GREENBAUM, D. and HOPE-STONE, H. F. (1959) *Lancet*, **1**, 73–75.

HALNAN, K. E. (1973) *British Journal of Radiology*, **46**, 550.

HARTVIGSEN, F. B. (1955) *Acta radiologica*, **44**, 311–324.

HERBERT, P. A. and MILLER, R. F. (1945) *American Journal of Pathology*, **21**, 233.

HILTON, G. and SUTTON, P. M. (1962) *Lancet*, **1**, 283–287.

HOPE-STONE, H. F. (1967) *British Journal of Diseases of the Chest*, **61**, 57–70.

HOPE-STONE, H. F. (1969) *British Journal of Radiology*, **42**, 770–783.

HOPE-STONE, H. F. (1970) *American Journal of Neurosurgery*, **32**, 1, 83–88.

HOST, H., ABRAHAMSEN, A. F., JORGENSEN, O. G. and NORMAN, T. (1973) *Scandinavian Journal of Haematology*, **10**, 373–378.

JELLIFFE, A. M. (1973) The British National Lymphoma Investigation (Invited discussion). International Symposium on Hodgkin's Disease, Stamford University School of Medicine (March 20–24, 1973). *National Cancer Institute Monograph 36*, 427.

JELLIFFE, A. M., MILLET, Y. C., MASTON, J. A. P., BENNET, M. H., FARRER BROWN, G., KENDAL, B. and KELLING, D. H. (1970) *Clinical Radiology*, **21**, 439–445.

JELLIFFE, A. M. and THOMPSON, R. D. (1955) *British Journal of Cancer*, **9**, 21–36.

JENKINS, R. D. T., PETERS, M. V. and BURTE, J. M. (1967) *American Journal of Roentgenology*, **100**, 222–226.

JENSEN, J. B. E. (1973) *British Journal of Hospital Medicine*, **104**, 402–409.

JONES, A. E. (1964) *British Journal of Radiology*, **37**, 727–744.

JONES, S. E., FUKS, Z., KAPLAN, H. S. and ROSENBERG, S. A. (1973) *Cancer*, **3**, 32, 682–690.

KAPLAN, H. S. (1962) *Radiology*, **78**, 553–561.

KAPLAN, H. S. (1972) *Hodgkin's Disease*. Harvard University Press, Cambridge, Mass.

KAPLAN, H. S. and ROSENBERG, S. (1966) *Cancer Research*, **26**, 1268–1276.

KAY, D. M. and MCCREADY, R. (1972) *British Journal of Radiology*, **45**, 450, 437–443.

KELLER, A. R., KAPLAN, H. S., LUKES, R. J. and RAPPAPORT, H. (1968) *Cancer* (Philadelphia), **22**, 482–499.

Lancet, *The* (1974) **1**, 122. Editorial.

LUKES, R. J. and BUTLER, J. J. (1966) *Cancer Research*, **26**, 1063–1081.

LUXTON, R. (1953) *Quarterly Journal of Medicine*, **27**, 215–247.

MACMAHON, B. (1957) *Cancer*, **10**, 1045–1054.

MCDONALD, J. S. (1969) *Clinical Radiology*, **20**, 447–452.

Medical Research Council Working Party (1968) *British Medical Journal*, **1**, 201–208.

Medical Research Council Working Party (1973) *British Medical Journal*, **2**, 377–384.

MILLET, Y. L., BENET, M. H., JELLIFFE, A. M. and FARRER BROWN, G. (1969) *British Journal of Cancer*, **23**, 683–692.

MOSS, W. T. (1969) *Therapeutic Radiology*, 3rd edn, Mosby, St Louis, Miss.

NICHOLSON, W., BEARD, E., CROWTHER, D., STANSFIELD, A., VORTAN, C., HAMILTON FAIRLEY, G. and BODLEY SCOTT, R. (1970) *British Medical Journal*, **3**, 7–10.

PERRY, S., THOMAS, L. B., JOHNSON, R. E., CARBONNE, P. P. and HAYNES, H. A. (1967) *Annals of Internal Medicine*, **67**, 424–441.

PETERS, V. M. (1968) in *Hodgkin's Disease*, ed. Mollander, S. W. Thomas, Springfield, Ill., 101.

PETERS, V. M. and MIDDLEMISS, K. C. H. (1958) *American Journal of Roentgenology*, **79**, 114–121.

PINKEL, D., SIMON, J., HASTIE, H. O. and AUR, R. J. A. (1972) *Paediatrics*, **50**, 246–351.

RAPPAPORT, H., WINTER, W. J. and HICKS, E. B. (1956) *Cancer*, **9**, 792–821.

SHEER, A. C. (1955) *American Journal of Roentgenology*, **90**, 439–443.

SMITHERS, D. (1973) *British Journal of Radiology*, **46**, 911–916.

STEWART, J. R., COHN, H. F., FUJARLE, F., HANCOCK, E. O. and KAPLAN, H. S. (1967) *Radiology*, **89**, 302–310.

SZUR, L., SYLVESTER, J. A. and BERKLAY, D. K. (1962) *Lancet*, **1**, 1373–1377.

THOMPSON, A. D. (1955) *British Journal of Cancer*, **9**, 37–46.

VIANNA, N. J., GREENWALL, P., POLNAN, A., MAARO, J. and DAVIS, U. (1972) *Annals of Internal Medicine*, **77**, 169–180.

YOFFEY, J. M. (1960) *Quantitative Cellular Haematology*, Thomas, Springfield, Ill., 18.

ZEIGLER, J. C. (1974) in *Malignant Disease in Children*, ed. Deeley, T. J., Butterworth, London, 360–371.

CHAPTER EIGHT

Carcinoma of the Breast

G. W. H. Jardine

As much ink has been spilt discussing, as blood has, treating, carcinoma of the breast, which is the commonest malignant disease of women with an overall high death-rate of about 50 per cent.

The present position regarding treatment is one of great uncertainty, not only with regard to the traditional roles of surgery and radiotherapy, but also in relation to the steadily increasing number of hormone preparations, increasingly effective cytotoxic chemotherapeutic agents or combinations of agents, and the prospect of immunotherapy in the foreseeable future. Even before these latter methods of treatment became available the relative positions of surgery and radiotherapy were hotly disputed in spite of numerous large and small, selected and unselected, controlled and uncontrolled series, which have often produced conflicting results.

This confusion and uncertainty has resulted, or so it seems, in a feeling that, if there is no obvious advantage in treating by any one method, then it does not matter how much care is taken in the application of the chosen method. This can have disastrous results on the wellbeing, even if only temporarily, of the individual patient.

In attempts to clarify this situation, clinical impressions have long been discarded in favour of 'trials' with large numbers of patients which are tabulated and subjected to various methods of statistical analysis. Even here there is much confusion, as exemplified by the overthrow of Bond's (1968) radiotherapeutic nihilism by Haybittle's (1968) re-analysis of the same series of patients. Unfortunately the mathematics of this is complicated and may be as far beyond many clinicians treating carcinoma as it is beyond the present author. This confusion has, in the United Kingdom, been exemplified by the conflicting views of McWhirter (1955) in Edinburgh and Paterson (1959) in Manchester with regard to the use of routine post-mastectomy irradiation. This particular controversy may be resolved by the current Kings College/Addenbrooks trial, at least in so far as it applies to the group of patients considered by that trial, but progress will be painfully slow as the natural history of the disease is such that five- or even ten-year survival figures may not be sufficient to reach a satisfactory conclusion.

It is disappointing that many, if not most, comparative series have relied on clinical and pathological classification, whereas the majority of those engaged in the treatment of breast cancer are well aware that there is a factor or, more likely, factors which are of much greater fundamental importance in determining the outcome of treatment than can be described in these terms. Any comprehensive protocol for the treatment of breast cancer must satisfactorily account and allow for the 'hopeless' case, with a long survival, treated by means which would not normally be expected to produce such a survival, and also the horrifying enhanced local recurrence seen by all radiotherapists (fortunately seldom) in an irradiated area, as described by Cole and Hanlan (1971).

Diagnosis

Before any treatment can be considered it should be a *sine qua non* that all possible clinical and pathological information about the tumour, its extent, and perhaps also about the patient's immune state should be available; yet, although no significant advance has been made for many years in clinical examination, it is amazing how often this is badly or incompletely carried out or recorded. Although the TNM classification of the International Union Against Cancer is now widely used, when notes are studied retrospectively it is often either found impossible to 'stage' the patient or, worse still, the records of different observers result in widely different stagings. It is only by meticulous attention and application that this can be avoided. As long as radiotherapy has been available so have diagnostic X-rays, yet still occasionally a patient is subjected to the mutilation of mastectomy without even a radiograph of the chest, let alone a skeletal survey, which should surely be the 'right' of all such patients.

In addition to clinical and routine radiographic examinations, there are now available mammography, thermography, infra-red photography, ultrasonography and radio-isotopic methods to aid diagnosis of both the presence and the extent of breast disease.

Mammography

This method of examination is now in routine use and of undoubted value as a diagnostic method to determine both the presence and the extent of breast cancer.

The multifocal nature of breast cancer in the same breast is well known, but Leader (1973) quotes different authors' accounts of incidence of bilateral cancers as ranging between one and 21·6 per cent when the whole life of patients is considered, and an even more surprising figure of 1–7 per cent for concurrent bilateral breast cancer. These figures alone would argue a strong case for mammography as a diagnostic and follow-up examination.

Thermography

Although this method of examination is free of any irradiation danger and has been used fairly extensively for mass screening techniques, it too frequently gives false positive or negative results to be used alone (Stark and Way, 1970).

A combination of clinical examination, mammography and thermography has been shown by Furnival *et al.* (1970) to produce a surprisingly high degree of accuracy. In patients presenting with symptoms they obtained the results shown in Table 8.1 by individual methods of examination.

Table 8.1. Diagnostic accuracy of breast investigation by individual methods (after Furnival *et al.* (1970))

	Correct results (%)	
	Malignant	Benign
Clinical examination (Single observer)	81·8	81·4
Thermography (Range of three observers)	41·6–53·2	11·7–38·6
70 mm mammography (Range of three observers)	39·0–61·0	47·6–58·3

When these methods were combined, the accuracy of diagnosis in malignancy rose considerably, as shown in Table 8.2.

Table 8.2. Diagnostic accuracy of breast investigation by multiple techniques (after Furnival *et al.* (1970))

	Correct diagnosis of carcinoma (%)
Clinical examination alone	81·8
Clinical examination + thermography	89·6
Clinical examination + mammography	90·9
Clinical examination + thermography + mammography	94·8

It would seem that, whenever possible, all these methods should be made available and used where breast cancer is to be treated.

Infra-red Photography

Jones and Draper (1970) compared this method of examination with thermography, and their results suggest that with regard to malignant, as opposed to benign, breast disease this method of examination has little to offer.

Ultrasonography

This relatively recent and little-used method of investigation in breast cancer is, according to Evans and Gravelle (1973), of some use in differentiating solid and cystic lesions, but with the apparatus available at present it is of little real value.

Radioisotopic Techniques

The above methods of investigation are related to the breast itself; although local recurrence can present many problems, the major stumbling-block to improving the depressing survival figures in breast cancer is that of distant metastases, and it is in the detection of skeletal metastases that radioisotopic techniques are of value. Galasko (1969) reported that 24 per cent of 'operative' patients had bone metastases. It is perhaps too early to accept this as a typical figure and assume that all abnormalities detected are the result of metastases but, even if the true detection rate should only be a fraction of this, it is a figure which gives much cause for concern. If such patients are excluded from radical treatment, survival will 'improve' in the operated group, although of course the overall survival of patients will be unaffected. What will happen, however, is that many doomed women will be saved a useless and psychologically disturbing mutilation.

The apparatus used consists of either rectilinear scanners or gamma cameras with one of a number of isotopes, and the accuracy of the results would seem to be related to the critical adjustment of isotope and dose, type of collimater and scan speed. In the hands of Merrick (1973), fluorin-18 gave results which led to the conclusion that adding X-ray examination gave a 'negligible' greater pick-up rate, that a rectilinear scan was better than a gamma camera picture, and ^{18}F better than strontium-85. However, Galasko and Doyle (1972), using ^{18}F and a gamma camera, reached the conclusion that radiography was a better detector of metastases in the ischeal and pubic regions only and that, to avoid 'false positives', concurrent radiographic examination was essential. Unfortunately, ^{18}F is, as a result of its 1·84 hour half-life, only available close to the site of production, but this is now of little significance: polyphosphates which form complexes with technetium-99m are now readily available, and this isotope can be used in any department undertaking this type of work. This, with the related technetium diphosphonate, gives results of greater resolution, at least as good as fluorine scanning and better than skeletal radiography (Charkes *et al.*, 1973; Silberstein *et al.*, 1973).

Treatment

Any disease which is progressive to death will invariably be treated; the decision not to treat is not only more difficult to take on the part of the therapist, of whatever sort, but may also be open to legal criticism. Park and Lees (1951) cast doubt on the effect of operative treatment in breast cancer and reached the depressing conclusion that treatment was but an incident in the course of the disease. Such a belief does not preclude slow improvement in survival rates, as programmes of screening and self-examination will result in the appearance of patients earlier in the natural course of the disease. This conclusion of Park and Lees was refuted by McWhirter (1960) who also pointed out that survival is directly related to the size of the primary tumour. He also made a plea for an 'auditing body' to whom all results would be submitted before publication, in an attempt to produce some degree of comparability between different series.

Perhaps if this suggestion had been acted upon there would now be less confusion about treatment, and the 'ping-pong' of published papers would not have persisted. It was McWhirter (1955) who, recognising the poor results, especially the high local recurrence-rate on the chest wall, of the then standard extensive operative procedure of Halsted – a method of treatment then already 60 years old, started the move to less radical treatment which continues today. McWhirter advocated the routine use of post-operative irradiation following simple mastectomy, but it was not long before this was itself challenged by Paterson (1959) and in 1963 by Kaae and Johansen, who, by analysing the results from seven different centres using different 'radical' treatments varying from supra-radical surgery as practised by Dahl-Iversen and Tobiassen (1963) to McWhirter's method, showed that there was no difference in results by using any of these different methods of treatment.

These results were more surprising at the time of publication than they are now in the light of current knowledge. If tumours of the breast are not as individual as the patients who have them, at least few would now accept cancer of the breast as a single entity and, with increasing awareness of the immune state, it is obvious that the hosts can offer different resistances to their tumours. If we allow even only two types of tumour in two different types of patient, we have four different groups which may require entirely different methods of management – what is correct for one perhaps being disastrous for another. If this is accepted, together with the fact that a quarter of patients have distant disease at the time of radical surgery, the conflicting results of treatment by different methods and in different areas are not surprising.

If mastectomy were an effective treatment there would be a strong case, in view of the bilateral incidence of tumours already mentioned, for bilateral mastectomy. Such a suggestion to a patient is greeted with horror, and often with downright refusal, but it is the author's experience that no patient who has subsequently had a second mastectomy has not volunteered, or agreed on direct questioning, that she would have preferred the double operation at the outset. The reason is simple: the patient feels more symmetrical, whether or not she wears a prosthesis.

Dahl-Iversen and Tobiassen (1963) showed that radical surgery was no better than restricted surgery, and Cole (1964) that routine post-operative irradiation (by the Manchester technique) produces no better results than omitting this procedure. In reaching this conclusion, however, she did add the proviso that careful follow-up was essential; this is often forgotten by our surgical colleagues who follow her teachings. The reason for the necessity for early detection of local recurrence is the much better result obtained if irradiation is carried out at this time, rather than when the tumour has locally advanced.

As all treatment for breast cancer produces morbidity, and the more extensive the treatment, whether surgical, radiotherapeutic, hormonal or cytotoxic, the greater is the morbidity, it is reasonable to consider whether mastectomy is in fact necessary. Mustakallio (1972), in a twenty-five-year follow-up of cases where the tumour was removed by wedge or local excision and the remaining breast tissue and related glandular areas were irradiated, gave results that were at the least no worse than those of other conventional methods of treatment; it seems surprising that this method is not more frequently used.

Bond (1972), studying figures from the Mayo Clinic, Edinburgh and Birmingham, showed axillary lymph node involvement to be a major factor in determining five-year survival. Unfortunately this is a difficult means of determining a treatment policy as the nodes have to be removed to determine their state, since 50 per cent of palpable nodes contain no tumour and 25 per cent of impalpable nodes are involved by tumour. Any such method of determining treatment would also have to consider the state of the internal mammary lymph nodes in addition to those in the axilla. Handley (1952) described 10 per cent of internal mammary involvement when axillary nodes were not involved and 48 per cent when they were.

Black and Asire (1969) showed that sinus histiocytosis in lymph nodes is associated with a good prognosis and it may be that irradiation of these reacting nodes is harmful to the patient.

What can be recommended out of all this apparently conflicting and inadequate evidence? Firstly, it would seem only right that every patient who is going to be subjected to radical treatment should have more extensive investigation then has been routine in the past. In addition to the older investigations, bilateral mammography, skeletal radiographic survey and skeletal radioisotope scan (these last two to be evaluated together) should be performed.

Those operable patients without any evidence of metastases should then be considered for treatment by the method of Mustakallio (1972). If the clinician feels he cannot treat by this means, then simple or local mastectomy should be the maximum surgery which is undertaken. The decision to give or to withhold immediate post-operative irradiation depends on the presence or absence of tumour on histological examination of pectoral or other lymph nodes obtained at the time of operation. If no irradiation is given, close follow-up at intervals (initially of not more than one month) is mandatory so that irradiation can be used early for local recurrence or lymph node enlargement.

There would not seem to be sufficient advantage in castrating premenopausal patients as part of their planned initial therapy to justify the extra psychological trauma which such a measure produces.

Palliative Irradiation

Although there is a place for 'toilet' mastectomy in the large fungating tumour in a large breast, most palliation is by means of irradiation. This includes those patients whose only contraindication to operation is a positive radio-isotope bone-scan when, apart from complete local removal of the tumour, or biopsy, to confirm the diagnosis, no surgery is required.

Most metastatic disease responds to irradiation more rapidly than to hormone therapy, especially with regard to painful bone deposits. In pathological fractures, irradiation with or without internal fixation is mandatory (Fig. 8.1). Spinal deposits with evidence of cord compression merit special attention as here, especially when there is any sign of bladder disturbance, there is a considerable degree of urgency: treatment should be instituted within twenty-four hours. Some neurosurgeons view this complication with a degree of despair which is not justified if treatment is started promptly (Hall and Mackay, 1973). Of patients with an incomplete block, shown by myodil examination, 35 per cent achieved satisfactory walking and bladder function. They also noted better and more rapid pain relief by laminectomy than by radiotherapy, even when paraplegia was complete, though a combination of both methods probably gives the best results. Even if the expectation of life is short, to maintain bladder function is of inestimable value to the morale of patients so afflicted, and makes terminal care so much easier that admission to hospital may not be necessary.

Intracranial deposits causing symptoms can be treated by irradiation but, even with the best wig available, epilation is, for a woman, a most distressing complication, and is inevitable with radiotherapy, albeit usually temporary. Such treatment, therefore, should be reserved for those who appear in the opinion of the therapist to have a relatively good prognosis, as usually with this type of metastatic spread expectation

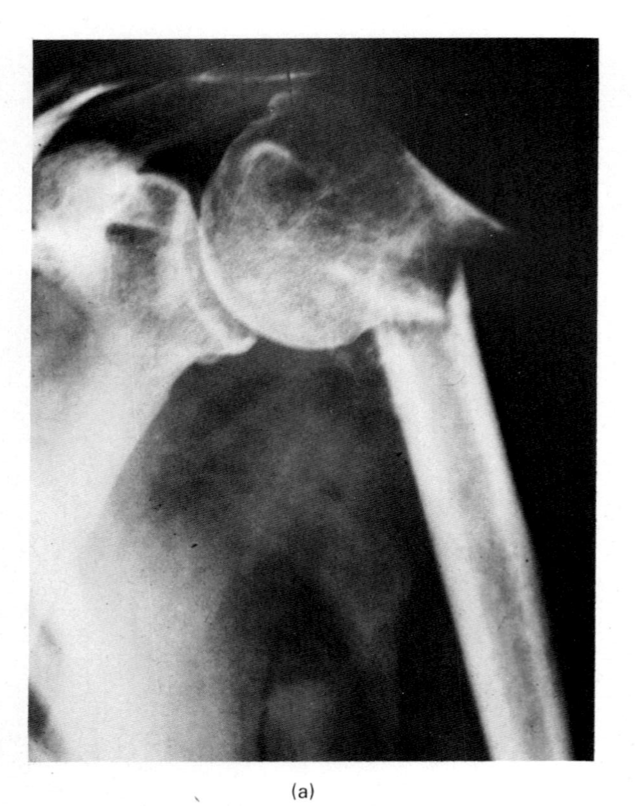

(a)

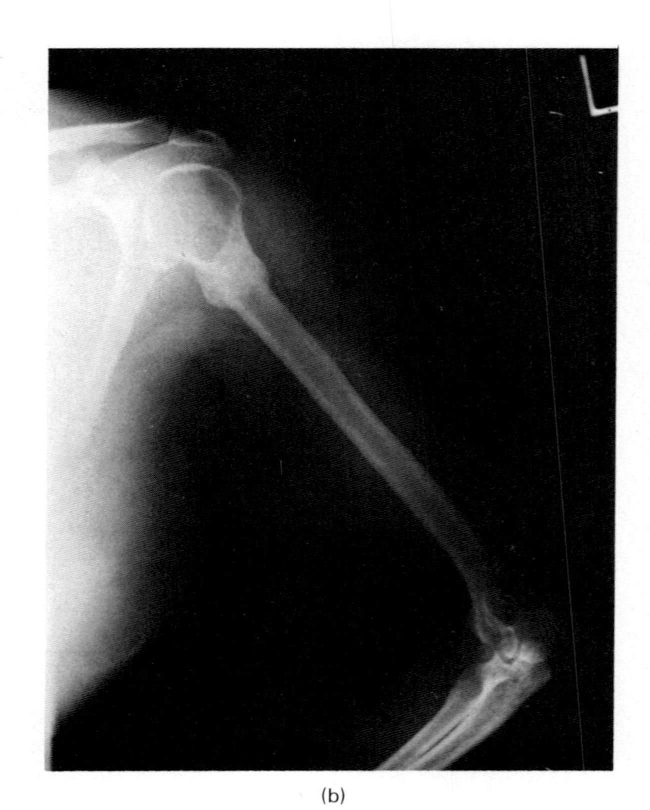

(b)

Fig. 8.1. Pathological fracture of humerus (a) before and (b) one year after palliative irradiation (3000 rad in ten treatments). No internal fixation was used.

of life is short. Retinal deposits causing visual disturbance can, however, be treated effectively by means of megavoltage irradiation with good effect and little upset to the patient. The danger of late cataract development can be ignored.

Locally advanced and ulcerated tumours can usually be healed by local irradiation taken to a moderate dose. Until such time as fungating tumours heal, much can be done to make the patient's lot more tolerable – not by applying layer after layer of ointment, but by frequent mechanical débridement to the point just short of producing bleeding and then applying locally a lotion such as gentian violet; but it must be stressed to those dealing with this, that the cleansing is more important than the application.

Hormone Therapy

There is at present no place for this type of therapy in the apparently curable patient, but even if metastatic disease is treated by irradiation it is usual practice at the same time to start some form of hormone therapy as the second line of treatment. As with primary treatment, there is much variation in the methods recommended by different clinicians, and a swing away from the extensive surgical approach such as adrenalectomy or hypophysectomy. The latter is now only generally used when there has been a relapse after a good, sustained response to more simple hormonal treatment as, although the immediate response is often dramatic, the recurrence of symptoms is frequently as dramatically rapid and disappointing.

In pre-menopausal patients there are few who would adopt any method other than castration as initial therapy and it is of little functional import whether this is surgical or radiotherapeutic, although the latter method avoids the necessity for an operation. In the patient ten or perhaps five years post-menopausal, the most common and probably best method is to use an oestrogen; Stilboestrol has long been the 'standard' drug, but its tendency to cause nausea and vaginal bleeding reduces its usefulness. Ethinyl-oestradiol may be less toxic. Tamoxifen (an anti-oestrogen) may come to replace stilboestrol as initial treatment in this group of patients, in view of its apparent equality of efficacy and lack of major side-effects.

The group of recurrent patients most difficult to treat is those in the immediate post-menopausal age-group, and here the choice is very much a personal one as the results of empirical therapy are little different from those using assessments of hormonal status. Norethisterone (SH420) by mouth, for soft-tissue deposits, and drostanolone propionate (Masteril) by intra-muscular injection, for bone metastases, are probably as good as any. Fluoxymesterone (Ultandren) has the advantage of being given orally and is not very virilising. Prednisone not only acts as a hormone but will increase the general sense of wellbeing; it is recommended for liver metastases which are almost always relatively unresponsive to other therapy. Nandralone phenylpropionate or diconate (Durabolin or Deca-Durabolin) are suitable alternatives in bone involvement and contribute to the sense of wellbeing. They appear to be slightly more effective if combined with prednisone.

When the patient in this pre- or post-menopausal group relapses, treatment along the lines of the intermediate group should be instituted.

Cytotoxic Chemotherapy

This newer method of treatment is rarely used as part of the initial attack on a tumour as it is, of course, toxic, and requires a considerable investment of time by patient and physician in monitoring blood-counts and administering drugs. Stoll (1969) has combined it with hormone therapy, but little use is now made of this technique. Cytotoxic drugs are most commonly held in reserve until hormone therapy has failed, but are probably indicated as first therapy for the slow, inexorable local *en cuirasse* type of recurrence.

As in other diseases treated by cytotoxic drugs, the tendency is away from the use of single agents towards multiple-pulsed therapy, but the dramatic results which have followed this type of treatment in Hodgkin's disease and acute lymphocytic leukaemia in children have not been seen in breast cancer. The régime of Hanham *et al.* (1971), using cyclophosphamide, methotrexate, vincristine and 5-Fu, is probably as good as any but, as with all such treatments, should only be undertaken by those experienced in it, there being no place for the occasional chemotherapist. Unfortunately, such chemotherapy has to be repeated at frequent intervals (3–4 weeks) for the rest of the patient's life and may represent a large fraction of a relatively short existence. Large numbers of such patients can strain the capacity of any oncological department. The relationship between a long disease-free interval to recurrence and good response to treatment does not appear to hold for cytotoxics as it does for hormone therapy.

Immunotherapy

Although this type of treatment is still almost exclusively experimental it is here that, at the present time, there would seem to be more hope for the 'breakthrough' which will fundamentally alter the outlook for cancer patients. Little evidence is available of tumour-specific antigens against solid tumours in man, other than for melanomata, but the indirect evidence of an immune factor is strong. In breast disease the presence of sinus histiocytosis is taken as evidence of a positive response and is associated with a better prognosis. The susceptibility of those suffering from malignant disease to infection and haemolytic anaemia is indirect evidence of an immune response which such patients lack. Patients with a depressed immune state do not react to tuberculin, and cannot be immunised against dinitrochlorobenzine (DNCB); perhaps it is on the basis of some such test that patients should be selected for different methods of treatment.

Attempts to promote an immune response to tumour can be non-specific, the patient's own immune system being stimulated to respond to his own tumour; this is being done by Mathé (1970) using BCG and Woodruff (1970) using *Corynebacterium parvum*. Specific response to tumour can be stimulated by the host's own tumour cells rendered non-viable by irradiation; Mathé's work has shown that this is undoubtedly effective in leukaemia, that the specific stimulation is better than the non-specific BCG and that the two together are better than either alone. It has also been shown in animal models that immunotherapy can result in rejection of tumour grafts only up to a certain maximum size, after which it becomes ineffective. It is this size-effect which would appear to be the cause of the overwhelming of the immune response in man, once a tumour passes a critical size; thus immunotherapy will be an addition to, not replacement for, standard therapy and the timing of it in relation to that therapy will need careful investigation, as shown by the work of Currie and Bagshawe (1970).

Psychological Aspects of Mastectomy

It is difficult for a male to comment on this feature of management of breast cancer, but there must now be few women who are not aware of the significance of a lump in the breast and, in particular, of mastectomy. As knowledge is more widely disseminated, patients adopt a more critical approach to any treatment offered. The therapist must be prepared to substantiate the need for any such treatment, especially if it involves mutilation. The word 'cancer' is sufficiently evocative without the added burden of mutilation by mastectomy. In the past, attempts to cure the disease by 'radical' means have been allowed to outweigh all other considerations.

Never more than today has the female breast been discussed and paraded as a sex symbol in advertisement, literature and television, with the inevitable result that its loss must be correspondingly psychologically traumatic. As exposure of the organ increases, the results of surgical removal become more difficult to conceal while leading a normal life. Much can and should be done, and is only too often not done, in the way of helping such patients. The immediate provision of a lightweight plastic foam prosthesis enables the patient to leave hospital after surgery with some semblance of a normal form, but too little attention is paid to providing the patient with the best prosthesis from the increasing selection available, and advising patients about the special swimwear which has been designed and produced for her. The usual 'appliance fitter' probably does not have enough time or specialised experience for this; the author has been greatly helped in one clinic by a nurse who herself has suffered mastectomy, and all breast clinics would benefit from similar first-hand experience.

An article in the magazine *Woman's Own* (Austin, 1973) relates one patient's feelings after mastectomy and her joy when, after five years, she was offered plastic surgery with insertion of a 'silastic' prosthesis. It is probable that most oncologists will have grave doubts regarding the wisdom of opening up tissue planes to carry out such an operation, but before denying this to any woman we must be able to provide an accurate assessment of the dangers of such a treatment. As with so many aspects of breast cancer treatment, adequate information is not available. It may well be that every woman subjected to mastectomy will eventually be able to have such a prosthesis inserted without any detriment to her chance of local recurrence or survival.

Techniques of Radiotherapy

Although there have been no dramatic improvements in the techniques since McWhirter's (1955) description of his four-field orthovoltage method, there have been and continue to be minor advances. In all radiotherapy planning, all field junctions and consequent danger of over- or under-dosage are to be avoided. The complicated irregular shape of the treated volume, which includes chest wall, internal mammary, supraclavicular and axillary lymph nodes, makes this almost impossible. This is not as great a disadvantage as might at first appear, as the requirements of chest wall and lymph node irradiation are different.

The chest wall and usually also the breast, if it has not been removed, are irradiated to prevent local recurrence or because of skin involvement. This being so, the dose has to be brought up to skin-level. Although orthovoltage irradiation produces maximum skin-dosage it is still inferior to megavoltage irradiation using bolus, on account of the greater gradient across the volume treated and the greater absorbed dose in cartilege. The technique of a 'glancing pair' of fields (with bolus), using megavoltage, is the present treatment of choice. If the separation of these fields and the shape of the chest wall allows, the internal mammary chain can be included.

When regional nodes are irradiated there is no expectation of skin-involvement by tumour, and a direct megavoltage shaped field can be used, the dose then not being limited by skin-reaction. Such a single field can be used to treat internal mammary, supraclavicular and axillary nodes, *en bloc*. One disadvantage of the lack of skin-reaction using this type of treatment is that it is easier to produce late damage to brachial plexus and artery as a result of the absence of any warning skin-changes.

The dosage employed varies greatly from clinic to clinic, depending

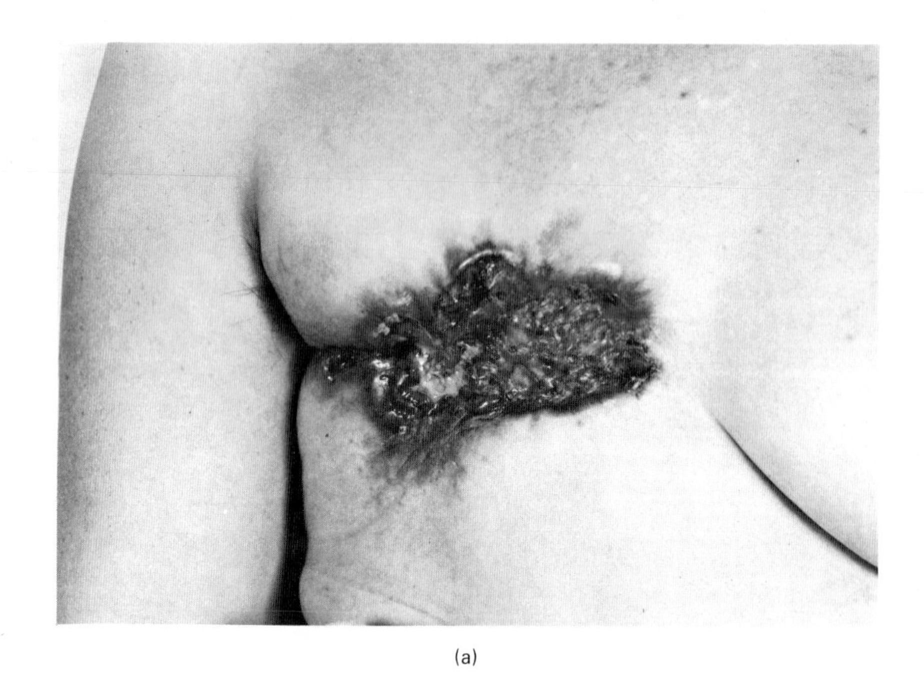

(a)

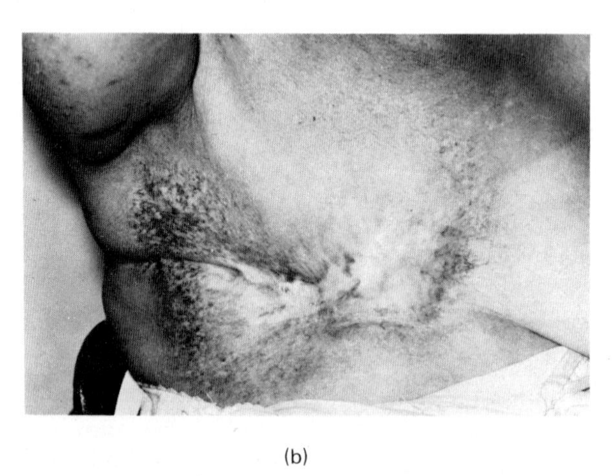

(b)

Fig. 8.2. Advanced breast cancer (a) before and (b) nine years after telecobalt irradiation: 4500 rad in twenty treatments achieved good local control.

on factors such as which part in the treated volume is taken as the reference point, overall time and frequency of irradiation. All such techniques are the outcome of experience on the part of the therapist. Of all the factors the most significant is probably the overall time of treatment, and this is often related to the pressure of work in the clinic; typical tumour doses are from 4000 rad in 15 treatments to 5000 rad in 25 treatments. Where the primary tumour is irradiated alone, doses of the order of 8000 rad have been given in 65 days by Montague (1970). These higher doses are used when treating larger masses of tumour, but may not be necessary (Fig. 8.2).

Interstitial irradiation has long been used and is still the method of choice for the late recurrence in a scar which is not operable but can still effectively be dealt with by a relatively small implant. It can be used even when previous beam-directed therapy has been given to the chest wall, provided account is taken of the skin change when prescribing the dose. The more diffuse nodular early recurrence around a scar carries a much worse prognosis, usually spreads fairly rapidly and is better treated by a similar technique to that used in post-operative chest wall irradiation.

Pierquin *et al.* (1971) have developed and used with some success an after-loading technique with iridium-192 wire which is applicable to breast cancer. It is particularly of value if this technique is used for the primary tumour mass and beam-directed therapy is used to treat the rest of the breast, including the iridium-irradiated volume. As this method of treatment conserves the organ it would appear to be worthy of a more extended trial (see Chapter 1). This technique may also be used for chest wall recurrence after previous irradiation (Fig. 8.3).

Electron irradiation of the chest wall is attractive to the radiotherapist as, with accurate measurement of chest wall thickness, possible with ultrasonics, the chest wall can be irradiated with less damage to the underlying lung than occurs with all other techniques. A study of this method of therapy has been carried out at the M.D. Anderson Hospital by Tapley and Fletcher (1970). In their series routine electron treatment was given post-operatively to a group of high-risk patients, identified by node involvement, large or fixed tumours and skin involvement. In this group they had a 10 per cent local recurrence rate.

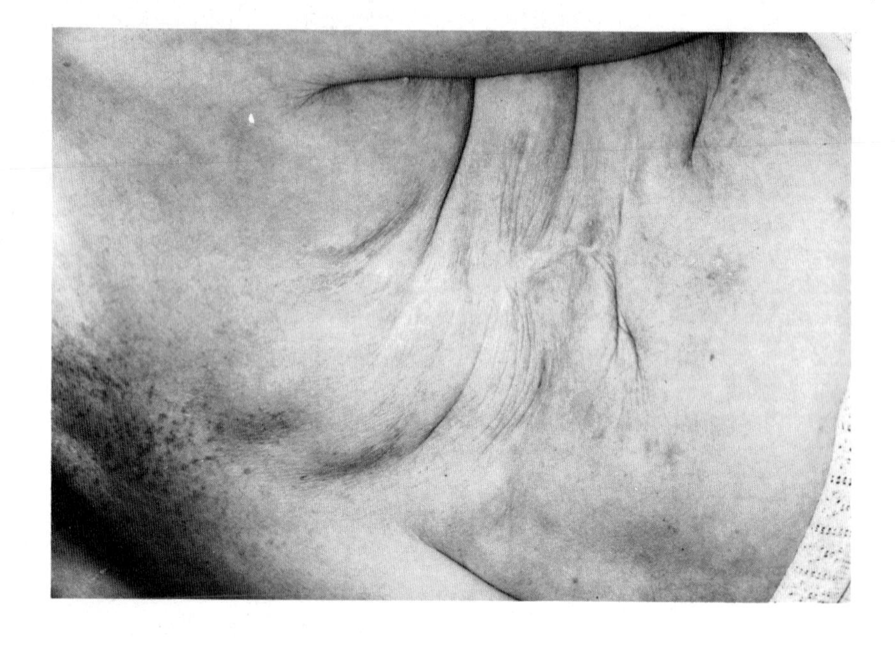

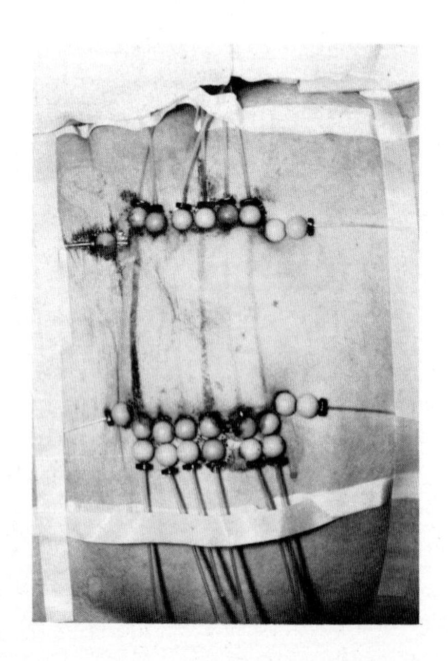

Fig. 8.3. Locally recurrent breast cancer showing
(a) treatment by iridium implant and
(b) result after nine months.

Where a waiting policy was adopted subsequent irradiation failed to control the recurrence in 51 per cent of cases.

Conclusions

Breast cancer is still an enigma which kills by distant spread, and therefore local treatment cannot produce cure when the tumour has already metastasised. For this reason a full and careful search to delimit the extent of local disease and spread should be made. This philosophy is summed up in the couplet by Robert Burns (1759–1795)

Then gently scan your brother man
Still gentler sister woman.

No radical treatment with all its attendant damage should be undertaken when it cannot cure. Effort must be directed towards a better system of classification which will include parameters not routinely considered at present, in order that better selection of the available methods of treatment can be made for each patient. It seems possible that immunotherapy may in the future have something to offer in the early treatment of breast cancer. Those treating this disease must realise that an enthusiastic approach is not sufficient, and seek more critically to apply the present relatively ineffective methods of treatment while seeking for better.

The use of surgery and radiotherapy may be declining, and hormone, cytotoxic and perhaps immunotherapy, increasing. Thus breast cancer should no longer be treated by one specialist, but by a team who subject no patient to treatment until all information available under the circumstances existing has been obtained. It is equally important that all information that may help in the future planning of better treatment should be obtained in every case.

References

AUSTIN, J. (1973) *Woman's Own*, 10 October, 60–66.
BLACK, M. M. and ASIRE, A. J. (1969) *Cancer*, **23**, 251–259.
BOND, W. H. (1968) *The Treatment of Carcinoma of the Breast*, ed.

Jarrer, A. S. Exerpto Medical Foundation for Syntax Pharmaceuticals Ltd, Maidenhead.

BOND, W. I. (1972) *Modern Trends in Radiotherapy.* Butterworth, London.

British Medical Journal (1973) **4**, 124. Editorial.

CHARKES, N. D., VALENTINE, C. and GRAVITZ, B. (1973) *Radiology*, **107**, 563–570.

COLE, H. and HANLAN, K. E. (1971) *Clinical Radiology*, **22**, 133–135.

COLE, M. (1964) *Breast Journal Surgery*, **51**, 216–220.

CURRIE, C. A. and BAGSHAWE, K. D. (1970) *British Medical Journal*, **1**, 541–544.

DAHL-IVERSEN, E. and TOBIASSEN, T. (1963) *Annals of Surgery*, **157**, 170–173.

EVANS, K. T. and GRAVELLE, I. H. (1973) *Mammography, Thermography and Ultrasonography in Breast Disease.* Butterworth, London.

FURNIVAL, I. C., STEWART, H. J., WEDDELL, J. M., DOVEY, P., GRAVELLE, I. H., EVANS, K. T. and FOREST, A. P. M. (1970) *British Medical Journal*, **4**, 461–463.

GALASKO, C. S. B. (1969) *British Journal of Surgery*, **56**, 757.

GALASKO, C. S. B. and DOYLE, F. H. (1972) *Clinical Radiology*, **23**, 295–297.

HANDLEY, R. S. (1952) *Proceedings Royal Society Medicine*, **14**, 565.

HANHAM, I. W. F., NEWTON, K. A. and WESTBURY, C. (1971) *British Journal of Cancer*, **25**, 462–478.

HAYBITTLE, J. L. (1968) *British Journal of Radiology*, **41**, 639.

HALL, A. J. and MACKAY, N. N. S. (1973) *Journal of Bone and Joint Surgery*, **55**, 497–505.

JONES, C. H. and DRAPER, J. M. (1970) *British Journal of Radiology*, **43**, 507–516.

KAAE, S. and JOHANSEN, H. (1963) *Annals of Surgery*, **157**, 175–179.

MATHÉ, G. (1970) *British Medical Journal*, **4**, 487–488.

MCWHIRTER, R. (1960) *Clinical Radiology*, **xi**, 144–149.

MCWHIRTER, R. (1955) *British Journal of Radiology*, **xxviii**, 128–137.

MERRICK, M. V. (1973) *British Journal of Radiology*, **64**, 968–971.

MONTAGUE, E. D. (1970) in *Breast Cancer, Early and Late*, M.D.

Anderson Hospital. Year Book Medical Publishers, Chicago, Ill., 191–198.
MUSTAKALLIO, S. (1972) *Clinical Radiology*, **23**, 110–116.
PARK, W. W. and LEES, J. C. (1951) *Surgery, Gynaecology and Obstetrics*, **93**, 129–152.
PATERSON, R. J. (1959) *Journal of Faculty of Radiologists*, **10**, 130–133.
PIERQUIN, B., CHASSAGNE, D. and COX, J. D. (1971) *Radiology*, **99**, 661–667.
SILBERSTEIN, E. B., SAENGER, E. L., TOFE, A. J., ALEXANDER, G. W. JR. and PARK, H. M. (1973) *Radiology*, **107**, 551–555.
STARK, A. M. and WAY, S. (1970) *Lancet*, **2**, 407–409.
STOLL, B. (1969) *Hormonal Management of Breast Cancer*, Pitman Medical, London.
TAPLEY, W. D. and FLETCHER, C. H. (1970) in *Breast Cancer, Early and Late*, M.D. Anderson Hospital. Year Book Medical Publishers, Chicago, Ill.
WOODRUFF, M. F. A. (1970) *British Medical Journal*, **4**, 486–487.

CHAPTER NINE

Tumours of the Colon, Rectum and Anus

G. Newsholme

In Western countries, growths of the lower bowel rank second only to those of the lung as a cause of death from cancer. In England and Wales, 15 804 men and women died of the disease in 1971 compared with 30 701 dying of lung cancer and 11 262 of cancer of the breast. During the past few decades there have been improvements in the results of surgery, partly due to better surgical techniques and partly to earlier diagnosis, but, in spite of this, most patients with carcinoma of the large intestine die of the disease. Slaney (1971), in a survey of the West Midland Region, found an overall five-year survival rate of only 20·5 per cent with a crude five-year survival rate of 42·5 per cent for those patients who could be treated by radical surgery.

These figures, while probably representative of this country and the USA as a whole, are considerably worse than those reported from some specialist centres where concentrated expertise is dealing with highly selected groups of patients. Hawley (1974) points out, for instance, that in District Hospitals perhaps 20 per cent are admitted as emergencies with intestinal obstruction or perforation, which worsens their prognosis, and one-third of the large group surveyed by Slaney had hopelessly advanced disease when first seen, in many cases dying soon afterwards. Failing the development of a simple screening test which would allow sub-clinical disease to be detected, and accepting that further improvement in surgical results is likely to be relatively small, it seems that progress will depend on the augmentation of surgery by some additional form of therapy.

Surgery is more likely to fail in patients whose tumours are anaplastic or poorly-differentiated histologically, and where the tumour has already metastasised to lymph nodes or has penetrated the full thickness of the bowel wall. Cancers arising in the lower two-thirds of the rectum below the peritoneal reflection are more likely than those of the upper third to infiltrate the pelvic viscera, reach lymph and blood vessels and thus to develop distal metastases. By contrast, growths which are well-differentiated histologically and have not infiltrated the full thickness of the bowel wall or spread to lymph nodes do well with surgery.

Any way of improving the prospects of the poor-risk group is greatly to be desired, but up to the present time no treatment is available which can approach the effectiveness of surgery. Increasing interest is being shown in the development of different methods of adjuvant therapy in the hope that such combined treatments will prove more effective than surgery alone.

Adjuvant Radiotherapy

It has been known for more than 60 years that carcinoma of the lower bowel sometimes responds to radiotherapy and Symonds (1914) was probably one of the first to describe adjuvant radiotherapy at any site when he reported a patient with a rectal growth treated by radium, resulting in marked shrinkage which made surgical removal possible some months later. Phillips (1942) and Williams and Horwitz (1956) have reported series of cases of carcinoma of the rectum treated by megavoltage radiotherapy at St Bartholomew's Hospital with considerable symptomatic relief in many cases, and a small number of long-term survivors following radiotherapy alone.

The slow acceptance of the value of radiotherapy has been due to the relative ineffectiveness of orthovoltage (250 kV) irradiation in this condition, combining as it does the disadvantages of poor penetration in depth, high skin-dose and increased absorption of radiation in the pelvic bones. It has been repeatedly confirmed by many radiotherapists that patients with inoperable or recurrent growths of the colon and rectum obtain worthwhile relief of symptoms with moderate doses of megavoltage radiotherapy (Urdaneta-Lafee *et al.*, 1972). The fact remains, however, that in spite of clear evidence that these tumours frequently respond, sometimes quite markedly, to radiotherapy, cure is infrequent even when dosage is high. Nevertheless, it should be stated that there is a definite place for the use of radiotherapy, given radically with intent to cure in certain patients unsuitable for surgery either because of their age and general condition or because of the extent of their disease.

Encouragement in the use of adjuvant radiotherapy has been given by radiobiologists working with cell cultures and experimental animals. *In-vitro* and *in-vivo* studies (Whitmore, 1964) have shown that it may require only 500–2000 rad to reduce a cell population to 10 per cent of its previous value, whereas 5000–7000 rad may be needed for virtual sterilisation of a tumour (or even higher doses if anoxic, more radioresistant, cells are present) and significant increases in cure-rate, when compared with the results of surgery alone, can be obtained for certain experimental tumours when a *non*-curative dose of X-rays is combined with surgery. It is assumed that this improvement is due to the considerably reduced fraction of viable cells present in the irradiated tissues, with a consequent reduction in the chance of local regrowth or dissemination post-operatively. Twenty to thirty per cent of the full therapeutic dose of irradiation has been shown to contribute significantly to the control of malignant tumours in many animal experiments. In colo-rectal cancer a clear distinction needs to be made between the lower-dose, adjuvant therapy suggested by radiobiological research, which may enhance surgical cure-rates in tumours already operable, and the high dosage (5000–6000 rad in 5–6 weeks) required to render an inoperable tumour surgically operable.

There is experimental evidence to suggest that adjuvant radiotherapy is less effective when given after, rather than before, surgery (Perez, 1970) and, clinically, radiotherapy is less well tolerated when given post-operatively. Irradiation after manipulation and surgical resection will not reach those malignant cells that have widely disseminated at operation and there is likely to be decreased oxygen tension in the area of the operation as a consequence of damage to small blood vessels, with a risk that any remaining cancer cells will thus be less sensitive to irradiation than are normal well-oxygenated cells.

The advantage of post-operative radiotherapy is, of course, that it can be planned in the knowledge of the operative findings. It would help greatly in weighing up the value of pre-operative irradiation and in judging when it should be used if some method were available of assessing tumour-spread and histological grading. To ask the patient, often elderly, to accept a prolonged course of irradiation in the knowledge that, when reactions to this have settled, he must submit himself to a considerable operation for a condition he knows or suspects to be malignant, is quite unjustifiable unless he can be assured that his chances of cure will be appreciably enhanced as a result.

Growths in the rectum and pelvic colon can be biopsied pre-operatively and some attempt at histological grading made (although examination of the whole tumour subsequently removed does not always give an identical result). The degree of local tumour-spread, however, and the extent of lymph node involvement can, at the present time, only be discovered at operation. Lower limb lymphography does not opacify the pelvic and mesenteric lymph nodes and is only able to demonstrate advanced spread which has reached the external iliac or para-aortic lymph nodes. ^{67}Ga concentrates in a number of different types of tumour, including poorly-differentiated adenocarcinoma (Vaidya *et al.*, 1970), but an isotope scan or gamma image of the abdomen following a tracer dose has a relatively limited value in relation to the pre-operative staging of bowel tumours. A staging laparotomy has been suggested and no doubt, if therapy could be developed until it was as effective in bowel cancer as radiotherapy and chemotherapy in Hodgkin's disease, the idea would become as generally accepted in suitable cases as it has become in the latter condition.

Figure 9.1 shows the relative frequency of occurrence at various sites in a series of large bowel cancers. Those involving the sigmoid colon and rectum comprise more than two-thirds of all growths of the lower intestine and it is perhaps fortunate in this respect that radiotherapy given to the pelvis and lower abdomen is better tolerated than when given to the upper abdominal contents. Most of the reported

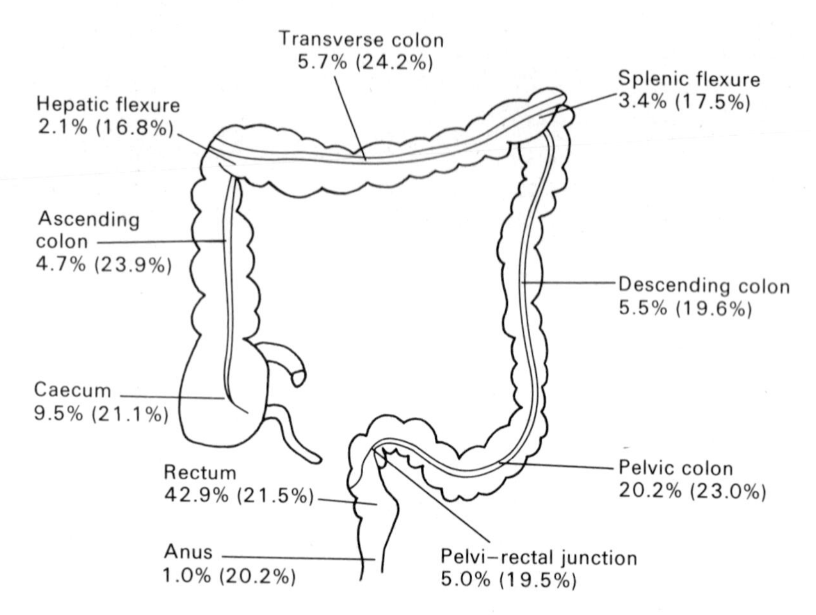

Fig. 9.1. Distribution of carcinoma of the colon and rectum in 10 918 cases from the Birmingham Region, 1960–65 (five-year survival rates shown in parentheses).

work in connection with adjuvant radiotherapy of this condition has been concerned with carcinoma of the rectum and pelvic colon.

Pre-operative Radiotherapy: Low-dosage Studies

In the United States moderate and low-dose radiotherapy, given pre-operatively, has been tried at the Memorial Hospital, New York, since 1939 (Stearns *et al.*, 1959) and more recently by the Veterans Administration Surgical Adjuvant Group (Dwight *et al.*, 1972). The intention has been, as previously mentioned, to reduce the fraction of viable cells present and thus reduce the chance of local re-growth or dissemination. The radiation field-size has been generally to the order of 20 × 20 cm, extending from the perineum approximately to the level of the fourth lumbar vertebral body, a dose of 2000 rad being given in ten treatments over two weeks. Experimental studies suggest that the benefits of radiation given in this way would be likely to cover only one or two generations of tumour cells and operation is therefore carried out, in most cases, within a few days of completing treatment.

Surgery presents no problem after radiation dosage of this magnitude and the whole régime appears to be well tolerated. The first report from the Memorial Hospital suggested that pre-operative irradiation given thus to more than 700 patients had a considerable influence on survival, since this irradiated group showed a ten-year survival of 27 per cent compared with a non-irradiated group of similar size of whom only 10 per cent survived for ten years following surgery only. The survey, however, was a retrospective one and a subsequent prospective trial (Stearns *et al.*, 1968) has failed to confirm the earlier results, underscoring again the fact that even a large series can provide misleading results unless prospective and randomised.

Pre-operative Radiotherapy: High-dosage Methods

High-dose pre-operative radiotherapy is being practised in a number of centres, the differing treatment volumes being used reflecting the uncertainty about the degree of tumour-spread and showing clearly our need for a method of pre-operative staging of the disease (Fig. 9.2).

Kligerman *et al.* (1972) use radiation fields which cover the whole of the pelvic contents and include the primary and pelvic side-walls with a narrower extension upwards to cover the lymphatic drainage of the rectum and pelvic colon to the origin of the inferior mesenteric artery at the level of L2. Using megavoltage radiotherapy a dose of 4000–4500 rad can be given in 4–4½ weeks. Although the fields extend upwards to the third part of the duodenum, treatment is said to be well tolerated. Diarrhoea frequently develops but can be controlled by simple measures without interrupting the course. In most cases surgery is possible four weeks later, when the radiation reactions have settled, without difficulty or increase in morbidity. Kligerman *et al.* report the use of this method in 15 cases, using 16 controls. No tumour cells could be found in operation specimens from four of the 15 irradiated cases and only three of the 15 were shown to have lymph node involvement, compared with 11 of the 16 controls. The results encouraged them to treat more patients along the same lines, but no conclusions as to the ultimate value of radiotherapy can be drawn until more cases have been treated and more time has elapsed.

A second approach to high-dose adjuvant radiotherapy is the irradiation of the primary only, without any attempt to cover lymph node drainage areas. Using a small radiation volume of the order of 10

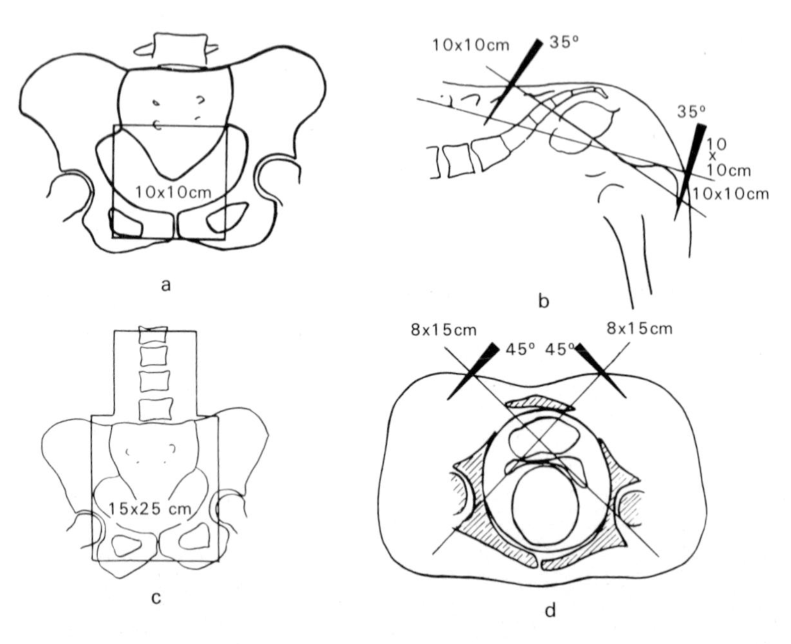

Fig. 9.2. Some of the treatment fields in use in radiotherapy of carcinoma of the rectum and pelvic colon.

a Allen (1970)
b Garrett (1971)
c Kligerman (1972)
d Rodriguez-Antunez (1973)

cm in diameter it is possible in the pelvis to give a dose of 5–6000 rad in as many weeks. Such therapy is usually well tolerated and obstructive symptoms, if present, usually improve during treatment, preliminary colostomy being avoided as far as possible. Allen and Fletcher (1970) using megavoltage radiotherapy and, for the most part, opposed 10 × 10 cm anterior and posterior pelvic fields have given, at the rate of 900 rad per week, a total of approximately 5000 rad, operation being carried out four to six weeks later when radiation reactions have settled. Experience shows that surgery at this stage poses no real difficulty and healing is not normally delayed. They report no evidence of local recurrence in the 51 cases in the series who have been irradiated, and then operated on, since 1960. Of 16 cases originally considered unresectable, eight regressed to a degree allowing surgery to be carried out after irradiation. Ten of the 51 had no gross tumour left following radiotherapy – five in whom no cancer could be detected in the operation specimen, and only *in situ* carcinoma in the other five. Involved lymph nodes were found in only ten of the 51 cases. These authors were, however, unable to find any difference in two-year survival between this group and an earlier, non-irradiated group of cases. The absence of local recurrences they consider significant, since the local recurrence rate after surgery alone is commonly about 20 per cent (Morgan, 1957).

Another method has been adopted by Rodriguez-Antunez *et al.* (1973), whose stated intention has been the prevention of dissemination of viable tumour cells at the time of operation – their cases were judged to be operable and there was no intention of reducing tumour bulk or trying to render an inoperable tumour removable. A daily tumour-dose of 800 rad for three days (total tumour-dose 2400 rad) was given on a cobalt unit using two posterior oblique pelvic fields with 45° wedge filters to produce uniform dosage within the treatment volume, usually about 15 cm in length. Surgery was carried out 10–15 days later without complications, apart from occasional delay in healing of the perineal wound. Of 70 cases for which five-year survival figures were available, 43 were found subsequently to be operable. In 26 of the operable cases the growth was found to be confined to the bowel and adjacent tissues and of this group 21 (81 per cent) survived free of recurrence for five years or more. The remaining 17 cases showed spread to lymph nodes and only four of these patients (23·5 per cent) survived for five years. Of the 13 with node involvement who died in this group, three died of local recurrence rather than distal metastases.

The aims of these various adjuvant radiotherapy régimes differ, as do their demands on the patients, varying from a brief course of treatment with operation in less than two weeks to one lasting five or six weeks with operation six weeks later. Treatment areas vary from 100 to 400 cm^2, or more.

Immunological Considerations

Cellular immunity to colon cancer has been demonstrated in a considerable proportion of patients with the disease (Stewart, 1969) and a favourable response reported in a number treated by immunotherapy (Griffen and Meeker, 1972). The possibility that radiotherapy might reduce the immune response and adversely affect the host–tumour relationship has to be considered. Nothing very definite emerges from a survey of the published work on adjuvant radiotherapy but it is of interest that Stearns *et al.* (1959) found a higher incidence of liver metastases in patients given pre-operative irradiation, although the possibility that the radiotherapy given might have altered the immune response was not discussed.

Palliative Radiotherapy

For the relief of symptoms due to inoperable or recurrent disease, radiotherapy is of definite value, particularly in the pelvis. Colostomy, as previously mentioned, can be avoided in many patients with inoperable growths of the rectum and pelvic colon, the tumour being treated locally to fairly high dosage (4000–6000 rad in 4–6 weeks) using small fields. More than half of those with recurrent pelvic disease, inoperable perineal masses, pain radiating to hips and legs, rectal bleeding, tenesmus and discharge can be helped.

To a lesser extent, symptoms due to intra-abdominal spread can be relieved, treatment then being directed to the site of the predominant symptom, often a bulky metastatic mass or painful liver deposit. In such cases, perhaps one-third will obtain worthwhile relief. Jaundice, unless accompanied by evidence of considerable damage to liver cells, is not a contraindication, but attempts to treat the whole abdomen are not justified. Symptoms due to metastases in bone or mediastinum can often be relieved, the response, as at other sites, being dependent to a considerable extent on the dose given.

Chemotherapy

At the present time the only drugs which have been shown to exert a significant effect on adenocarcinoma of the bowel are the fluorinated pyrimidines of which 5-Fu has been most used. Appreciable tumour regression and clinical improvement occurs in approximately 20 per cent of patients treated. The drug is dangerous and death from haematological failure well-known following the earlier recommended method of giving short intensive courses. This method of administration has been found to be no more effective and far less safe than weekly intravenous injections of 15 mg/kg body weight (maximum single dose 1·0 g). The dose may be increased to 20 mg/kg body weight after four weeks, weekly injections continuing until mild toxic symptoms appear (aphthous stomatitis, pharyngitis, oesophagitis, diarrhoea or fall in white cell and platelet count). It is also possible to give 5-Fu by mouth; 15 mg/kg body weight orally in fruit juice each day for six days, then once weekly, has produced similar results to those of intravenous therapy and it is suggested that the response of liver metastases may be enhanced by absorption of the drug into the portal circulation (Lahiri *et al.*, 1971). Although occasional responses to other drugs such as methotrexate and the vinca alkaloids occur, combination chemotherapy using multiple drugs and high-dose intermittent therapy has not proved of value in colonic carcinoma.

Adjuvant Chemotherapy

The treatment of cancer by a combination of radiotherapy and cytotoxic agents is increasingly popular, but hopes that such combinations would improve the results of radiotherapy given alone have so far, in carcinoma of the colon at any rate, been disappointed. Bleehen (1973) points out that the majority of drugs when combined with radiation probably kill tumour cells and normal cells in an additive manner. In such cases the improved tissue-tolerance to radiotherapy when used on its own would allow an increase in the dose given and achieve the same end-result as the combined treatment.

Some drugs may truly potentiate the radiation effect – the combination being more effective than the individual treatments and producing proportionately more cell-death for a given dose of radiation. The potentiation by the drug may be due partly to the production of temporary mitotic arrest and cell-cycle synchronisation, which implies that the timing of the delivery of subsequent radiotherapy may be critical if it is to act at the most sensitive part of the cell-cycle. A number of trials of the combined use of 5-Fu and radiotherapy for bowel cancer has been reported, none so far with conclusive results. Moertel *et al.* (1969), for instance, in a double blind trial, showed a significant improvement in mean survival of patients with gastro-intestinal cancer when 5-Fu was added to a particular radiotherapy régime, but, as pointed out by Bleehen, it may well be that a rather higher dose of radiation given alone would have produced the same result.

Surgery and Chemotherapy

The use of systemic 5-Fu after operation does not appear to influence results when surgical clearance has been adequate and chemotherapy could be considered truly adjuvant, but may possibly improve the outlook for cases with residual disease after surgery (Higgins *et al.*, 1971). Another approach, practised by Rousselot *et al.* (1968) for more than eight years, has been the injection of 5-Fu at operation into the bowel segment containing the tumour to be resected, in the belief that it may prevent the spread of tumour cells by lymphatics or veins during operation. The segment is first isolated by tapes which surround both gut and marginal vein, and clamping of the pedicular vessels is delayed to allow time for drug-absorption. Their results are inconclusive but suggest improved survival in patients whose operation specimens subsequently demonstrate node involvement.

From the foregoing it is clear that, although there is some hope that the local recurrence rate may be reduced by using pre-operative radiotherapy, there is so far no proof that combined methods of treatment improve survival in cancer of the large intestine. Progress in this direction can only be made by using properly controlled clinical trials, although Scott (1973) considers that the number of permutations and combinations of therapy, dosage and timing is so great that answers will not be obtained without resorting to animal experimentation, in spite of the difficulty of relating the results to the clinical situation.

The types of case which carry a poor prognosis are well-known and, if such cases could be identified and the extent of spread of their disease determined before treatment, the search for effective combinations of therapy could be narrowed considerably and unnecessary treatment of good-risk patients avoided. There is no doubt, too, that new and more effective chemotherapeutic agents are greatly needed in this condition.

Anus

Anal cancer is relatively uncommon, accounting in the Birmingham region for slightly more than one per cent of all cases of cancer of the large intestine and anus (Table 9.1). Growths can be divided into those arising below and those arising above the dentate line. the embryological junction of the proctodeal inpouching and the post-allantoic gut.

Table 9.1. Incidence of Carcinoma of Colon, Rectum and Anus, Birmingham Region, 1959–68

	Total cases registered	*Male*	*Female*
Colon	10280	4442	5838
Rectum (including pelvi-rectal junction)	8034	4591	3443
Anal canal	113	44	69
Anal margin	97	43	54

Anal margin tumours arising below this line are mainly squamous-celled carcinomas of relatively low grade, metastasising late, if at all, to the inguinal nodes and behaving in general like skin cancers elsewhere in the body. Tumours arising at or above the dentate line, *anal canal* carcinomata, tend to metastasise early to the mesenteric and pelvic lymph nodes as well as invading the immediately subjacent internal haemorrhoidal venous plexus and peri-rectal tissues. The dentate line is a band of epithelium of varying width at, or just above the level of the anal valves, the cells of which are transitional between the stratified squamous epithelium below and the cuboidal epithelium of the lower rectal mucosa above. Most anal canal tumours arise from this unstable transitional zone (Morson, 1960) and are squamous-celled growths of relatively poor differentiation. A few are transitional celled or 'basaloid' in type; Klotz *et al.* (1967) describe no fewer than 373 cases of transitional cloacogenic carcinoma of the anal canal which can be separated histologically from squamous-celled carcinoma and may carry a rather poorer prognosis.

Treatment

It is difficult for any one centre to accumulate enough cases to evaluate treatment methods, but a review of the literature of the last few years shows an increasing preference in favour of surgery for both anal margin and anal canal growths. Radiotherapy is of less value in the primary treatment of anal tumours than in dealing with squamous carcinoma at other sites, because of the intolerance of the anal tissues to radiation. The dividing line between a curative dose and that producing painful radionecrosis, stricture-formation and destruction of sphincter function is narrow.

Anal margin tumours, when small, are preferably treated by wide local excision, but the inguinal lymph nodes are not dissected unless they are considered, either initially or subsequently, to be involved (aspiration cytology of doubtful nodes may on occasion be helpful). Anal canal tumours, on the other hand, are treated by abdomino-perineal resection of the rectum, including a wide perineal dissection and, in women, excision in many cases of the posterior vaginal wall. Extensive infiltrating anal margin tumours are probably best treated in this way also.

Failes and Morgan (1973) report 16 patients surviving for five years out of a total of 65 with anal canal growths (25 per cent) finding, in spite of radical excision, that perineal and pelvic recurrences are common in those dying of the disease. This suggests that a case can be made out for the use of pre-operative radiotherapy in these cases. Some encouragement for this view can be seen in the work of Hickey *et al.* (1972), who claim it to be beneficial in the treatment of large tumours. When pre-operative radiation is planned, an initial abdominal exploration is carried out to assess spread, in particular to the liver, and colostomy done at a slightly higher level than normal to avoid the radiation field. A dose of 4000 rad in four weeks is given, followed by radical surgery one month later.

Radiotherapy, quite apart from its possible pre-operative value, is used in the palliative treatment of inoperable or recurrent disease and may have a small part to play in the treatment of localised tumours of the anal margin which can be accurately and adequately covered by a single-plane radium-needle implant. The hazard to sphincter-control of local excision, in certain cases, may very occasionally justify the use of radiotherapy in this way as the primary treatment. Williams (1962) treated successfully three such patients (two of them over 80 years old) seen over a twenty-year period.

References

ALLEN, C. V. and FLETCHER, W. S. (1970) *American Journal of Roentgenology*, **108**, 136–140.

BLEEHEN, N. M. (1973) *British Medical Bulletin*, **29**, 54–58.

DWIGHT, R. W., HIGGINS, G. A., ROSWIT, B., LE VEEN, H. H. and KEEHN, R. J. (1972) *American Journal of Surgery*, **123**, 93–102.

FAILES, D. and MORGAN, B. P. (1973) *Diseases of the Colon and Rectum*, **16**, 397–401.

GARRETT, M. J. (1971) *Clinical Radiology*, **22**, 521–523.

GRIFFEN, W. O. and MEEKER, W. R. (1972) *Surgical Clinics of North America*, **52**, 839–845.

HAWLEY, P. R. (1974) *British Journal of Hospital Medicine*, **11**, 211–216.

HICKEY, R. C., MARTIN, R. G., KHEIR, S., MACKAY, B. and GALLAGER, H. S. (1972) *Surgical Clinics of North America*, **52**, 943–950.

HIGGINS, G. A., DWIGHT, R. W., SMITH, J. V. and KEEHN, R. J. (1971) *Archives of Surgery*, **102**, 339–343.

KLIGERMAN, M. M., URDANETA, N., KNOWLTON, A., VIDONE, R., HARTMAN, P. V. and VERA, R. (1972) *American Journal of Roentgenology*, **114**, 498–503.

KLOTZ, R. G., PAMUKLOGLU, T. and SOUILLIARD, D. H. (1967) *Cancer*, **20**, 1727–1745.

LAHIRI, S. R., BOILEAU, G. and HALL, T. C. (1971) *Cancer*, **28**, 902–906.

MOERTEL, C. G., CHILDS, D. S., REITMEIER, R. J., COLEY, M. Y. and HOLBROOK, M. A. (1969) *Lancet*, **ii**, 865–867.

MORGAN, C. N. (1957) *Proceedings of the Royal Society of Medicine*, **50**, 1050–1052.

MORSON, B. C. (1960) *Proceedings of the Royal Society of Medicine*, **53**, 416–420.

PEREZ, C. A. (1970) in *Frontiers of Radiation Therapy and Oncology*, vol. 5, ed. Vaeth, J., Karger, Basel and New York, 20.

PHILLIPS, R. (1942) *Proceedings of the Royal Society of Medicine*, **35**, 768–770.

RODRIGUEZ-ANTUNEZ, A., CHERNAK, E. S., JELDEN, G. L. and HUNTER, T. W. (1973) *Radiology*, **108**, 689–690.

ROUSSELOT, L. M., COLE, D. R., GROSSI, C. E., CONTE, A. J., GONZALEZ, E. M. and PASTERNACK, B. S. (1968) *American Journal of Surgery*, **115**, 140–147.

SCOTT, O. (1973) *British Medical Bulletin*, **29**, 59–62.

SLANEY, G. (1971) in *Modern Trends in Surgery*, **115**, 140–147.

STEARNS, M. W., DEDDISH, M. R. and QUAN, S. H. Q. (1959) *Surgery, Gynaecology and Obstetrics*, **109**, 225–229.

STEARNS, M. W., DEDDISH, M. R. and QUAN, S. H. Q. (1968) *Diseases of the Colon and Rectum*, **11**, 281–284.

STEWART, T. H. M. (1969) *Cancer*, **23**, 1368–1387.

SYMONDS, C. J. (1913–14) *Proceedings of the Royal Society of Medicine*, **71**, 152.

URDANETA-LAFEE, N., KLIGERMAN, M. M., KNOWLTON, A. H. (1972) *Radiology*, **104**, 673–677.

VAIDYA, S. G., CHAUDRI, M. A., MORRISON, R. and WHAIT, D. (1970) *Lancet*, **ii**, 911–914.

WHITMORE, G. F. (1964) *American Review of Nuclear Science*, **14**, 347.

WILLIAMS, I. G. (1962) *Clinical Radiology*, **13**, 30–34.

WILLIAMS, I. G. and HORWITZ, H. (1956) *American Journal of Roentgenology*, **76**, 919–928.

CHAPTER TEN

Gynaecological Neoplasms

N. Howard and D. O'Connell

There have long been differences of opinion on the treatment of carcinoma of the cervix uteri, some centres favouring radiotherapy as the primary treatment, others preferring surgery. Even when surgery is performed, pre-operative radiotherapy is commonly used in the form of intracavitary irradiation. It is, however, agreed that the treatment of choice for carcinoma of the corpus uteri is by surgery, but again many centres employ pre-operative radiotherapy. Such intracavitary irradiation is widely used, either alone or combined with surgery. This is at present a major cause of stray radiation to staff and patients in hospital.

It is usually achieved by the use of ^{226}Ra, in tubes, packets or ovoids. The first popular technique originated in Paris in the early 1900s, the radium being inserted in cork and remaining *in situ* for five days. A later modification – the 'Stockholm technique' – utilises a metal intrauterine tube and flat silver boxes which are placed in the lateral fornices. A very popular and still widely used modification of the Paris technique – the 'Manchester' method – uses ovoids in the lateral fornices.

There has been great and widespread interest in attempts to reduce exposure from intracavitary irradiation. Indeed, the Faculty of Radiologists and the British Institute of Radiology have set up a working party on radium substitutes and after- and remote-loading techniques. Substitutes for radium which are being used are ^{137}Cs, ^{60}Co, and ^{192}Ir. These may be used as direct substitutes for radium and, although none is entirely suitable, caesium is probably the most popular, and will help to reduce the chances of stray radiation.

After-loading devices are used in several ways (Henschke, 1960; Henschke *et al.*, 1966; Chassagne, 1972). The Curietron was developed in Stockholm and uses conventional dosimetry and time (Walstam, 1965). The advantages derive from the absence of radioactive hazard, allowing manipulation of the source containers and their accurate positioning in relation to the tumour and other adjacent normal structures. This is achieved, we think, most effectively of all by the introduction of the machine known as the 'Cathetron' (O'Connell *et*

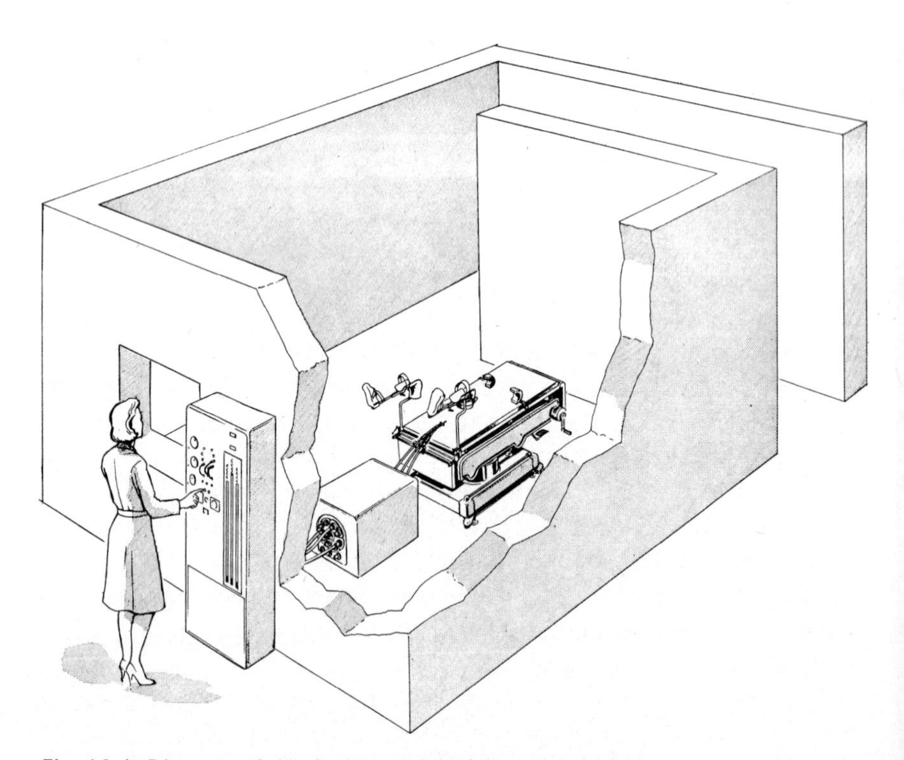

Fig. 10.1. Diagram of the Cathetron in a fully-protected room.

al., 1965; O'Connell, Howard, Joslin, Ramsey and Liversage, 1967; Liversage *et al.*, 1967; O'Connell, Howard and Joslin, 1967; Joslin *et al.*, 1967; Liversage, 1966, 1973). The Cathetron, unlike most other after-loading, remotely-controlled devices, makes use of a high dose-rate, employing ^{60}Co sources. It reduces the treatment time to only a few minutes instead of several hours or days, and allows the use of a fully-protected treatment room (Fig. 10.1). This new technique for the treatment of carcinoma of the uterus will be discussed in terms of the rationale of its introduction and design, its physical and radiobiological basis and its clinical use.

We should point out that the Cathetron is used in the treatment of tumours of the oesophagus, antrum and other cavities, and the skin, but these will not be discussed in this chapter.

Intent

The idea of after-loading was based on the necessity for protection of personnel from radiation hazard. In 1963–4 the possibility of using high dose-rates in after-loading for clinical purposes was identified, the specification written, and the system designed and developed by Charing Cross Hospital Radiotherapy Department, and TEM Ltd, Crawley. The necessary money for the prototype was generously provided by the Sembal Trust. Subsequently at our request, the Ministry of Health (now DHSS) supplied money for six machines, and set up a working party under Sir Brian Windeyer. This party approved the design and the prototype was completed. There have been no fundamental changes in design since that period, but improvements have been made in the design of parts such as the catheter stabilisers and the rectal spacers. The necessary preliminary clinical work was done at Charing Cross Hospital and involved considerable new work with regard to ethics, radiobiology, and safety factors, both mechanical and radiological.

All low dose-rate systems, intracavitary radium and caesium, the Cervitron and the Curietron suffer from a common drawback; personnel and other patients receive some dose of radiation. Even when employing sophisticated equipment such as the Curietron and Cervitron, where the nurse can withdraw the sources to the safe at the touch of a button, measurable doses of radiation may be received. Gynaecological radium is the major source of stray radiation in hospitals and this hazard is in practice related to one factor – the dose-rate at which the system operates.

If one uses high-intensity sources, times are reduced to minutes instead of a day or days and treatment can be given in a protective room, thereby completely eliminating the radiation hazard. At Charing Cross Hospital radiation received by personnel during set-up and treatment is so low that it is not measurable even by thermo-luminescent-dosimetry.

This system, the only one of its type, has several advantages apart from the lack of measurable radiation hazard to personnel.

1. Anaesthetics. We give three general anaesthetics for our system of radium over a period of three weeks; none is given for the Cathetron system (apart from the initial assessment), merely Pethidine or Valium for the nulliparous and the nervous. (This also reduces the admittedly small hazard of Halothane jaundice which we have seen twice in radium cases.)

2. For the above reason, and because of the short treatment times, patients can be and are dealt with on an outpatient basis. Very few have been inpatients.

3. Because there is no hazard, there is no hurry to place the source applicators. One inserts the catheters, and only when they are in the ideal position, as judged by direct vision and by rectal dose readings from monitoring sources, does one leave the room and cause the treatment sources to be motored from the safe into their respective catheters.

4. Joelsson and Bäckström (1969) showed that in using gauze packing (whether dry or greasy) to lift the vaginal radium sources off the rectum, there was an average increase of 26 per cent (50 per cent in two cases) in the rectal dose-rate between the beginning and the end of treatment. This is because of compression of the packing during succeeding hours by the weight of the ovoids. With a short treatment time, solid spacers can be tolerated by the patient and will allow a constant dose-rate to the anterior rectal wall (Fig. 10.2). Accurate model reconstruction of the relative positions of the Cathetron sources

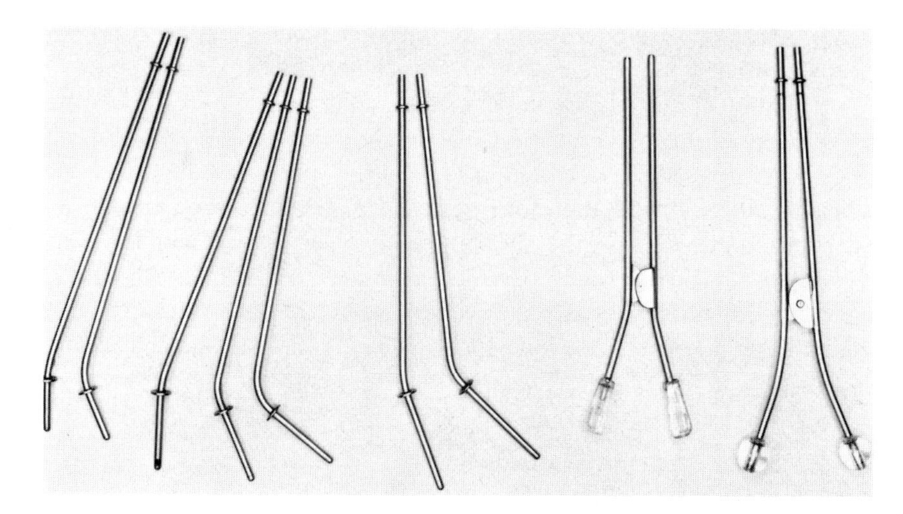

Fig. 10.2. Catheters, showing spacers and ovoids.

from six consecutive insertions showed that there was little change in their positions. Similar reconstruction of radium insertions shows that it is uncommon to achieve and maintain symmetrical and reproducable accuracy with sources which are not firmly stabilised by an external agency. This external stabilisation can be tolerated by the patient for only a limited period, but without it the sources tend to wander. With low dose-rates, therefore, one would expect variation from the original set-up in the uterus and vagina. With high dose-rate sources, they remain where placed for the short period necessary for the treatment.

Design

Any new treatment technique involves problems of design, dosage and clinical assessment and must be compared with current concepts and existing techniques. At Charing Cross Hospital it has been the practice for many years, for the treatment of carcinoma of the cervix, to use the Manchester distribution of radium sources (Tod and Meredith, 1953), but with a slightly increased loading allowing a total dose of 6000 rad to be given to point A in three 24-hour insertions spaced one and two weeks apart or, pre-operatively, a single 48-hour insertion for both cervix and body of uterus.

Irradiation for extensive involvement of the vagina by tumour was carried out by means of a cylindrical perspex vaginal colpostat, loaded to give a dose of the order or 6000 rad at 0·5 cm in 6 days.

The Cathetron was therefore designed to produce the same dose-distribution, to reduce the difficulties involved in introducing new techniques and to allow comparison of the new techniques with a well-established method. Three stainless steel catheters are accurately positioned in the patient – one in the uterine cavity and one in each fornix,

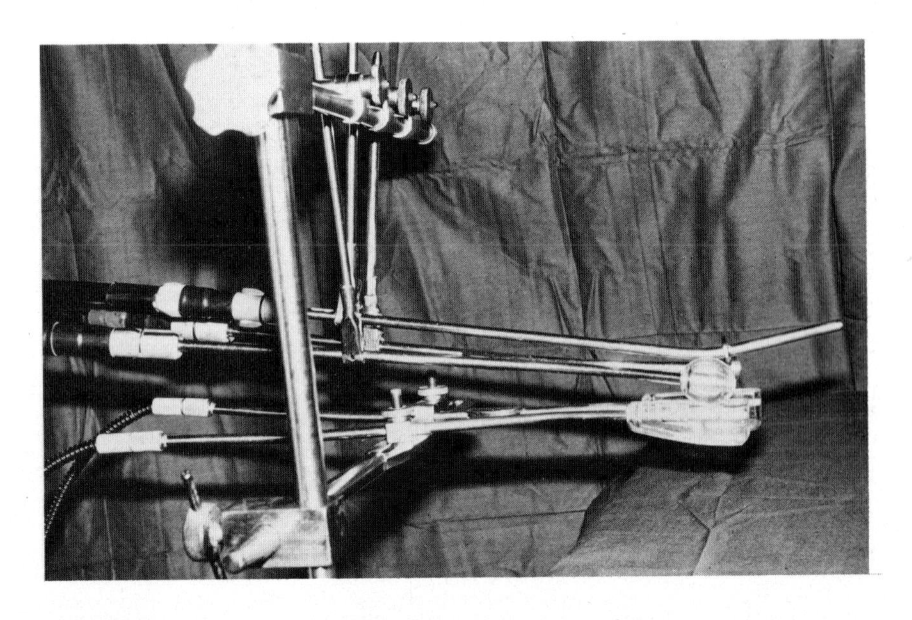

Fig. 10.3. Treatment set-up, showing solid Perspex spacers.

and each sitting on a solid perspex spacer to separate it from the rectum (Fig. 10.3). The pre-selected sources, attached to drive cables, are driven out of the storage container to the ends of the stainless steel catheters placed within the patient. The sources are driven out independently by three separate electric motors and are automatically returned

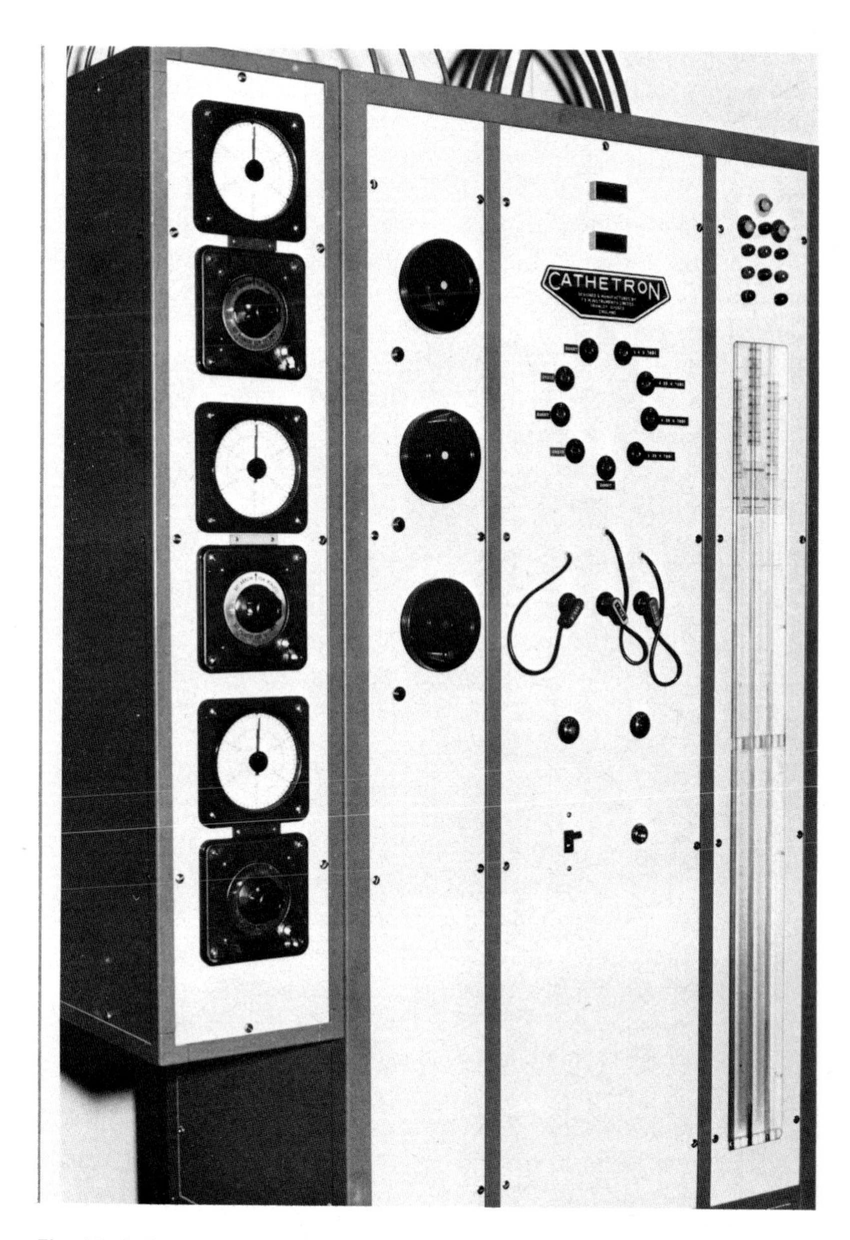

Fig. 10.4. Control panel.

to the storage container at the end of the pre-set treatment time. Indicators are mechanically linked to the source pencils and show their positions in their traverse at any moment. The sources are brought to rest at the end of the catheters by mechanical stops and springs, and may be drawn back a prescribed distance from the ends of the catheters by an over-riding manual control, should this be required (Fig. 10.4). Count-up and count-down times measure the amount of time–dose to be given and the amount actually given. In the event of a power failure the sources are automatically returned to the storage container by a gravity-controlled mechanism. A system of mechanical and electrical interlocks ensures safety in that it is impossible to expose a source unless all connections are completed correctly. A door interlock switch is incorporated in this circuit.

Design of Catheters and Source-pencils

Three slender steel catheters are used, one in the uterine canal and one in each fornix. The latter are enclosed in perspex ovoids to distend the vagina, reduce the surface dose, and enlarge the volume of tissue to be treated. The proximal ends of the catheters may be pressed together to separate the ovoids. There are three sizes of ovoid to match the Manchester system: small 2·0 cm, medium 2·5 cm and large 3·0 cm diameter.

The uterine tube catheters are fitted with stainless steel flanges at 10·25, 8·25, 4·25 or 2·4 cm from their closed ends. Above the flange the catheters are bent through angles of 0°, 20°, 40°, 60° or 80° round a radius of curvature of 3 cm, and are then straight for the remainder of their length. A uterine tube catheter is selected to suit the requirements of the individual patient. A reference line on the wall of the catheter at the junction with the cable allows the orientation of the uterine tube to be checked after insertion.

The angles chosen were developed as a result of many trial runs using perspex catheters in patients at the time of radium insertions. A selection is therefore available so that distortion and damage to tissues is avoided. The catheters, of rigid stainless steel, are all 33·75 cm long, 6·4 mm outer diameter and 0·5 mm wall thickness. The overall dimensions of all the source-pencils are identical, as are the drive cables, so

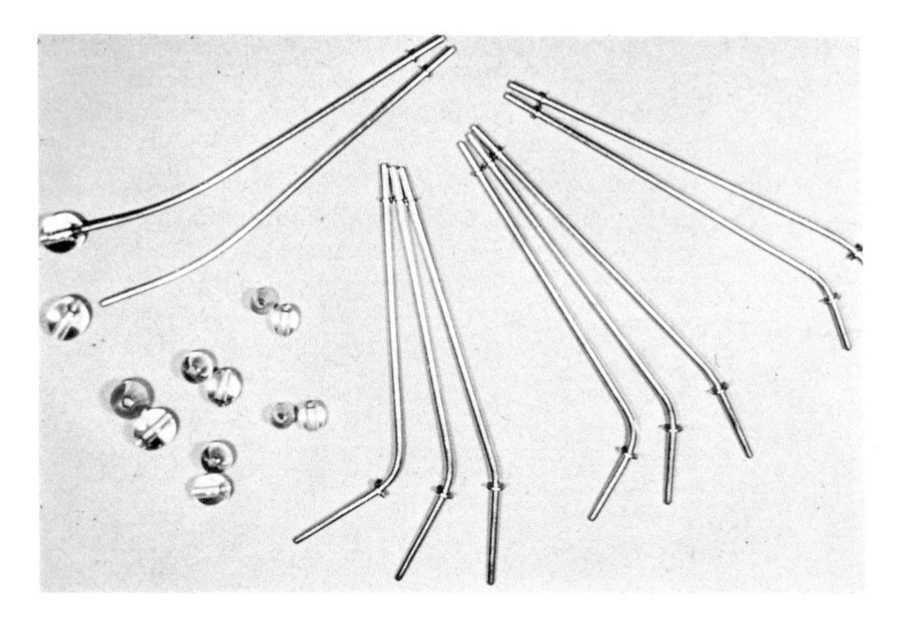

Fig. 10.5. Selection of catheters and ovoids.

that any catheter will accept any combination of source-pencil and drive cable. Some of the catheters available are shown in Fig. 10.5; the catheter diameter is no wider than that of existing uterine radium tubes, so that the degree of dilatation of the cervical canal needs to be no more than is currently necessary for radium (Hegar No. 7). The required overall length catheter was assessed in patients by using model catheters, but in the light of clinical experience it is now considered that the overall length could be reduced by a few centimetres.

Each source-pencil contains a number of stainless steel cylindrical source-capsules which have hemispherical ends. Their overall length is 8·0 mm, outer diameter 3·2 mm and wall thickness 0·5 mm. Each capsule contains a ^{60}Co solid cylindrical source of length 4·75 mm and diameter 1·6 mm. The cobalt is clad in nickel of thickness of 0·26 mm. In order to make up a source-pencil, the capsules and spacers required are loaded into a closed-ended helical spring 12 cm long made from cylindrical steel wire of diameter 0·61 mm. Before fixing this source-pencil to a section of flexible steel cable, a short length of compression spring is introduced. The latter is stronger than the outer spring which becomes extended 6 mm on final assembly. This is an aid to source-position accuracy.

The Radiochemical Centre (Amersham) supply the ^{60}Co sources, assemble the source-pencils and load them into the storage container (Fig. 10.6), which consists essentially of a lead sphere 53 cm in

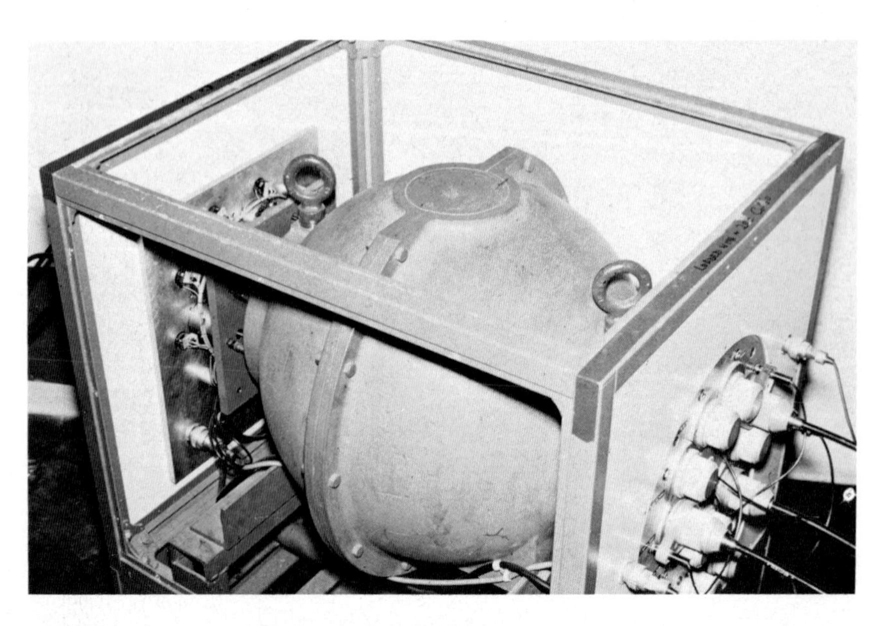

Fig. 10.6. Storage container for cobalt sources.

diameter. Nine stainless steel tubes (curved to prevent direct leakage of radiation) pass through this sphere and, when in the safe position, one source-pencil assembly rests in each tube so that the active portion lies near the centre of the sphere. The rear end of each source-pencil assembly just protrudes at the rear of the outer casing of the storage container and, by being coupled to any one of the three drive-cables, the source may be driven forward along the supply tube and into an attached catheter.

The feasibility of using ^{137}Cs sources was considered but, at the time the sources were ordered, and still today, the maximum activity that the Radiochemical Centre could safely insert into a standard source-capsule was only about 250 Ci, equivalent to about 90 mg of radium. Two such capsules could be placed in an ovoid source-pencil to give a total of 180 mg radium equivalent per ovoid. Thus, with caesium, dose-rates would be only nine times greater than with the radium sources in use at Manchester, and the time to deliver 1000 rad to point A would be approximately two hours. This time was not acceptable for the reasons already mentioned.

The Radiobiological Basis of the Cathetron

It seemed obvious, during the initial concept of and discussion about the Cathetron, that it would be impracticable to leave the sources *in situ* for the usual 24 hours of the Manchester system. The patient could not remain in the lithotomy position and connected to the machine for 24 hours, whether conscious or anaesthetised. The loading of the apparatus was designed to deliver the dose usually given by a 24-hour radium insertion in 15 minutes – that is, one hundred times faster. There was little clinical evidence, or indeed theoretical or experimental evidence, available at that time to allow an assessment to be made of the biological effects of doses delivered in a few minutes instead of 24 hours. While there is little dose-rate effect in the range 1–600 rad/min, an appreciable dose-rate effect exists at dose-rates less than 10 rad/min. (Thomson and Tourtelotte, 1953; Mitchell, 1960).

Measurements of the LD_{50} for mice by Joslin *et al.* (1967) confirmed that there was a dose-rate difference. They found that in mice the RBE for a single fifteen-minute irradiation compared with a single 24-hour irradiation was 1·6 for 30-day death and 1·8 for 4-day death.

Theoretical calculations (Liversage 1966, 1967) suggested that the relative biological efficiency of a fractionated high dose-rate régime involving N fractions, compared with a low dose-rate continuous treatment lasting t hours, would be approximately equal to one if $N = t/4$ (e.g. 12 fractions at high dose-rate, or continuous irradiation lasting 48 hours, would require approximately the same total dose to produce equal effects). This theory predicted that the RBE would be greater than 1 if N were less than $t/4$, and that RBE would increase as the number of fractions was decreased.

Because of the uncertainties involved, and in order not to prejudice the patients' chance of cure and to prevent any undue morbidity, it was decided that initially radical treatments should not be given on the Cathetron but that its use should be confined to pre-operative treatments at levels less than radical, to be followed by Wertheim's hysterectomy.

The standard Charing Cross pre-operative radium treatment is to give 4000 rad to point A in 48 hours, or about 8000–10 000 rad to the upper vaginal wall. Calculations bases on cell-survival theory predicted that we should give the same dose, i.e. 4000 rad if we gave twelve fractions, but that we should give less than 4000 rad if we gave less than twelve fractions. How much less depended on which cell-survival curve was considered to be applicable to the tissues of interest. The calculations were thus performed for a number of different cell-survival curves. Predictions based on Barendson's cell-survival curve are closer to the clinical results than predictions based on any other cell-survival curve considered.

For the Cathetron we chose six fractions as the most suitable number. From our clinical observations of vaginal reaction, it has now been established that six doses of 500 to 550 rad (total 3000–3300 rad) to point A in eleven or twelve days on the Cathetron produce approximately the same vaginal reaction as 4000 rad to point A from a single 48-hour radium insertion (i.e., under these conditions, an RBE of 1·2 to 1·3).

Carcinoma of the Cervix and Body of Uterus

A non-randomised trial was begun which consisted of a comparison between the effects of Cathetron irradiation with those of low-dose radium treatments. In effect, we were comparing in the short term the morbidity associated with each type of treatment, and in the long term the curative effects. It was obviously of considerable importance to be sure that we did not cause any harm to patients.

The radium equivalent was 4000 rad to point A in 48 hours, with our standard distribution of loading, i.e. 50 mg in the uterine tube and 25 mg in each ovoid. With the Cathetron we proceeded to give between 3000 and 3600 rad in six fractions to point A, over twelve days, using a similar distribution of radiation. This constituted a pre-operative treatment to each group of patients, after which we proceeded to Wertheim's or extended hysterectomy for carcinoma of the cervix and body respectively.

The degree of morbidity associated with each type of treatment varied considerably. Table 10.1 indicates the differences, and it would seem that the results in the series treated with the Cathetron were superior to those in the radium series.

Of the Cathetron group, there were six instances of morbidity affecting the operation: three of excessive bleeding, two of adhesions and one vesico-vaginal fistula. Post-operative complications included five cases of wound prolapse and one of pulmonary embolus. One remote complication was an incisional hernia.

There was more trouble with the radium-treated patients. Seven cases of fibrosis caused modification of the intended Wertheim's operation, and one case of haemorrhage necessitated ligature of the internal iliac vein. Post-operatively, there were two cases of fatal haemorrhage, two of deep vein thrombosis, two of wound sepsis, one of ileus and one of intestinal obstruction. There were seven cases of remote complications: uretero-vaginal fistulae, two; pelvic fibrosis, one; urinary stress incontinence, two; lymphocysts, two.

Although one hesitates to draw conclusions from what is necessarily a partially controlled trial, nevertheless there seems to be a difference between the two groups. It would seem that this is due to the fact that the Cathetron system allows accurate and ideal placement of the sources, the set-up being maintained throughout each treatment, which lasts about ten minutes. By contrast, radium sources are necessarily placed as speedily as possible and it may not therefore be as easy to achieve an ideal situation. As Joelsson and Bäckström (1969) have shown, over 24 hours the posterior vaginal packing decreases in thickness and therefore the ovoids tend to wander, and unless the uterine tube is stitched into position it tends to emerge. Over 48 hours, the situation deteriorates still further. It would seem that there is a

Table 10.1 Complications following pre-operative treatment by Cathetron and by low-dose radium

Treatment stage	*Cathetron*	*Radium*
Radiotherapy	nil	1. Fibrosis delayed operation for 250 days
Operation	*Average 2·0 pt blood transfusion* 1. Bleeding limited operation to extended hysterectomy instead of Wertheim 2. Bilateral salpingo oophorectomy only possible due to fibrosis 3. Bladder perforation healed in three months	*Average 3·18 pt blood transfusion* 1. Rectal perforation/colostomy 2. Resection rectum/ re-implanted ureter 3. Excised and re-implanted ureter 4. Excised and re-implanted ureter 5. Bladder perforation/healed 3/52 6. Bleeding internal iliac vein ligated ('Fibrosis' quoted cause in first five)
Post-operative	1. Abdominal wound dehiscence 2. Abdominal wound dehiscence 3. Abdominal wound dehiscence 4. Abdominal wound dehiscence 5. Abdominal wound dehiscence 6. Vaginal vault dehiscence 7. Pulmonary embolus (non-fatal)	1. Wound sepsis 2. Wound sepsis 3. Wound sepsis and partial dehiscence 4. Ileus 5. Partial intestinal obstruction 6. DVT/anticoagulation 7. DVT/anticoagulation 8. DVT/anticoagulation/Fatal haemorrhage 25th day 9. Fatal haemorrhage right common iliac vein 9th day
Remote	1. Incisional hernia	1. Uretero-vaginal fistula 2. Uretero-vaginal fistula 3. Fibrosis – non-function kidney 4. Urinary stress incontinence 5. Urinary stress incontinence 6. Abdomino-pelvic lymphocysts (required surgical drainage) 7. Inguinal lymphocyst (surgically drained) 8. Intestinal obstruction

clear-cut advantage in using the Cathetron here; one can give the same, or a higher, relative dose to point A, without increasing morbidity.

Table 10.2. Residual Carcinoma in Hysterectomy Specimen

	Cervix	*Endometrium*
Cathetron	11/18	18/28
Radium	8/13	20/24

Note: Attempts to separate 'viable' and 'non-viable' tumours are not useful or meaningful.

In this trial, the hysterectomy specimens were examined consistently by two pathologists in an endeavour to ascertain the degree of residual carcinoma. As may be seen from Table 10.2, in treatment to the cervix the difference in results was minimal, but for the body of the uterus pre-operative Cathetron treatment gave a greater number of cases where the tumour was eliminated from the primary site. A large dose may be given to the cervix by either method, and while the radium dose may be deficient it is still high enough to kill the tumour. On the other hand, the apparently less successful results of radium treatment of carcinoma of the body may be explained by a reduction of dose to the wall of the uterus due to displacement of sources, which does not happen with the Cathetron.

Carcinoma Involving the Vagina

Irradiation of tumours in the vagina, primary or secondary, or treatment of the vaginal vault following surgery for carcinoma of the body of uterus, has for over seventy years been carried out by the insertion of radium into the cavity. For over twenty years, the most popular method has been by using a cylindrical perspex colpostat, loaded along its central axis with radium tubes (Dobbie, 1953). It usually contains 50 mg and is inserted, often under general anaesthesia, and held in place by a suture through the labia. The dose is of the order of 6000 rad at 0·5 cm in 6 days, during which time the patient remains in hospital and in bed. The dose is predetermined in the light of past experience, and is hopefully correct for the tumour in that particular patient, but allows no flexibility.

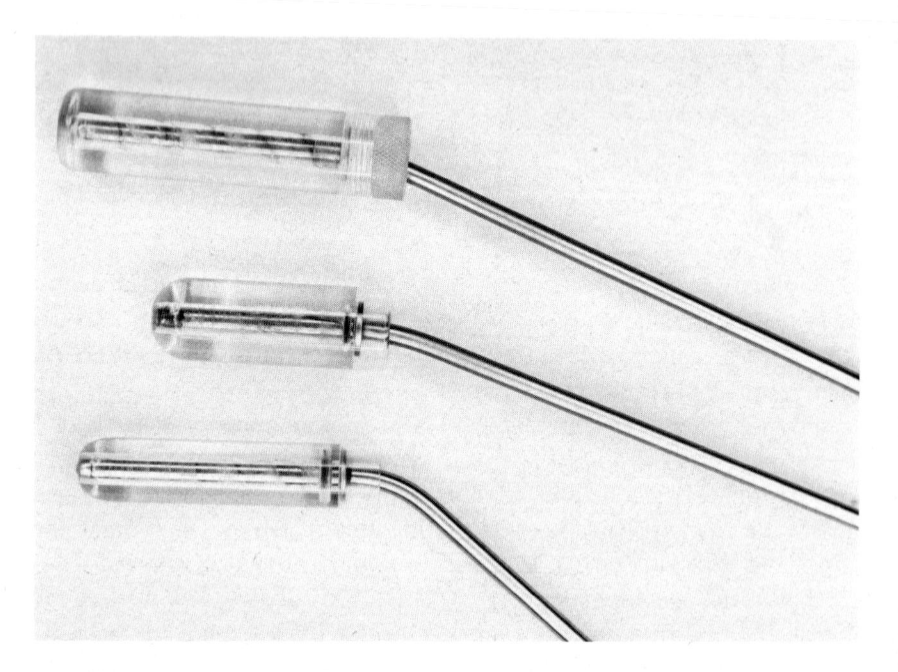

Fig. 10.7. Colpostat.

In the Cathetron system, the colpostat used is based on the radium method (Fig. 10.7). The patient is treated from home and needs no general anaesthesia or analgesia. Treatments are given every few days, delivering doses of between 500 and 1000 rad at 0·5 cm in each fraction. Treatment times are generally for a few minutes and seldom longer than 15 minutes. The total dose depends on reaction and response, as does the fractionation of dosage. Patients are treated in a fully-protected room, there being no radiation exposure to personnel.

Clinical Applications

Since 1966, we have treated 60 patients with tumour in the vagina from a variety of causes. The vagina is treated by intra-cavity irradiation:

(a) for primary tumours of the vagina;
(b) as adjuvant therapy in the radiation treatment of Stage III or Stage IV carcinoma of the cervix where the lower vaginal wall is involved;
(c) for recurrence in the vagina of a tumour from any site;
(d) post-operatively, for carcinoma of the body of uterus.

Primary Carcinoma of the Vagina

Primary carcinoma of the vagina is a rare disease; there were 120 deaths in the United Kingdom in 1971 (Registrar General, 1971). We have treated nine patients between 1966 and 1973, of whom five died between seven months and 28 months after Cathetron irradiation. However, four patients have survived between 17 months and 6½ years. The numbers are too small for statistical analysis, but the results are encouraging: the other advantages have been described already.

The first two of these patients were treated in 1966 and 1967 with seven fractions in 15 days to a dose of 3000 rad, and eight fractions in 16 days to a dose of 4400 rad. The second patient, though alive and well and apparently cured, had a necrotic ulcer at the introitus which caused much suffering. It was treated symptomatically and eventually healed – but took two years to do so. Apart from the reasons stated above, this patient provided another reason for our preference for a longer overall time. She herself is now delighted with the result, is leading a normal married life, and remains on good terms with her doctors!

We have recently treated a patient with a very rare lesion of the vagina. This lady of 73 presented in February 1973 with a profuse and irritating vaginal discharge. She was seen by several gynaecologists and had several examinations under anaesthetic, and several biopsies. All showed chronic inflammation only, but the patient's suffering steadily increased. It was eventually thought, in despair, that an hysterectomy would be necessary to stop the discharge and find the diagnosis. One last biopsy was taken and showed a lymphosarcoma. Cathetron irradiation was started on 10 October 1973, using an 8 cm colpostat and 6·25 cm source. Insertion on the first two occasions was difficult, but as the tumours shrunk and the discharge diminished it became very simple. At the end of treatment on 8 November 1973, after five fractions and 3750 rad at 0·5 cm in 30 days, there was no tumour and virtually no discharge. She died ten months later of disseminated disease.

Adjuvant Therapy

Cathetron and vaginal irradiation has been used as an adjuvant to treatment in ten patients with Stage III carcinoma of the cervix and two patients with Stage IV tumours. Of those with Stage III tumours, four are alive between 20 months and $5\frac{1}{2}$ years, and five are dead, having survived between 7 months and 2 years and 9 months. One patient was pregnant and died post-operatively. One Stage IV patient is alive after $2\frac{1}{2}$ years and the other died after fifteen months.

In all these patients, other forms of treatment – external irradiation and sometimes radium – were also used, as one would expect with these extensive tumours, but the Cathetron colpostat was most useful in clearing vaginal extension of tumour in some cases. If the tumour extends into the lower third of the vagina it is beyond the reach of a conventional radium insertion and difficult to clear with external irradiation.

Secondary Vaginal Deposits

Twenty-three patients with secondary deposits in the vagina have been treated by the Cathetron colpostat. As might be expected, most died, surviving between 3 months and 3 years and 9 months (eight out of eighteen survived more than one year). However, four are alive, one with tumour, between 7 months and 2 years. Of these secondaries, nine originated in the corpus uteri, seven in the cervix, two in the bladder, and one in the urethra, colon, rectum and ovary; in one the primary was unknown.

Carcinoma of Body of Uterus

Twelve patients have been treated post-operatively for carcinoma of body of uterus. Although our gynaecological colleagues and we our-selves prefer pre-operative irradiation, this is not always possible, and sometimes the carcinoma is found unexpectedly at histological examination of the operative specimen. In one patient the narrowness of the introitus and vagina made pre-operative intra-cavity irradiation impossible.

Of these twelve patients, ten are alive, well and free of disease for periods from six months to six years and ten months. Seven patients were treated more than two years ago. Two patients were also treated with cobalt irradiation to the pelvis. Two patients died 13 and 14 months after treatment. One, who also had cobalt therapy to the pelvis, had a Grade IV tumour.

The dose and fractionation used varied from 500 rad at 0·5 cm in one fraction, when used with cobalt, to 4500 rad on six fractions in four weeks. Unlike Joslin, who originally worked with us at Charing Cross Hospital and helped us with the introduction of the Cathetron, but who now prefers successive daily treatments of the order of 3000 rad in five fractions in five days (Joslin and Smith, 1971), we tend to use once-weekly fractions of 500 or 700 rad, four to six fractions, and an overall time of three to five weeks. We find that this is more convenient for outpatients (and for staff), and dosage can be readily and accurately adjusted to the reaction, which is much more difficult if the treatment is completed within a few days.

Our thanks are due to Dr W. E. Liversage for constant help and criticism, to Miss P. Turnbull for the plates, and to Miss C. E. Paxton for typing and re-typing the chapter without complaint.

References

CHASSAGNE, D. (1972) in *After-loading in Radiotherapy*, ed. Simon, N. Conference Proceedings, New York, May 1971, 53–59.

DOBBIE, B. M. W. (1953) *Journal of Obstetrics and Gynaecology of the British Empire*, **60**, 702–705.

HENSCHKE, U. K. (1960) *Radiology*, **74**, 834.

HENSCHKE, U. K., HILARIS, B. S. and MAHAN, G. D. (1966) *American Journal of Roentgenology*, **96**, 45–51.

JOELSSON, I. and BÄCKSTRÖM, A. (1969) *Acta radiologica (Therapy, Physics, Biology)*, **8**, 343–359.

JOSLIN, C. A. F., RAMSEY, N. W. and ANDREWS, H. J. (1967) *British Journal of Radiology*, **40**, 627–630.

JOSLIN, C. A. and SMITH, C. W. (1971) *Clinical Radiology*, **22**, 118–124.
LIVERSAGE, W. E. (1966) *British Journal of Radiology*, **39**, 338–349.
LIVERSAGE, W. E. (1967) *British Journal of Radiology*, **40**, 394–395.
LIVERSAGE, W. E. (1973) *Proceedings of the Royal Society of Medicine*, **66**, 940–941.
LIVERSAGE, W. E., MARTIN-SMITH, P. and RAMSEY, N. W. (1967) *British Journal of Radiology*, **40**, 895–904.
MITCHELL, J. S. (1960) *Studies in Radiotherapeutics*. Blackwell, Oxford, 234.
O'CONNELL, D., HOWARD, N. and JOSLIN, C. A. (1967) *British Journal of Radiology*, **40**, 895–904.
O'CONNELL, D., HOWARD, N., JOSLIN, C. A., RAMSEY, N. W. and LIVERSAGE, W. E. (1965) *Lancet*, **2**, 570–571.
O'CONNELL, D., HOWARD, N., JOSLIN, C. A., RAMSEY, N. W. and LIVERSAGE, W. E. (1967) *British Journal of Radiology*, **40**, 882–887.
REGISTRAR GENERAL (1971) *Statistical Review for England and Wales*. HMSO, London.
THOMSON, J. F. and TOURTELOTTE, W. W. (1953) *American Journal of Roentgenology*, **69**, 826.
TOD, M. and MEREDITH, W. J. (1953) *British Journal of Radiology*, **26**, 252–257.
WALSTAM, R. (1962) *Physics in Medicine and Biology*, **7**, 225–228.
WALSTAM, R. (1965) *Acta radiologica*, Suppl. 236.

CHAPTER ELEVEN

Tumours of the Male Urogenital Tract

C. R. H. Penn

The management of urogenital malignancy offers considerable opportunities for the close liaison between urologists, radiologists, pathologists and radiotherapists. These opportunities present both in the essential initial assessment of nature and extent of tumour and in the combination of treatment modalities. Facilities for joint assessment of new cases and joint follow-up are of great value in improving the care of these patients, particularly with carcinoma of the bladder.

Testis

Testicular tumours account for 1–2 per cent of all malignant tumours of men, with an annual incidence of 2–3 per 100 000 men (Blandy, 1966). The commoner testicular tumours can be subdivided into the seminomas and the teratomas. The former present classically between the age of 30 and 40, while the latter present 10 years earlier, in the 20s. Both lesions tend to spread early via lymphatics, shortly followed by blood stream.

Many attempts at histological classification of these lesions have been made. That most widely accepted in the United Kingdom is the British Testicular Tumours Panel and Registry (TTPR) Classification

(Pugh, 1973). In the United States the classification of Dixon and Moore (1952) is widely used and the divergences between these classifications, as summarised in Table 11.1 for the more common tumours, account for the difficulty in evaluating the European and North American approaches to these lesions.

Table 11.1. Comparison of British and United States classifications of commoner testicular tumours (after Blandy *et al.* (1970))

TTPR			DIXON and MOORE	
Seminoma			Seminoma pure	Group I
Teratoma				
Teratoma differentiated	(TD)		Teratoma pure or with seminoma	Group III
Malignant teratoma intermediate				
—	MTIA		Teratoma pure or mixed	Group IV
—	MTIB	MTU*		
Malignant teratoma anaplastic	(MTA)	MTU*	Embryonal carcinoma	Group II
Malignant teratoma trophoblastic	(MTT)		Chorion carcinoma	Group II
Combined tumour				
Seminoma and teratoma			Teratoma with seminoma	Group III

*Malignant teratoma undifferentiated (Pugh, 1973)

Staging

The TNM system of staging testicular tumours is summarised in Table 11.2.

Blandy's staging system is summarised in Table 11.3. It appears to have considerable relevance in determining treatment policy and is fairly well correlated with results obtained. There is considerable assumption of occult metastases in this classification but there is satisfactory evidence that this is justified.

Table 11.2. TNM system of staging testicular tumours (UICC, 1973)

T_0	No evidence of primary tumour
T_1	Tumour occupying less than one half of the testis and surrounded by a palpably normal gland
T_2	Tumour occupying one half or more of the testis but not producing enlargement or deformity of the testis
T_3	Tumour confined to the testis but producing enlargement or deformity of the testis
T_4	(a) Tumour extending to epididymis only
	(b) Tumour extending to other structures
N_a	Regional nodes impossible to assess
N_0	No deformity of regional nodes on lymphography
N_1	Regional nodes deformed on lymphography
N_2	Fixed palpable abdominal nodes
M_0	No evidence of distant metastases
M_1	Distant metastases present, including lymph nodes outside the abdomen

Table 11.3. Staging of testicular tumours (after Blandy *et al.* (1970))

Stage I	T_1–T_4, N_0, M_0: assume occult metastases in abdomen and pelvis (T_4 tumours necessitate different local treatment from T_1–T_3 lesions)
Stage II	T_1–T_4, N_1–N_2, M_0: assume occult metastases in mediastinum and supraclavicular fossae
Stage III	T_1–T_4, N_1–N_2, M_1
IIIA	Involved nodes in supraclavicular fossa: assume occult metastases in mediastinum and abdominal nodes
IIIA	Involved nodes in supraclavicular fossa and mediastinum: assume occult metastases in abdominal nodes
IIIB	Metastases in lung fields alone: assume occult metastases in mediastinum, supraclavicular fossae and abdominal nodes
IIIC	All the above areas demonstrably involved

Investigation

Orchidectomy is an essential first stage in establishing the diagnosis of a possible testicular tumour. It is the only way of providing an exact histological diagnosis and further removes a source of metastases. Since an intact tunica albuginea provides a very effective barrier to involvement of the scrotal lymphatics by the tumour, it is mandatory that the testicle is exposed through an inguinal incision. If this precaution is observed and there has been no previous surgery to the scrotum and tunica, such as an orchidopexy, it is possible to spare the scrotum and contralateral testis in post-operative treatment and thus avoid sterilisation. Once the scrotum is incised the prognosis is considerably worse, due to early lymphatic involvement (Blandy *et al.*, 1970).

Full radiography of the chest is essential, including lateral views and tomograms of the mediastinum. Whole lung tomography is indicated if there is any suspicion of intrapulmonary lesions. The para-aortic nodes should be investigated with at least an intravenous pyelogram which should demonstrate ureteric displacement from involvement of these nodes.

Lymphography can be of considerable value in the management of testicular tumours. It permits more definite staging where a positive lymphogram would indicate irradiation of the mediastinum and the supraclavicular fossae as well as the pelvic and para-aortic nodes. It also permits more accurate treatment planning, particularly in the region of the para-aortic lymph nodes where the margin between treating nodes and avoiding kidneys is often very narrow.

A pre-treatment lymphogram permits observation of the response of involved nodes to irradiation; persistence of these nodes, particularly in teratoma, may necessitate retroperitoneal node dissection.

Lymphography also opens up the possibility of intra-lymphatic radiotherapy, although the traditional difficulties in using this technique to deal with formed masses of tumour, and the good results already obtained with conventional radiotherapy for the more sensitive tumours, make this of doubtful value.

A further radiological technique which has been advocated is inferior vena cavography. This demonstrates large masses of lymph nodes by virtue of their compression of the inferior vena cava, but otherwise appears rather less sensitive than lymphography. It may be of value where a large mass of lymph nodes has caused a complete lymphatic block and it is desired to investigate the state of the nodes above the level of the block.

The blood count and electrolyte and urea estimation are of value, particularly in view of the contemplated wide-field irradiation. Hormone studies, such as the pregnancy test, have been associated for some years with the investigation of testicular tumours, particularly the teratomas, and there is evidence that a positive AZ test is an indicator of a poor prognosis. Blandy *et al.* (1970) found a high incidence of MTIB and MTA lesions, usually with metastases, associated with the positive pregnancy test, although a negative test was of no prognostic significance.

Table 11.4. Treatment Policy for Testicular Tumours

Stage I	T_1–T_{4a}, N_0, M_0: simple orchidectomy and post-operative DXT to pelvic and para-aortic nodes, sparing scrotum and contralateral testis.
Stage I	T_{4b}, N_0, M_0, and if the scrotum has been opened surgically: orchidectomy and removal of involved scrotum, and post-operative DXT to pelvic, para-aortic and inguinal nodes and scrotum (of necessity treating contralateral testis).
Stage II	T_1–T_{4b}, N_1, M_0: initial management as above followed after one month by prophylactic irradiation of mediastinum and supraclavicular fossae for seminomas, and for teratomas, if the abdominal nodes have responded well.
Stage IIIA	Irradiate mediastinum and supraclavicular fossae first. Review after one month and treat pelvic and para-aortic nodes at that time if no further distant metastases have developed and blood count permits.
Stages IIIB+C	Seminoma: attempt irradiation of all areas shown to contain tumour, possibly supplementing by cytotoxic drugs.
Stages IIIB+C	Teratoma: treatment is essentially palliative with irradiation to areas causing symptoms, possibly supplemented by cytotoxic drugs or hormones.

Treatment Policy

A suggested treatment policy is summarised in Table 11.4. It adopts an essentially European approach in withholding surgical dissection of the pelvic and para-aortic lymph nodes in teratomas of Stages T_1–T_3, N_0–N_1, M_0. No prospective controlled study has been undertaken to compare routine dissection and post-operative irradiation of these nodes with post-operative radiotherapy alone.

The problem of comparison is further complicated by most of the surgical series being reported from the United States, while most of the radiotherapy-alone series are from Europe, and the different histological classifications apply. However, Hope-Stone *et al.* (1963) restaged the then available London Hospital material according to the criteria of Dixon and Moore and achieved a five-year survival of 11 out of 16 (68·7 per cent) for teratoma Group IV. This can be compared with the surgical series of Patton *et al.* (1960), who achieved a five-year survival of 36 out of 66 (54·5 per cent).

A more recent review of the London Hospital series by Chapman *et al.* (1973) yielded a five-year survival of 33 out of 37 (89 per cent) for all cases graded as MTIA. These cases were treated without node dissection and these lesions appear to be reasonably comparable with the cases submitted to surgery in the North American centres, when one considers the high incidence of distant metastases in the MTIB and MTA grades. Further, the American series report a lower incidence of seminomas than the European series, the difference amounting to some 30 per cent; it is felt that if one-third of the patients in the European series did in fact have genuinely radioresistant lesions, the results should be substantially worse overall than the North American series, which they are not.

A radical orchidectomy involves major surgery of access with associated morbidity. Patton *et al.* (1960) report up to 27 per cent of patients as having an inoperable tumour once this access has been achieved. If successful surgery is performed, 75 per cent of patients are made impotent (Walsh *et al.*, 1971). Most of these patients receive post-operative radiotherapy, and in this context the surgery delays treatment, and carries with it a theoretical risk of adhesions which predispose to post-irradiation ulceration or necrosis of the small bowel.

Radical retroperitoneal node dissection may, however, be of considerable value in patients where, following radiotherapy, the lymphangiogram fails to show satisfactory regression of abdominal or pelvic lymph nodes, and where there is still no evidence of metastases above the diaphragm.

Radiotherapy Technique

The primary treatment of T_1–T_3, N_0 lesions, where the scrotum has not been breached surgically, aims to treat the pelvic and para-aortic lymph nodes of both sides in continuity (Fig. 11.1). This is simply achieved by a pair of parallel and opposed fields, shaped like an inverted T, and extending from the level of T9 above to the junction of the upper two-thirds and lower one-third of the obturator foramen below. The lateral extremities of the lower part of the field extend 2·5 cm wide of the margin of the true pelvis on each side, while the upper part of the field is narrowed to spare the kidneys. This part of the field particularly is most easily planned individually if a pre-operative lymphogram has been performed. In any case an IVP taken at the same time as the marker films is necessary to ensure that the kidneys are spared. The lower margin of the field is carefully adjusted to shield the scrotum, and lead blocks are used to shield the opposite testis. Treatment is delivered with a progressively rising dose over the first few fractions, and experience suggests that this precaution greatly increases the tolerance of the gastrointestinal tract and the bone marrow to the wide-field irradiation. Blood counts are monitored three times a week and the dose per fraction modified in the light of these.

In general, the proposed dose of 3000 rad for seminoma is delivered in four weeks or less. For teratomas the mid-line dose aimed for is 4000–4500 rad, and this is usually delivered in about five weeks. Dose on the remaining testicle is measured using a lithium fluoride dosemeter; experience with the London Hospital series has suggested that gonad doses of 50–200 rad only need be expected. If the primary tumour was T_{4b}, or if previous surgery has been performed on the scrotum or tunica, it is necessary to extend the lower part of the field to include both groups of inguinal nodes and the whole scrotum.

For lesions with N_1–N_2 more individually-planned fields are needed and it may be necessary for these fields to overlie part of one or both kidneys. Here again IVP marker films taken while the lymphogram

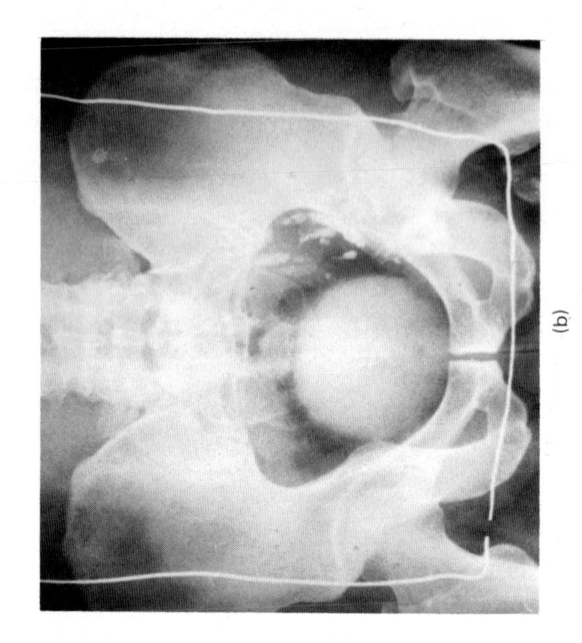

(b)

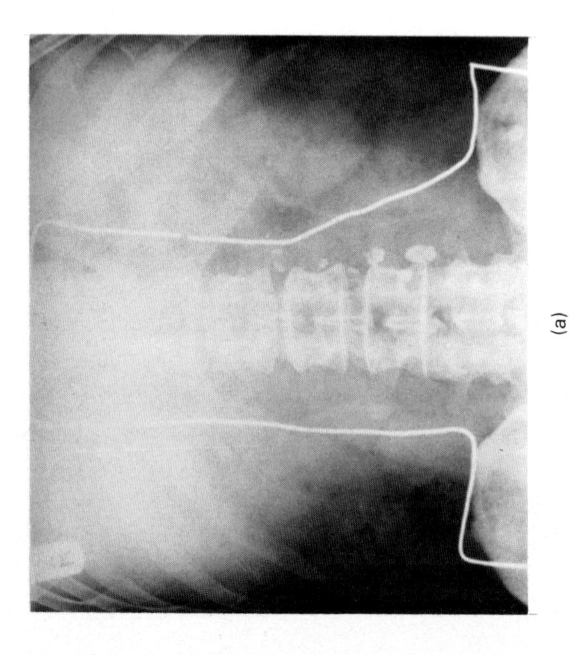

(a)

Fig. 11.1. a Marker film of upper end of treatment volume in post-operative irradiation of seminoma. Note adjustment to field to cover involved node. b Lower end of treatment volume in the same case.

contrast persists provide the simplest way of encompassing tumour with minimal damage to normal structures. Repeat X-rays of the abdomen after 2000 rad may suggest that there is sufficient shrinkage present for the fields to be further trimmed to reduce the volume of kidney taken to beyond tolerance.

For Stage II (T_1–T_4, N_1, M_0) tumours, prophylactic irradiation of the mediastinum and supraclavicular fossae using parallel and opposed anterior and posterior T-shaped fields should be given. This can be started one month after the completion of initial treatment, provided the blood count has returned to normal levels. The dose aimed for is 3000 rad in four weeks for seminoma, 4000 rad in 4 to 5 weeks for teratoma.

The treatment of disseminated pulmonary metastases from seminoma merits the use of 'chest bath' irradiation. Here large anterior and posterior opposed fields are used, accurately tailored to cover the lung fields, the mediastinum and the supraclavicular fossae. Because of the problems of pneumonitis and post-irradiation fibrosis, which would be lethal with the whole lung volume involved, the tumour-dose should not exceed 2500 rad delivered over a period of four weeks in 20 fractions, with a slow build-up of dose per fraction as before.

Side-effects

Normal tissues at risk include the preserved testis, the kidneys, the gastrointestinal tract, the marrow and the spinal cord. Sparing the opposite testis is felt to be justified: bilateral lesions occur in less than 2 per cent of cases (Whittle, 1957) and some of these have developed despite prophylactic irradiation of the opposite testicle. Regular follow-up with examination of the remaining testicle is obviously of value in this context; successful treatment of a new primary developing at that site has been reported (Blandy *et al.*, 1970). The preservation of fertility is obviously of value to an otherwise healthy young man, and is not considered unethical since the MRC Report (1956) suggests that the dose of 50–200 rad to the remaining testicle would add only 0·1 per cent to the present level of 7–8 per cent genetic mutations at the first generation. However, Smithers *et al.* (1973) suggest that contraceptive precautions are taken for a year after treatment.

The tolerance of the kidneys has been suggested as 2250 rad

delivered over five weeks (Luxton, 1953), and shielding as large a proportion as possible of the renal parenchyma beyond this dose is vital.

It is not possible to shield substantial volumes of gut and bone marrow. Treatment of the gut will result in nausea, anorexia and diarrhoea in a proportion of cases, but this is minimised by using a slow build-up of dose per fraction and can be usefully palliated with Torecan, Maxolon or pyridoxine for the former and mist. kaolin et morphine or Lomotil for the latter. Bone marrow depression by wide-field irradiation is a greater hazard: blood counts must be recorded frequently and dose-rate adjusted, or even treatment stopped, if the total white cell count falls below 3000 and the platelet count below 100 000. The use of anabolic steroids such as Deca-Durabolin or Anapolon may be of value in this context.

In some cases a very rapid fall in blood count may prevent the treatment of the whole of the para-aortic and pelvic nodes in one volume. Here, treatment may have to be divided by treating the para-aortic nodes first and subsequently treating the pelvic nodes with a matching field after the bone marrow has recovered. It is, however, difficult to match one field to the other without a gap or an overlap. A gap may allow tumour to escape treatment, while an overlap may damage the spinal cord, where tolerance has been described as 4500 rad in 5 weeks for the length of cord involved in this treatment volume (Boden, 1948). (See Chapter 4.)

Cytotoxic Drugs

A wide range of cytotoxic drugs used singly and in combination have been used in the management of metastatic testicular tumours. Useful regression of disease can be achieved in 50 per cent of cases (Foley *et al.*, 1972) although long-term response may only occur in 10 per cent (Bloom and Hendry, 1973).

Probably the most encouraging work with combined chemotherapy has been the use of VAM (vincristine, actinomycin D and methotrexate) with MTA teratomas. This is fairly ineffective on MTIA lesions. For disseminated lymphomas involving testis COP (cyclophosphamide, vincristine and prednisone) may be used. Bagshaw (1968) has treated MTT lesions with a régime similar to that for choriocarcinoma in women, using methotrexate with folinic acid rescue and actinomycin D.

Single-agent chemotherapy using Procarbazine has been advocated for seminoma as equally effective as combined treatment, simple to administrate and almost entirely non-toxic (Blandy *et al.*, 1970).

Hormone Therapy

With the fairly disappointing results of chemotherapy in disseminated testicular tumours in mind, the recent report by Bloom and Hendry (1973) of three cases out of a series of 16 who responded to hormone therapy in the form of medroxy progesterone acetate (Provera), 100 mg t.d.s. orally, is of great interest. One of these patients is alive and disease-free at 7 years from starting hormone therapy. This treatment is almost completely free from side-effects and merits further investigation.

Results

The London Hospital results for testicular tumours treated since 1950, using treatment techniques essentially similar to those described above, have recently been reviewed by Chapman *et al.* (1973). Crude five-year

Table 11.5. Testicular Tumours: Crude five-year Survivals (after Chapman *et al.* (1973))

Lesion	*Available for Review*	*Survival*	%
Seminoma	87	75	86
MTIA	37	33	89
MTIB	14	4	29
MTA	12	2	17

survivals for those available for review at that interval are summarised in Table 11.5. There is a remarkably good five-year survival for the MTIA teratomas when compared with the other teratomas, and this in a series where retroperitoneal node dissection has not been carried out as a routine.

Renal Parenchyma

The commoner malignant tumours at this site are the adenocarcinoma in adults and the nephroblastoma in children. Tumours of the renal pelvis are discussed later with other lesions of urothelium.

Adenocarcinoma (Grawitz's Tumour)

Adenocarcinoma accounts for $2\frac{1}{2}$ per cent of adult malignancies. It occurs most commonly in the fifth or sixth decades with a sex ratio of male to female of approximately 3:1. The tumour shows varying degrees of differentiation, the more anaplastic lesion showing earlier invasion of perirenal tissues, draining lymph nodes and renal vein, than the well-differentiated. Overall, however, it is very variable in behaviour and some tumours grow slowly to a very considerable size without yielding metastases, while others metastasise early and widely.

In general the main factors affecting prognosis appear to be the grade of the tumour and the presence or absence of renal vein involvement, although a low-grade tumour with renal vein involvement probably carries a better prognosis than a high-grade tumour with no renal vein involvement. Particularly remarkable is the development of occasional solitary metastases which occur more often with this primary than any other malignancy, and which are occasionally amenable to curative treatment. Also, a number of patients may present with symptoms remote from the kidney, in particular with hypertension, polycythaemia, or 'pyrexia of unknown origin'.

Staging and Investigation

The UICC TNM staging is similar for all renal carcinomas and is summarised in Table 11.6.

Considerable information about the nature of the primary lesion can be obtained by a combination of intravenous pyelography with nephrotomography and renal arteriography. The accuracy to be expected of the pre-operative assessment is highly relevant to the choice of treatment policy. It has been widely reviewed (Folin, 1967; Evans, 1968) and lies between 95 and 100 per cent.

Table 11.6. TNM Staging of Renal Tumours (UICC, 1973)

T_0	No evidence of primary tumour
T_1	No enlargement of kidney Minimal calyceal abnormality on urography
T_2	Kidney enlarged but mobile *or* Gross deformity of one or more calyces on urography *or* Displacement of ureter
T_3	Kidney enlarged and mobility limited without complete fixation *or* Urography shows deformity of the pelvis of the kidney *or* There is evidence of vascular compression
T_4	Kidney enlarged and with complete fixation
N_x	Regional lymph nodes impossible to assess
N_0	No deformity of regional nodes on lymphography
N_1	Regional nodes deformed
M_0	No evidence of distant metastases
M_{1a}	Single metastases only
M_{1b}	Multiple metastases
P_1	Tumour infiltrating only the parenchyma of the kidney
P_2	Tumour extending beyond the kidney but not infiltrating intrarenal or extra-renal veins or lymph vessels
P_3	Tumour infiltrating intrarenal or extrarenal veins and/or lymphatics

A full chest series, blood count, mid-stream urine, electrolyte and urea estimation are needed.

Lymphography will demonstrate involved regional nodes, permitting more accurate staging, and may permit more individual adjuvant radiotherapy.

Treatment Policy

Surgery, where feasible, is the mainstay of treatment of the primary lesion and locally inoperable lesions are rarely controlled by irradiation alone. There is, however, considerable support for the addition of irradiation to surgery either pre-operatively, post-operatively or both.

Until recently, British practice has concentrated on post-operative radiotherapy for all lesions more extensive than T_1. Riches *et al.* (1951), reviewing 1746 cases from 67 centres, reported five-year survivals improved from 30 to 49 per cent and ten-year survivals from

17 to 27 per cent by the addition of post-operative irradiation to nephrectomy. A similar improvement was reported by Bratherton (1964), but a retrospective survey by Peeling *et al.* (1969) showed no advantage from post-operative irradiation in their series, where only the more advanced cases tended to be referred for treatment.

Pre-operative irradiation has been advocated by Riches (1968), who reports three long-survivors (20, 15 and 7 years) of a series of 11 cases, all with high-grade tumours with renal vein involvement. At the present time a multi-centre trial organised by the Institute of Urology attempts to compare low-dose pre-operative irradiation, with additional post-operative treatment if indicated, with higher-dose post-operative treatment alone. Results are not yet available from this, and the whole concept of pre-operative irradiation involves administration of treatment without a tissue diagnosis.

Single metastases in soft tissues are often amenable to surgical removal and occasionally this can be curative. Other metastases should be irradiated for palliation.

There is increasing interest in hormone therapy for metastases from adenocarcinoma of the kidney. Bloom (1971) reports a response to medroxy progesterone acetate (Provera), 100 mg t.d.s., in 16 cases out of 80 (20 per cent). At least two of the patients in this series who failed on Provera obtained useful palliation from testosterone.

Treatment Technique

For pre-operative treatment, opposed anterior and posterior fields are used to irradiate the renal bed and the para-aortic lymph nodes. The fields will cross the mid-line but the opposite kidney must be spared. IVP marker films are used. The tumour-dose is 3000 rad in 15 fractions over 3 weeks. Surgery is undertaken 3 to 4 weeks after completion of treatment.

If the tumour was not P_1 at operation, a similar dose is given post-operatively. On this occasion it is necessary to spare the spinal cord, as the sum of the two treatments is beyond cord tolerance. A convenient technique is that of Bratherton (1964), using ipsilateral anterior oblique, posterior oblique and lateral wedged fields.

If no pre-operative treatment has been given, post-operative irradiation can use similar anterior and posterior fields to the pre-operative treatment. The dose, however, is 4000 to 4500 rad in 20 fractions over 4 weeks.

Nephroblastoma (Wilms's Tumour)

These tumours contain elements of malignant epithelium and connective tissue and are thought to represent embryonic renal tissues. Almost all present in infancy or early childhood with an average age at onset of three years, becoming extremely rare after seven years. They form 20 per cent of childhood malignancies and are characterised by early and rapid spread through the renal parenchyma into the perirenal tissues and early invasion of the lymphatics and blood stream. There is a particularly high early incidence of pulmonary metastases.

The TNM staging of nephroblastoma is the same as for hypernephroma. Pre-treatment investigation is essentially the same although the more sophisticated angiographic techniques are not usually used.

Treatment Policy

Surgery is again the mainstay of treatment of the primary lesion and is the only way of providing a definitive diagnosis. Before the development of the transperitoneal approach, pre-operative irradiation was sometimes essential to permit surgical removal of the larger tumours. Today, the transperitoneal approach with early ligation of the renal pedicle permits removal of relatively large tumours without great difficulty. Radiotherapy is used post-operatively, usually combined with chemotherapy except in children under one, where the prognosis is generally considered to be very good and treatment technically difficult.

The best reported result prior to the introduction of adjuvant chemotherapy was the 47 per cent two-year survival achieved by Gross (1953) using early and radical post-operative irradiation, which was superior to anything achieved previously by surgery alone.

Typical results achieved by post-operative radiotherapy and chemotherapy are those of Stone and Williams (1969), who report a two-year survival of 54 per cent from a combination of post-operative irradiation and actinomycin D. At the present moment a Medical

Research Council trial is in progress comparing the less toxic vincristine with actinomycin D, in this context.

Treatment Technique

The primary treatment is laparotomy with surgical exploration of the tumour. If this confirms the diagnosis, nephrectomy with early clamping of the renal pedicle is performed, and actinomycin D 15 μg per kg body weight is given at the time of operation. This is followed by three similar doses over the next 3–6 days. Post-operative radiotherapy is commenced within a fortnight of the day of operation.

The volume to be irradiated is a matter of some dispute. Pearson *et al.* (1964) suggest that the whole abdomen should be irradiated, shielding only the unaffected kidney. If the tumour was resectable and there was neither spill at operation nor evidence of disseminated metastases in the abdomen, a more localised field may be preferable to treat the renal bed and draining lymphatics only. In practice this involves a volume extending from the dome of the diaphragm above to 2–3 cm below the lower pole of the kidney below. The medial edge of the field extends to 1 cm to the opposite side of the spine. A tumour-dose of 3000–3500 rad in 20 fractions over four weeks with rising input is usually well tolerated, although it must be remembered that this volume represents a large proportion of the child's total body volume and bone marrow depression may be considerable, particularly following actinomycin D. Maintenance chemotherapy, after the completion of radiotherapy, is now advocated, and the MRC trial régime calls for either intermittent actinomycin D or intermittent vincristine for almost two years from presentation. These prolonged course of injections can be very trying for the child.

Side-effects

The side-effects of irradiation of one flank in a young child have received considerable attention. Neuhauser *et al.* (1952) report that a secondary scoliosis with atrophy of the muscle in the irradiated flank is almost inevitable in these cases. This complication, however, appears to be very rarely recorded in British or European literature, although symmetrical loss of height may occur (Pearson *et al.*, 1964).

Urothelium

The lining of the renal pelvis, the ureter, the bladder and the urethra is similar throughout, being formed of transitional epithelium. It is becoming increasingly recognised that a carcinoma of one of these structures may only represent part of an overall disease process. In a Royal Marsden Hospital (1970) series of 274 cases of carcinoma of the bladder submitted to total cystectomy, 38 cases had tumour in the penis or urethra at the time of surgery, and a further 29 cases had growths in one or other ureter. A further 8 cases developed tumour in the ureter or renal pelvis after adequate control of the bladder lesion. This concept of urothelial disease has considerable implications in the initial assessment, treatment and follow-up of patients suspected of carcinoma of the bladder.

Urothelial carcinoma accounts for 3 per cent of deaths due to malignant disease. It commonly presents after the age of 40 with increasing incidence with age thereafter. The sex ratio is 3 males to 1 female. Predisposing factors include chemicals (particularly aromatic amines), cigarette-smoking, chronic inflammation, stone-formation, maldevelopment, diverticula and schistosomiasis.

The commonest histological type of tumour is the transitional cell carcinoma which may appear macroscopically as papillary or solid and may be single or multiple. Squamous carcinoma also occurs, although adenocarcinoma of other than urachal origin is excessively rare. Transitional cell carcinoma can be graded according to the pleomorphism of the cells and their mitotic activity.

Tumour spread appears to be initially by local growth or seedling deposits to other parts of the urothelium followed by sub-mucosal spread in the lymphatics with later spread to the iliac and para-aortic lymph nodes. Blood-stream spread, particularly to lung, liver and bone, is relatively late.

Staging

The UICC staging of carcinomas of the renal pelvis is essentially the same as that of carcinomas of the renal parenchyma and the relative rarity of tumour deposits in urethra and ureter has resulted in no staging system yet being internationally agreed. Accurate and reproducible staging of bladder carcinoma is, however, widely recognised as essential for adequate management, and the UICC staging system is based on a combination of clinical and radiological assessment and biopsy, as summarised in Table 11.7.

Table 11.7. TNM Staging of Bladder Carcinoma (UICC, 1973)

TIS	Tumour confined to mucosa (carcinoma *in situ*)
T_1	Invasion of sub-mucosa
T_2	Invasion of superficial muscle
T_3	Invasion of deep muscle or perivesical tissue
T_4	Infiltration of pelvic side walls or adjoining organs
N_x	Lymph nodes not assessed
N_0	Negative lymph nodes on lymphography
N_1	Positive lymph nodes on lymphography
M_0	No distant metastases
M_1	Distant metastases present

Investigation

The use of urine cytology as a means of screening populations at risk has received considerable interest recently. This has been quite widely applied in the cable and rubber industries and has led to the detection of many tumours at an early stage with a possible improvement in survival rates. Similarly, in a symptomatic patient it can be a useful initial investigation, as is urine culture, blood count, and electrolyte and urea estimation. Initial radiological assessment includes a chest X-ray and IVP.

In all suspicious cases a formal cystoscopy and examination under anaesthetic is indicated; if tumour is seen, biopsy down to muscle permits adequate assessment of tumour stage and grade. Modern developments with fibre-optics have made this a simpler and more accurate procedure.

For established cases, vesical arteriography and lymphography have recently been advocated. The former has not yet proved its worth, but the latter provides a further means of detecting extra pelvic spread of disease which would preclude curative surgery. It may also permit more individual planning of irradiation for T_3 tumours.

Treatment Policy

The primary management of tumours of the renal pelvis, ureter and urethra is surgical. Nephro-ureterectomy is advocated for lesions of the renal pelvis and ureter, and either direct resection for small urethral tumours or cysto-prostato-urethrectomy for more extensive lesions at this site. Occasionally, post-operative irradiation may be useful for adherent tumours of ureter or renal pelvis, or if the peri-urethral lymphatics are involved. It may also be considered for bilateral lesions or new primary lesions in the remaining kidney, although its use in these circumstances carries a high risk of irradiation nephritis and there is increasing interest in surgery for both sides followed by renal transplantation. Carcinoma of the bladder, however, offers many possible combinations of irradiation and surgery.

Smaller tumours of Stages TIS and T_1 confined to the bladder can usually be controlled by closed cystodiathermy, which has become more reliable with recent technical improvements, particularly fibre-optics. Multiple tumours are frequently very difficult to control in this way; external irradiation to the bladder alone, intravesical epodyl or colloidal gold and Helmstein's bladder dilatation technique have all been used. The last shows considerable promise in these circumstances, also for recurrent haematuria following irradiation and in T_4 tumours not suitable for radiotherapy (England *et al.*, 1973).

T_2 lesions, 4 cm in diameter or less, respond well to open cystodiathermy followed by implantation of radioactive tantalum or iridium wire or gold grains. Dix *et al.* (1970) report a five-year survival of 78 per cent for papillary differentiated carcinoma treated in this way, although a number of their cases had T_1 lesions and might have been controlled by closed resection alone.

An occasional T_2 lesion will be suitable for partial cystectomy if it is sited either at the vault of the bladder or in a diverticulum: the lesion should be single, with a sharp margin between the tumour and normal bladder mucosa, and the rest of the bladder should be normal. A margin of at least one inch is advocated (Wallace, 1968). If these criteria can be achieved, results from this technique are very satisfactory; however, it is rarely possible to find a suitable lesion and it is very probable that this technique is practised more often than it should be.

More extensive T_2 and T_3 lesions confined to the bladder may be considered for radiotherapy alone, surgery alone, or a combination of the two. Well localised megavoltage treatment of these lesions can be well tolerated and interferes neither with the normal passage of urine nor with sexual potency. A trial is at present being organised by the Institute of Urology to compare the results of pre-operative radiotherapy to the true pelvis, followed by elective total cystectomy at an interval of four weeks, with radical radiotherapy alone. At the present moment no statistically significant results are obtainable from this.

T_4 tumours, by virtue of their fixation to pelvic side wall, are locally inoperable; here palliative radiotherapy is the mainstay of treatment, although five-year survivals are very rare. A Helmstein vesical dilatation may relieve haematuria, and a nerve block or cordotomy pelvic pain.

Radiotherapy Technique

For implantation of T_2 lesions the choice of material today lies between radioactive iridium or tantalum 'hairpins' and gold grains. The hairpins provide a geometrically more satisfactory implant, but the long half-life of the wire necessitates the removal of the implant at a later date, requiring the hairpins to be drawn down the urethra with occasionally traumatic results. The actual implantation of the wire also takes rather longer to perform, with additional radiation hazard to the surgical team. The use of gold grains, with their short life of 2·7 days, permits a permanent implant and the actual implantation by a gold-grain gun or trocars and cannulae can be very quickly accomplished. A dose of 6000 rad is given as a permanent implant.

The volume to be irradiated for more extensive T_2 and T_3 lesions is in dispute. The technique advocated in the Institute of Urology trial irradiates the whole true pelvis to 4000 rad in 20 fractions over four weeks, followed either by surgery or by a further 2000 rad in 10 fractions over two weeks, localised to the primary tumour with a small margin. An alternative approach using radiotherapy alone yields apparently equal results from delivering 5000–5500 rad in 20 fractions over four weeks to the tumour and margin alone.

Irradiation of the pelvis uses a pair of anterior and posterior megavoltage fields extending from the lower border of L4 above to the lower margin of the obturator foramen below, and laterally to just beyond the pelvic side walls (Fig. 11.2a). The more localised fields to

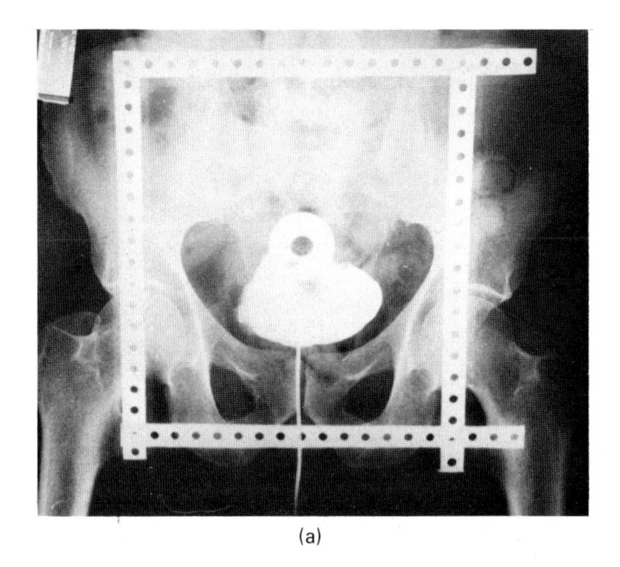

(a)

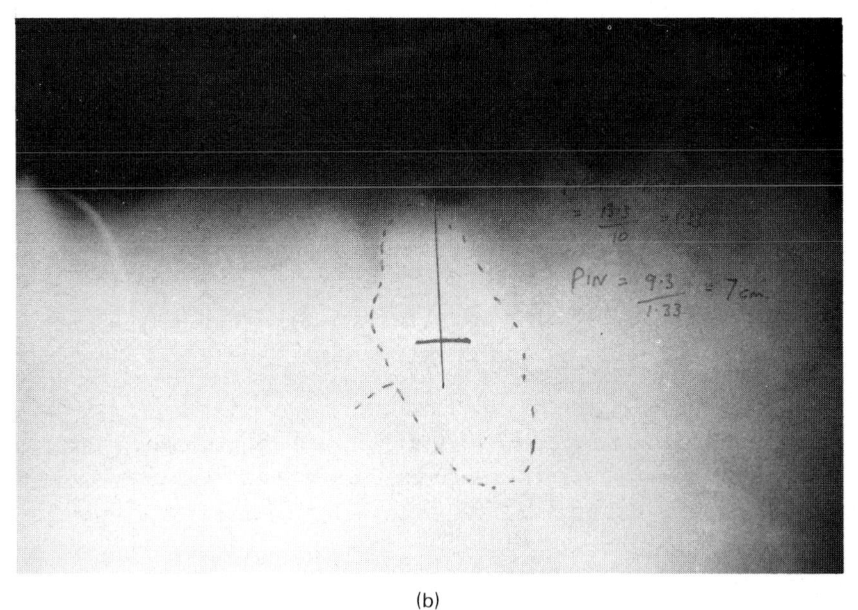

(b)

Fig. 11.2. a Anteroposterior marker film showing true pelvic fields for irradiation of T_3 tumours of the bladder.
b Shoot through lateral marker film in the same case. Note marker rings on anterior abdominal wall.

the primary require cystogram localisation and planning of fields to minimise the dose to the rectum. Particularly important in this technique is the shoot through lateral film with the anterior skin-mark outlined with lead and either a ladder of lead marks or a lead ring of standard diameter used to check on magnification (Fig. 11.2b). From this cystogram the depth of the centre of the treatment volume is obtained, and from this either a 3-static-fields technique or a rotation technique can be developed.

Prostate

Clinical carcinoma of the prostate is the third commonest malignancy in adult males and there is an even higher incidence of carcinoma of the prostate discovered as an incidental finding at post mortem or patients dying of other conditions. The majority of patients with clinical carcinoma present late in life but substantial numbers present in middle age and it may occur at any age over forty.

Most of the lesions are adenocarcinomas of varying degrees of differentiation and tend to arise from the outer group of prostatic glands (Franks, 1969). Thus urinary symptoms occur later than with benign prostatic enlargement. The tumours vary considerably in their behaviour. In the older patients they may remain as a latent nodule with no evidence of growth or dissemination for some years. In the younger patient there may be rapid local spread with involvement of local lymphatics and early blood-stream dissemination, resulting chiefly in bony metastases.

Staging

The TNM staging is summarised in Table 11.8. An alternative system is that of the Veterans Administration Co-operative Urological Research Group (Blackard, 1974) which is widely accepted and appears relevant to treatment policy and prognosis. This is shown in Table 11.9.

Investigations

Examination under anaesthetic, cystoscopy and biopsy are essential to establish the diagnosis and stage the local lesion. A blood count should be made, electrolytes, urea and prostatic serum acid phosphatase should be estimated and a skeletal survey and full chest X-ray series

Table 11.8. TNM Staging of Prostatic Carcinoma

T_x	Incidental finding of carcinoma in operative specimen
T_0	No evidence of primary tumour
T_1	Tumour occupying less than one half of the prostate and surrounded by palpably normal gland
T_2	Tumour occupying one half or more of the prostate but not producing enlargement or deformity of the gland
T_3	Tumour confined to the prostate but producing enlargement or deformity of the gland
T_4	Tumour extending beyond the prostate
N_x	Nodes impossible to assess
N_0	No deformity of regional nodes on lymphography
N_1	Regional nodes deformed on lymphography
N_2	Fixed palpable abdominal nodes
M_0	No evidence of distant metastases
M_1	Distant metastases present
M_{1a}	No metastases other than bone
M_{1b}	Metastases other than bone present

Table 11.9. VACURG staging of prostatic carcinoma

VACURG stage	*TNM equivalent*			*Incidence* (%)
I	T_x	N_0	M_0	5
II	T_1–T_3	N_0	M_0	7
III	T_4	N_0	M_0	48
IV	T_0–T_4	N_0–N_1	M_0–M_1	40

undertaken. If radical surgery or irradiation is under consideration a lymphogram must be undertaken to exclude involved abdominal nodes.

Treatment Policy

Stage I lesions (T_x, N_0, M_0) will have been discovered at simple prostatectomy and probably no further action is indicated, apart from follow-up and oestrogen for symptomatic recurrence or metastases. In patients under sixty and with more extensive Stage I or poorly-differentiated lesions, radical prostatectomy may be considered, but no significant improvement in survival has yet been reported for this (Blackard, 1974).

Stage II lesions (T_1–T_3, N_0, M_0) may be considered for radical local treatment and it is in the fit patient under sixty-five in this stage that radical prostatectomy is most likely to be considered. Less than 5 per cent of patients will be suitable, and the high incidence of incontinence and impotence make the procedure unattractive.

For the older patient, conservative surgery in the form of a trans-urethral resection will rapidly relieve the symptoms of obstruction and provide a histological diagnosis. It can safely be supplemented by oestrogens in this age-group. Barnes and Ninan (1972) report a 60 per cent ten-year survival by this method. In the younger patient oestrogen failures are more common and the cardiac risks are more significant. Here an alternative to radical surgery in Stage II is transurethral resection followed by radical radiotherapy. Ray *et al.* (1973) report a 72 per cent five-year survival in a series of 160 patients treated in this way, which equals the results of radical prostatectomy.

Stage III (T_4, N_0, M_0) and Stage IV (T_0–T_4, N_0–N_1, M_0–M_1) lesions have been treated with palliative intent only. The original VACURG study (Mellinger *et al.*, 1967) demonstrated that the reduction of deaths from prostatic carcinoma achieved by oestrogens was offset by an increase in cardiovascular deaths. It is felt that oestrogens are best withheld until there are significant symptoms or definite evidence of progression of disease. Localised symptoms can be treated by local treatment, such as trans-urethral resection for urinary obstruction or palliative irradiation for localised bony metastases. Orchidectomy offers little advantage over oestrogens in primary management, except where there is a high risk of cardiovascular complications.

High-dose radiotherapy has been used with radical intent for Stage III lesions (Ray *et al.*, 1973). However, the dosage used, 5500 rad in 27 fractions over 5½ weeks to the whole pelvis, followed by supplementary 1500 rad to the prostate, has caused many complications.

Patients with advanced disease meriting treatment but refractory to oestrogens may benefit from castration. Adrenalectomy or hypophysectomy can improve 50 per cent of cases relapsing following oestrogen, and the latter can simply be achieved by an yttrium implant to the pituitary (Fergusson, 1965). Other alternatives include palliative radiotherapy, cytotoxic drugs such as fluorouracil, and estracyt, a nitrogen mustard derivative of oestradiol which is metabolised to active nitrogen mustard in prostatic tissues (Jonnson and Hogberg, 1971).

Radiotherapy Technique

Radical radiotherapy for the Stage II lesion requires very well localised treatment and the close proximity of the treatment volume to the rectum presents the biggest difficulties in treatment planning. In practice, it is necessary to treat the anterior one-third of the rectum while sparing the posterior two-thirds.

A localising cystogram is used, similar to that described above for bladder carcinoma but supplemented by barium in the rectum (Fig. 11.3). Mantell (1974) advocates two anterior and oblique wedged fields

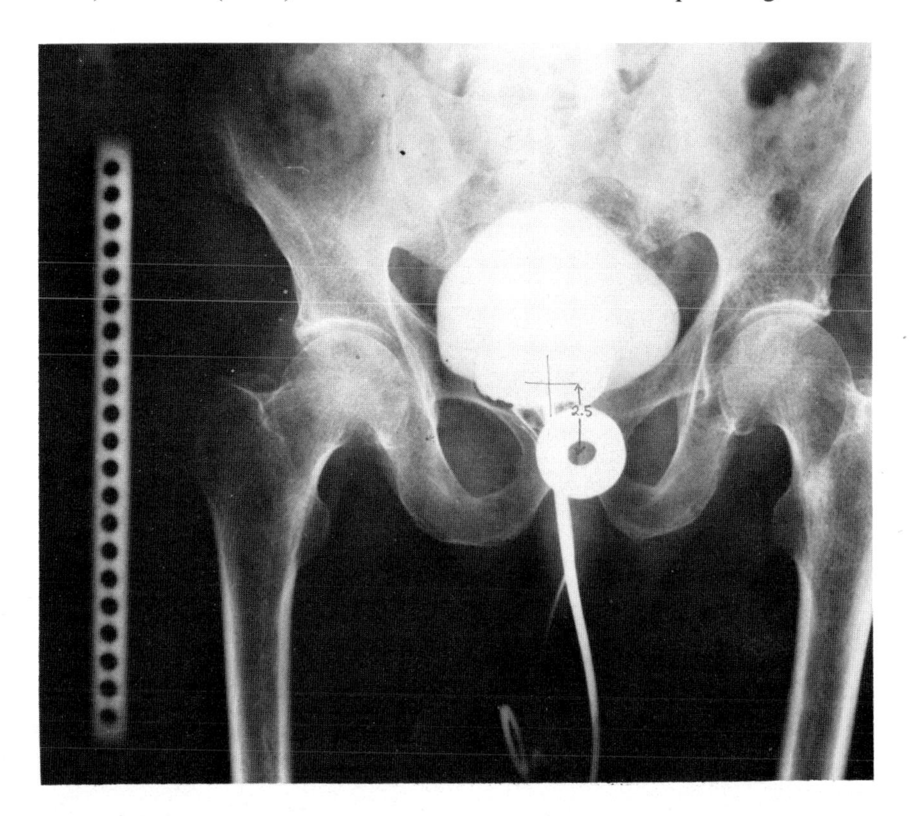

Fig. 11.3. a Anteroposterior marker film for irradiation of T_2 carcinoma of prostate.

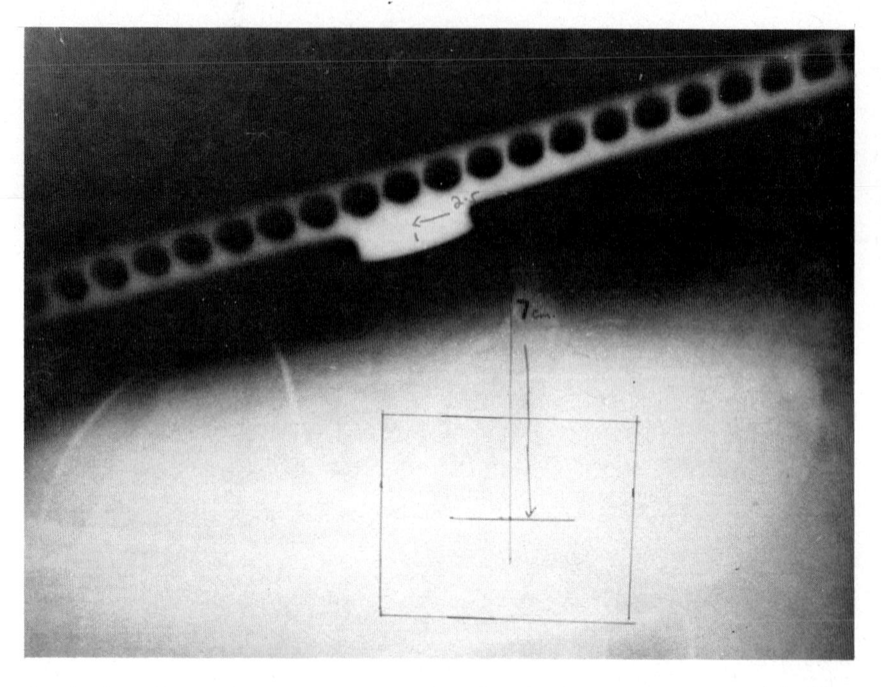

Fig. 11.3. b Shoot through lateral marker film in the same case as (a). Note barium in rectum.

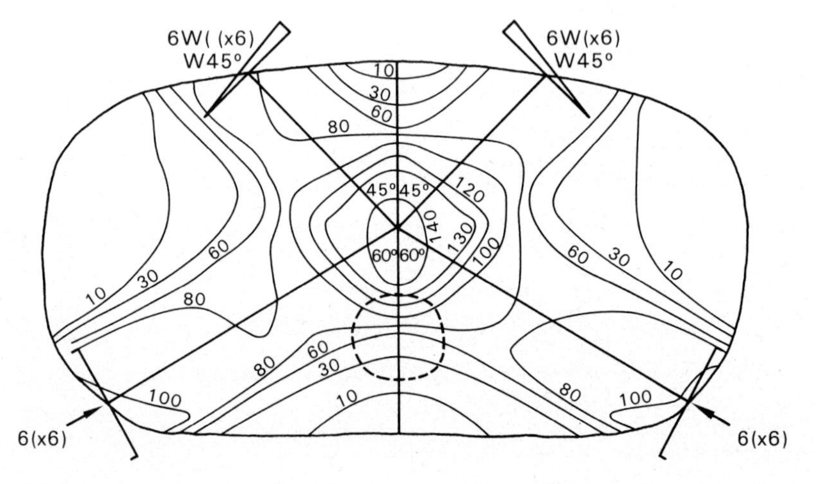

Fig. 11.4. Isodoses for four-field irradiation of T_2 carcinoma of prostate (plan courtesy Dr H. F. Hope-Stone).

supplemented by two posterior and oblique plain fields to provide the best dose-distribution (Fig. 11.4). Tumour dose is 5500 rad in 20 fractions over four weeks.

Penis

Almost all malignancies of the penis are squamous carcinomas although other rarer lesions include urothelial transitional cell carcinoma in the penile urethra and intra-epidermal carcinoma *in situ* or erythroplasia of Queyrat. Penile carcinoma is rare in Europe and North America and accounts for less than 0·2 per cent of male deaths from malignant disease. It effectively never occurs in those circumcised in infancy and classically presents in the fifth and sixth decades. It arises in the glans or the inner surface of the prepuce and may spread widely over the surface before commencing deep invasion to the erectile tissue and the urethra.

Enlarged inguinal nodes are a frequent finding although this is almost as often due to secondary infection as to metastases. The TNM system of staging is summarised in Table 11.10 and minimum investigations include full clinical assessment, biopsy of the primary and a chest X-ray.

Table 11.10. TNM Staging of Carcinoma of Penis (UICC, 1973)

TIS	Carcinoma *in situ*
T_0	No evidence of primary tumour
T_1	Tumour 2 cm or less in largest dimensions – strictly superficial
T_2	Tumour 2–5 cm in greatest dimensions – minimal infiltration
T_3	Tumour more than 5 cm or with deep infiltration including urethra
T_4	Tumour infiltrating neighbouring structures
N_0	No palpable nodes
N_1	Movable unilateral nodes
	N_{1a}: nodes not considered to contain growth
	N_{1b}: nodes considered to contain growth
N_2	Movable bilateral nodes
	N_{2a}: nodes not considered to contain growth
	N_{2b}: nodes considered to contain growth
N_3	Fixed nodes
M_0	No evidence of distant metastases
M_1	Distant metastases present

Treatment Policy

For lesions in Stages T_1 and T_2, N_0, M_0, surgery and irradiation yield equal results. Duncan and Jackson (1972), using irradiation, report 18 out of 20 cases free from recurrence after a mean period of three years. This is essentially comparable with the 55 per cent crude three-year survival overall, obtained by Frew *et al.* (1967) from a surgical series containing 24 cases out of 46 with lesions in Stages T_1–T_3, N_0, M_0. Radiotherapy involves a longer treatment with more initial side-effects than surgery, but avoids mutilating operation and psychological trauma. Amputation is feasible for late recurrence and is easier than irradiation for recurrence following surgery.

T_1 lesions on the glans can occasionally be treated with single direct fields using superficial X-rays. More extensive T_1 and T_2 lesions are treated either with a mould or with beam-directed irradiation. These two techniques are directly compared by Duncan and Jackson (1972). The radium mould group had 24 recurrences in 45 cases, and seven strictures but no necroses. The recurrences and two of the strictures required salvage surgery. The beam-directed group of 20 cases had only two recurrences but six strictures and two necroses. Both recurrences and both necroses required subsequent surgery. The survival rate at three years was about the same, being 80 per cent in the former group and 90 per cent in the latter. They conclude that the use of beam-directed irradiation involves less hazard to staff than the moulds, and gives a higher control-rate at the price of slightly greater morbidity.

T_3 and T_4 tumours require primary amputation of the penis if operable. Inoperable lesions may derive useful symptomatic relief from palliative irradiation. Mobile metastatic nodes (N_{1b} and N_{2b}) require block dissection in the absence of distant metastases. Frew *et al.* (1967) advocate a delay at least until the primary has healed to permit enlarged nodes secondary to infection in the primary to regress spontaneously, and thus minimise unnecessary block dissection. Fixed metastatic nodes (N_3), imply a poor prognosis but can be usefully palliated by irradiation. Newaishy and Deeley (1968) obtained complete regression in 47 per cent of cases, and some response in a further 24 per cent. Their one-year survival was 33 per cent and there were no survivors at two years.

Radiotherapy Technique

The use of radium in moulds has largely been replaced by iridium wire, which is easier and safer to handle. An inner shell is constructed to fit the patient and over this is slid an outer shell containing the active wire. The active volume extends beyond the tip of the penis and for 2–3 cm on the perineal side of the lesion.

Treatment is given intermittently with the patient removing his own mould, and is completed in 7–10 days with the mould worn for about ten hours a day. With this fractionation 6000 rad is delivered to the skin and 5000 to the urethra. Exceeding this urethral dose carries a high incidence of stricture formation.

A sophisticated variant of the classical mould has been described by Mantell and Morgan (1969) for the TIS lesions. An individual mould is cast from silastomer rubber and inert yttrium oxide. The whole is then activated in a pile to yield a beta-emitting plaque. Two applications each of 1500 rad are used.

Beam-directed treatment requires homogeneous irradiation of the same volume as that covered by the mould. A wax block is prepared, split into two halves to contain the penis accurately. This serves to maintain a constant volume treated, compensate for varying separation, and abolish skin-sparing. Opposed 5 × 6 to 8 × 6 cm lateral telecobalt fields are used. A mid-line dose of 5000 to 5500 rad in 20 fractions over four weeks is advocated. Inoperable metastatic nodes are treated with direct fields on telecobalt. An incident dose of 4000 rad in 20 fractions over four weeks gives adequate palliation (Newaishy and Deeley, 1968).

References

BAGSHAW, K. (1968) Personal Communication to Hope-Stone, H. F., cited in Blandy *et al.* (1970) q.v.

BARNES, R. W. and NINAN, C. A. (1972) *Journal of Urology*, **108**, 897–900.

BLACKARD, C. E. (1974) *British Journal of Hospital Medicine*, **11**, 357–372.

BLANDY, J. P. (1966) *Hospital Medicine*, **1**, 133–138.

BLANDY, J. P., HOPE-STONE, H. F. and DAYAN, A. D. (1970) *Tumours of the Testicle*. Heinemann, London.

BLOOM, H. J. G. (1971) *British Journal of Cancer*, **25**, 250–265.

BLOOM, H. J. G. and HENDRY, W. F. (1973) *British Medical Journal*, **3**, 563–567.

BODEN, G. (1948) *British Journal of Radiology*, **21**, 464–469.

BRATHERTON, D. G. (1964) *British Journal of Radiology*, **37**, 141–146.

CHAPMAN, R. H., BLANDY, J. P., HOPE-STONE, H. F., POLLOCK, D. and DAYAN, A. D. (1973) *Proceedings of the Royal Society of Medicine*, **66**, 1044–1047.

DIX, V. W., SHANKS, W., TRESSIDER, G. C., BLANDY, J. P., HOPE-STONE, H. F. and SHEPHEARD, B. G. F. (1970) *British Journal of Urology*, **42**, 213–228.

DIXON, F. J. and MOORE, R. A. (1952) *Atlas of Tumour Pathology*, Fascicles 31B and 32. US Armed Forces Institute of Pathology, Washington, DC.

DUNCAN, W. and JACKSON, S. M. (1972) *Clinical Radiology*, **23**, 246–248.

ENGLAND, H. R., RIGBY, C., SHEPHEARD, B. G. F., TRESIDDER, G. C. and BLANDY, J. P. (1973) *British Journal of Urology*, **45**, 593–599.

EVANS, J. (1968) *Journal of the American Medical Association*, **204**, 3, 223–226.

FERGUSSON, J. D. (1965) *Congress of the International Society of Urology*, **13**, 2, 329–333.

FOLEY, J. F., LEMON, H. M., MILLER, D. M. and KESSINGER, A. (1972) *Journal of Urology*, **108**, 439–442.

FOLIN, J. (1967) *Acta radiologica* (Supplement), **267**, 7–96.

FRANKS, L. M. (1969) *British Journal of Hospital Medicine*, **2**, 575–582.

FREW, I. D. O., JEFFERIES, J. D. and SWINNEY, J. (1967) *British Journal of Urology*, **39**, 398–404.

GROSS, R. E. (1953) *Surgery in Infancy and Childhood*. W. B. Saunders, Philadelphia.

HOPE-STONE, H. F., BLANDY, J. P. and DAYAN, A. D. (1963) *British Medical Journal*, **1**, 984–989.

JONNSON, G. and HOGBERG, B. (1971) *Scandinavian Journal of Urology and Nephrology*, **5**, 103–107.

LUXTON, R. W. (1953) *Quarterly Journal of Medicine*, **22**, 215–242.

MANTELL, B. S. (1974) Personal communication.

MANTELL, B. S. and MORGAN, W. Y. (1969) *British Journal of Radiology*, **42**, 855–857.

Medical Research Council (1956) *Hazards to Man of Nuclear and Allied Radiation*. HMSO, London.

MELLINGER, G. T., BAILAR, J. C. and ARDUINO, C. J. (Veterans Administration Cooperative Urological Research Group) (1967) *Surgery Gynaecology and Obstetrics with International Abstracts of Surgery*, **124**, 1011–1017.

NEUHAUSER, E. B. D., WITTENBURG, M. H., BERMAN, C. Z. and COHEN, J. (1952) *Radiology*, **59**, 637–650.

NEWAISHY, G. A. and DEELEY, T. J. (1968) *British Journal of Radiology*, **41**, 519–521.

PATTON, J. F., SELTZMAN, D. N. and ZONE, R. A. (1960) *American Journal of Surgery*, **99**, 525–532.

PEARSON, D., DUNCAN., W. B. and POINTON, R. C. S. (1964) *British Journal of Radiology*, **37**, 154–160.

PEELING, W. B., MANTELL, B. S. and SHEPHEARD, B. G. F. (1969) *British Journal of Urology*, **41**, 23–31.

PUGH, R. C. B. (1973) Paper read at Institute of Urology Seminar.

RAY, G. R., CASSADY, J. R. and BAGSHAW, M. A. (1973) *Radiology*, **106**, 407–418.

RICHES, E. W., GRIFFITHS, I. H. and THACKRAY, A. C. (1951) *British Journal of Urology*, **23**, 297–356.

RICHES, E. W. (1968) *Journal of the American Medical Association*, **204**, 3, 230–231.

Royal Marsden Hospital (1970) Series presented in Clinical Oncology Course.

SMITHERS, D. W., WALLACE, D. M. and AUSTIN, D. E. (1973) *British Medical Journal*, **4**, 77–79.

STONE, J. and WILLIAMS, I. G. (1969) *Clinical Radiology*, **20**, 40–46.

Union Internationale Contre Le Cancer (1973) *TNM Classification of Malignant Tumours*. Geneva.

WALSH, P. C., KAUFMANN, J. J., COULSON, W. F. and GOODWIN, W. E. (1971) *Journal of the American Medical Association*, **217**, 309–312.

WALLACE, D. M. (1968) *Hospital Medicine*, **1**, 831–838.

WHITTLE, R. J. M. (1957) *British Journal of Radiology*, **30**, 7–12.

CHAPTER TWELVE

Bone Tumours

G. Newsholme

Tumours of Bone

Primary malignant tumours of bone are rare, occurring far less frequently than metastatic growths. Between 1959 and 1968 a total of 130 677 cases of malignant disease was registered in the Birmingham region but only 406 (little more than 0·3 per cent) of these arose primarily in bone. More than half of these tumours are osteosarcomata (64 per cent in this series). Table 12.1, using figures taken from McKenna *et al* (1966), shows the relative frequency and peak age of

Table 12.1. Relative frequency and peak ages of incidence of bone sarcomata (McKenna *et al*., 1966)

	Total cases	*Median age of incidence*	*5-year survival* (%)
Osteosarcoma	258	17	13·2
Chondrosarcoma	139	38	28
Fibrosarcoma	60	38	31·7
Parosteal (juxtacortical) fibrosarcoma	22	30	81·8
Paget's sarcoma	33	60	—
Sarcoma in irradiated bone	22	—	22·7

incidence of different types of bone sarcoma which they found on reviewing a large series at the Memorial Hospital, New York.

The question of biopsy of these bone tumours is still a matter of discussion and individual judgement. In many bone tumours different areas of the growth show varying histological appearances and the pathologist would, ideally, like to see a large and representative section of the tumour extending down to the centre of the bone. The disadvantage of a large open biopsy in malignant cases is not so much the often-mentioned risk of general dissemination of tumour cells as the local possibilities of haematoma formation, infection, fungation of the tumour through the incision, flexion contracture of joints and even fracture through a bone further weakened by tissue removal. It has been shown that tumour cells, surprisingly, appear in greater numbers after manipulation or palpation of an osteosarcoma than during biopsy (Foss *et al.*, 1966) and that the demonstration of circulating tumour cells under these circumstances seems to have no prognostic significance.

In some cases aspiration cytology and drill biopsy may provide adequate information, especially in differentiating primary and secondary growths in bone. In others they may be helpful in deciding how best to carry out a more adequate tissue removal using punch, trephine or open biopsy through a small incision.

Osteosarcoma

Histologically, osteosarcomata are characterised by the formation of osteoid tissue and bone by the tumour cells. In addition to a stroma of undifferentiated spindle cells, cartilage and fibrous tissue are often present and may predominate in some cases. The prognosis for all these variants is similar and subdivision on histological grounds is not thought useful. Most of them occur between the ages of 10 and 20 years, in the metaphyses of the long bones, especially round the knee joint. Osteosarcomata may arise in abnormal bone such as Paget's disease (Fig. 12.1) and areas of radiation osteitis. They do not differ histologically but occur usually after middle age and involve the long bones less frequently; Paget's sarcoma has a particularly bad prognosis. The WHO international histological classification of bone

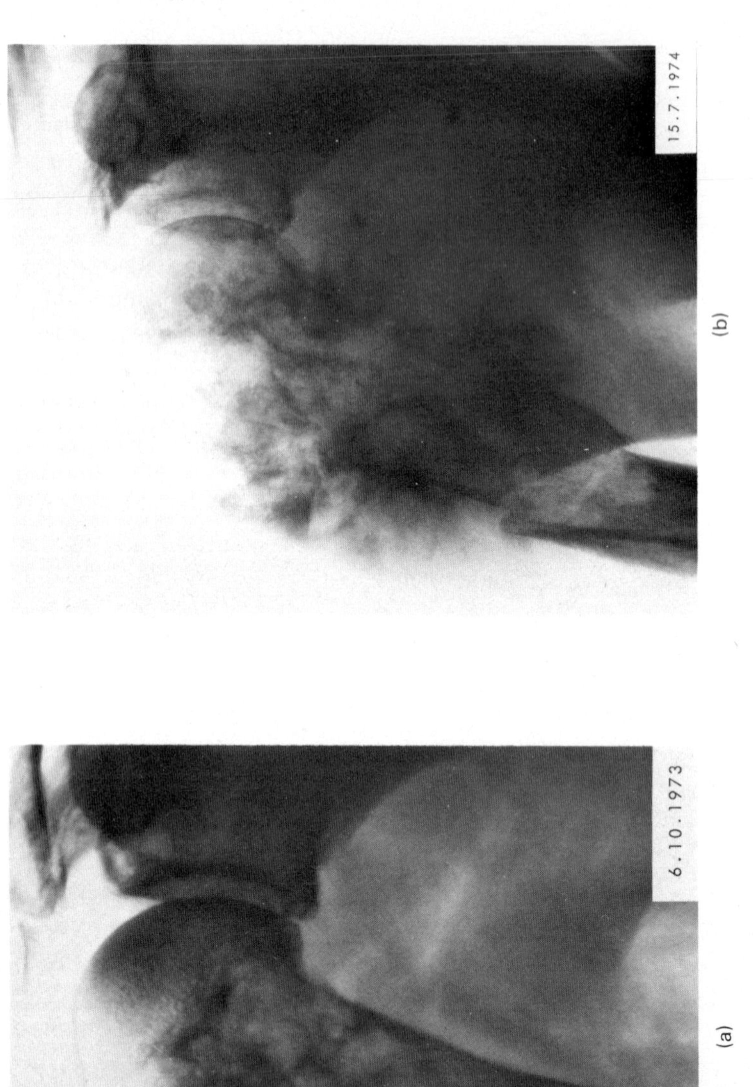

Fig. 12.1 Paget's disease of the humerus (confirmed by biopsy) in a man aged 65, showing (b) development of osteosarcoma with pathological fracture nine months later.

tumours (1972) lists the rare juxtacortical (parosteal) osteosarcoma separately, because of its distinctive pathology. Growth is slower and prognosis considerably better than for the commonly-occurring type.

The word 'osteogenic' has caused confusion, being assumed by some (with etymological correctness) to mean 'bone-producing' and by others to carry the wider connotation of 'arising from bone'; it seems wiser to avoid its use. Four out of five of all cases of osteosarcoma die within two years of metastatic spread, almost always to the lungs. The outlook is better for patients between the ages of 10 and 30. Younger patients tend to do badly, as do the elderly, in many of whom the sarcoma is associated with Paget's disease. The outcome is also related to the site. Tumours of the long bones in general are not so dangerous as those of the flat bones. Amputation, when possible, at a level above that of the joint of the bone involved remains the standard treatment. Although less radical surgery with amputation through the bone 10 cm or so above obvious tumour has its advocates, skip areas in the medullary cavity undoubtedly occur and there is an increased risk of stump recurrence.

Osteosarcoma shows some response to radiotherapy and Woodard and Coley (1947) showed that this response was dose-dependent; tumours given 6000 to 9000 rad in two to three months underwent regression in many cases, with pain relief in most and occasional complete disappearance. This is the only form of treatment possible for tumours arising in difficult sites such as the spine or skull, when radiotherapy is given to local tissue tolerance levels. Cade (1955) urged the use of radiotherapy as the initial treatment in all cases of osteosarcoma, amputation then being reserved for those failing to respond and for the more fortunate minority in whom no pulmonary metastases had appeared four to six months later.

The timing of the operation remains a difficult decision, but by using this method of delaying it, about half are spared what will prove in retrospect to be an unnecessary amputation. There is no evidence to support the suspicion that viable tumour cells may metastasise to the lungs during the waiting period. In Britain about one-third of patients with osteosarcoma are treated by primary amputation and the remainder by methods similar to that used by Cade, although elsewhere in the world the proportion of primary amputations is considerably higher.

The MRC working party on bone sarcoma (Sweetnam, 1972) found that those treated by primary amputation did no better in terms of survival, whereas in the group treated initially by radiotherapy many were saved operation.

A possible disadvantage of the Cade method which still needs consideration, however, is that patients spared amputation because of the early development of metastases may later suffer much distress due to local recurrence. Little information on this aspect is available although the experience of Jenkin *et al.* (1972) suggests that it is important. They found that lung metastases did not cause major symptoms until the terminal stages, but the morbidity associated with an active primary was severe – recurrence of activity in a bone tumour being as distressingly apparent to the patient as it is to his doctor. Pain, limited joint movement and forced inactivity because of the risk of fracture all spoil the quality of the remaining months of life. The other consideration is that a considerable fraction of their short life-span must be spent by these young patients either undergoing irradiation in bed in hospital or travelling several times a week to hospital for radiotherapy.

Lung Metastases

Lung deposits which remain solitary are rare, but the possibility of excision should always be considered in cases where the primary tumour has been dealt with radically and successfully. Sweetnam (1972) reported that 8 out of 12 patients operated on for excision of a solitary pulmonary metastasis were alive at follow-up on average some $6\frac{1}{2}$ years later.

About one-third of amputation specimens after irradiation to full dosage (Lee and Mackenzie, 1964) show complete tumour disappearance, but the use of similar doses to irradiate established diffuse lung metastases would be out of the question since at even much lower dose-levels severe radiation pneumonitis can develop. Because the great majority of patients die of lung metastases a case can be made, nevertheless, for prophylactic irradiation of the lungs at the time of first diagnosis. A level of dosage which lung tissue can tolerate safely might, at this early time, prevent circulating tumour cells from successfully colonising and growing. It seems probable that most of the tumour cells which can be demonstrated in the circulation in patients with bone sarcoma are, in fact, eliminated from the body, and possible that in the case of the lungs this process might be enhanced by quite low-dosage irradiation. Newton (1972) reported the results in 13 patients with osteosarcoma of the limb bones given 1950 rad to both lungs in $2\frac{1}{2}$ weeks as part of their initial treatment. Preliminary figures suggest a considerable delay in the appearance of lung metastases and encourage the continuation of this trial, to which has since been added the drug ICRF 159 (Le Serve and Hellmann, 1972). Jenkin *et al.* (1972) gave, electively, 1500 rad in two weeks to the lungs of six patients with osteosarcoma, combined in four of them with actinomycin D. All six developed diffuse lung metastases within six months without significant lengthening of the disease-free interval between initial treatment and the appearance of metastases, as compared with a large group of unirradiated patients.

Chemotherapy

Of available chemotherapeutic agents, methotrexate in high dosage (given intermittently and combined with Citrovorum 'rescue') and Adriamycin are two which have been shown to produce a response in patients with disseminated osteosarcoma. Jaffe *et al.* (1973) report that methotrexate in doses between 100 and 200 mg per kg body weight followed by Citrovorum factor injections resulted in the disappearance of pulmonary metastases in two out of ten patients and partial regression of pulmonary metastases and bone metastases in two others – two dying, however, as a direct result of the therapy itself. Cortes *et al.* (1972) treated 13 patients with bony metastases from osteosarcoma with Adriamycin, producing appreciable improvement in five of them and achieving one complete remission.

Rosen *et al.* (1974) used a combination of both drugs and obtained varying degrees of regression for more than one month in seven out of thirteen patients with recurrent osteosarcoma, five out of six with bone pain obtaining relief. They suggest that combination chemotherapy might be valuable as an adjuvant in the primary treatment of the disease.

Immunological Aspects

Osteosarcoma can be shown to contain tumour-specific antigens and the presence of antibody in the serum of the majority of patients with this disease has been demonstrated by Reilly *et al.* (1972). Both passive immunity, produced by the injection of tumour-specific antisera prepared in animals, and active immunisation with tumour-specific antigens are ineffective (Marsh *et al.*, 1972). Marcove *et al.* (1972), however, have used a vaccine made of lysed osteosarcoma cells in patients following amputation, with preliminary results which suggest some lengthening of the disease-free interval between surgery and the first demonstration of pulmonary metastases and encourage continuation of this trial.

Attempts have also been made to stimulate cell-bound rather than humoral antibodies, since these appear to be the most important mediators of the immunological surveillance mechanism against solid tumours. Enneking (1972) reports the results in 22 patients of injecting sensitised white cells obtained from volunteers into whom slices of the patient's own tumour had previously been implanted subcutaneously. Although the clinical course was not modified in four of the patients who had already developed lung metastases, the overall results so far suggest a modest increase in the length of survival.

Survival Figures

The long-term survival in patients with bone sarcoma and the question of whether pre-operative radiotherapy has any influence on the outcome still remain matters of debate and disagreement. Conclusions drawn from small numbers of cases, difficulty in comparing unlike series, lack of histological detail and unwitting case selection have certainly played some part in this. Allen and Stevens (1973), for instance, state that radiotherapy followed by delayed elective amputation has resulted in improved survival in osteosarcoma, suggesting that this improvement may be due to the preservation and enhancement of an immune response by avoiding early surgery – dismemberment possibly lowering 'host-resistance' and immunity. Encouraging results in a series of ten patients are described (six patients alive and well from 30 to 114 months after diagnosis) and similar good results quoted in four other reported series (three of them small). While the suggestion is interesting, it is difficult to accept a premise made on the basis of so few cases, all of whom were between 9 and 20 years of age, had potentially operable tumours and no evidence of distal metastases.

Mention is also made of Ferguson's (1940) retrospective survey of over 400 cases from the Bone Sarcoma Registry in the American College of Surgeons. He found that patients in whom amputation for bone sarcoma had been delayed for six months or more after the initial diagnosis did twice as well, in terms of survival, as those undergoing earlier surgery, concluding that a more favourable quiescent stage of the disease was reached by such a delay. McDonald and Budd (1943) have already pointed out that no less than 30 per cent of the five-year survivors recorded by the Registry showed a favourable, fibrosarcoma type of histology with a corresponding reduction in the proportion of less favourable osteosarcoma cases. Ferguson's results are explained by natural selection, the six-month waiting period already having weeded out many of the poor-risk patients.

Lockshin and Higgins (1968), reviewing the literature of the last half-century, came to the conclusion that reported variations in survival of osteosarcoma could be attributed to lack of comparability between series, especially with regard to histology, tumour site and variations in study design. They found no conclusive evidence in favour of pre-operative radiotherapy, but were, of course, considering survival rather than the quality of palliation received by the majority of patients who ultimately die. The overall five-year survival figure for osteosarcoma is quoted by them as being about 15 per cent and that for bone sarcoma as a whole, about 20 per cent.

The results of treatment of osteosarcoma seem to have changed little in the course of the last few decades. Whether it will prove possible to salvage more cases of this distressing disease by prophylactic lung irradiation, adjuvant radiotherapy and other means, remains to be seen. Perhaps the greatest hopes for further improvement lie in the directions of adjuvant chemotherapy and immunotherapy.

Chondrosarcoma

Chrondrosarcoma is one of the primary tumours of bone least responsive to radiotherapy. Histologically characterised by the formation of cartilage but not bone, it usually occurs between the ages of 30 and 60 years, being uncommon under 20 years of age. It involves the pelvis, shoulder girdle and ribs more frequently than osteosarcoma, although femur and humerus are also among the more common sites. Treatment is essentially surgical. Chondrosarcoma is of slower growth than osteosarcoma and, while far less likely to produce lung metastases or other distal spread, has a marked tendency to recur locally so that wide surgical clearance carries a considerably better chance of cure than in osteosarcoma.

Fibrosarcoma

This is a less frequently occurring tumour, composed of collagen fibres without cartilage or bone, which has also a better prognosis than osteosarcoma, from which it may sometimes be difficult to differentiate histologically without an adequate biopsy. It involves the long bones, especially upper tibia and lower femur, and usually affects patients between the ages of 20 and 60 years. Its response to radiotherapy is rather better than that of osteosarcoma and, while treatment is essentially surgical, there is perhaps more justification than with osteosarcoma for considering radiotherapy as the primary treatment, especially for those tumours involving the upper limb.

Giant Cell Tumour

Giant cells feature more or less prominently in the histological appearance of quite a number of bone lesions, even including osteosarcoma. Most of those with which giant cell tumour of bone can be confused are relatively benign, e.g. reparative granuloma of the jaw bones, aneurysmal bone cyst (which seldom occurs in patients over twenty years of age) and the 'brown tumour' bone foci of hyperparathyroidism. When these benign conditions are excluded, giant cell tumour of bone is seen frequently to be an aggressive growth which can sometimes be extremely malignant in biological behaviour.

The separation of these tumours into three grades by Jaffe *et al.* (1940), mainly on the basis of the appearance of the stromal cells, has not been bettered, but it is nevertheless not possible at the present time to predict reliably the clinical behaviour of the tumour from its histological structure alone.

A considerable number of tumours in Grades I and II recur,

especially those treated by curettage and radiotherapy, and a few of these apparently benign lesions later develop lung metastases. The less common Grade III tumours showing sarcomatous-looking stroma are, however, more frankly malignant in behaviour; Campbell and Bonfiglio (1972), for instance, report that of 14 patients with giant cell tumours who died of their disease, 9 had Grade III tumours.

Complete excision of the tumour is the treatment of choice and is possible for tumours involving the fibula and ulna. With bone graft replacement, complete excision of the tumour is also possible – for instance, when the lower end of the radius or upper humerus is involved. At other sites, such as the lower femur and upper tibia, curettage and replacement of the tumour by bone chips is usual and the alternative of resection, bone graft and arthrodesis only resorted to in the event of recurrence. Cases in Grade III are treated by an amputation if possible, otherwise irradiation to tissue tolerance.

Neither the indications for radiotherapy nor the optimal time–dose relationship are clearly established. It is the only treatment practicable for tumours involving the sacrum, spine and skull base and is an alternative method to curettage for those which cannot be excised.

The use of radiotherapy has to be considered in relation to the possible risk of the development of a sarcoma years later in the bone irradiated, and the more debatable risk of the tumour itself becoming malignant as a result of irradiation. The incidence of undoubted post-radiation sarcomas, usually many years after treatment, is variably reported in different series and many of the cases reported up to the present time have been irradiated with orthovoltage (250–300 kV) X-rays, often using several courses of treatment to moderate dosage. Orthovoltage irradiation implies a dose in the bone approximately double that received by the soft tissue, each apparently moderate course giving quite a high dose to the bone itself. It is possible that megavoltage radiotherapy (which delivers only about 10 per cent more radiation energy to bone than to soft tissue) given in a single course of 4000–4500 rad over one month, as originally suggested by Tudway (1959), may prove more effective and less dangerous. Because of this, at present unquantified, risk of producing malignant change the present practice is to reserve radiotherapy primarily for tumours at those sites inaccessible to surgery, such as sacrum and spine.

Marrow Tumours

The remaining primary tumours of bone to be considered are those deriving from bone marrow rather than from bone itself, among which can be included Ewing's sarcoma, primary lymphomata of bone (reticulosarcoma, Hodgkin's disease, lymphosarcoma) and myeloma. Only Ewing's sarcoma and primary reticulosarcoma of bone will be discussed here.

Ewing's Sarcoma

Electron microscopy and tissue culture methods have now firmly established Ewing's sarcoma as a tumour in its own right although the histological differentiation of round-celled tumours of bone remains difficult. The growths from which it must be particularly differentiated are primary reticulosarcoma of bone and metastatic neuroblastoma (myeloma seldom presents problems because of the characteristic appearance of the cells and the associated protein changes in the blood and urine). Intracellular glycogen can be seen in stained sections of most cases of Ewing's sarcoma and although it is present in a few cases of neuroblastoma most of these can be differentiated clinically by the presence of catecholamines in the urine. Formation of the cells into rosettes (by no means always present, however) is characteristic of neuroblastoma, whereas reticulosarcoma shows a prominent reticulin network. Nevertheless, in about 20 per cent of malignant round-celled tumours of bone the attempt to reach a final diagnosis must be made on clinical rather than laboratory evidence (Price, 1972). Neuroblastoma occurs mainly in children under the age of five years, Ewing's sarcoma in older children and young adults with a mean age of 15 years and reticulosarcoma of bone, although occurring at all ages, characteristically affects older people.

Ewing's sarcoma is rare, representing perhaps 5 per cent of all primary bone tumours, and involves especially the pelvic bones, femur and tibia. Although any bone may be affected, the spine appears to be involved seldom. Fever, weight loss and anaemia occur in quite a number of cases. X-rays usually show a considerable soft tissue mass in addition to marked destructive changes in the bone (Fig. 12.2). 'Onion-skin' layering may be seen (Fig. 12.3). Secondary spread to the lungs

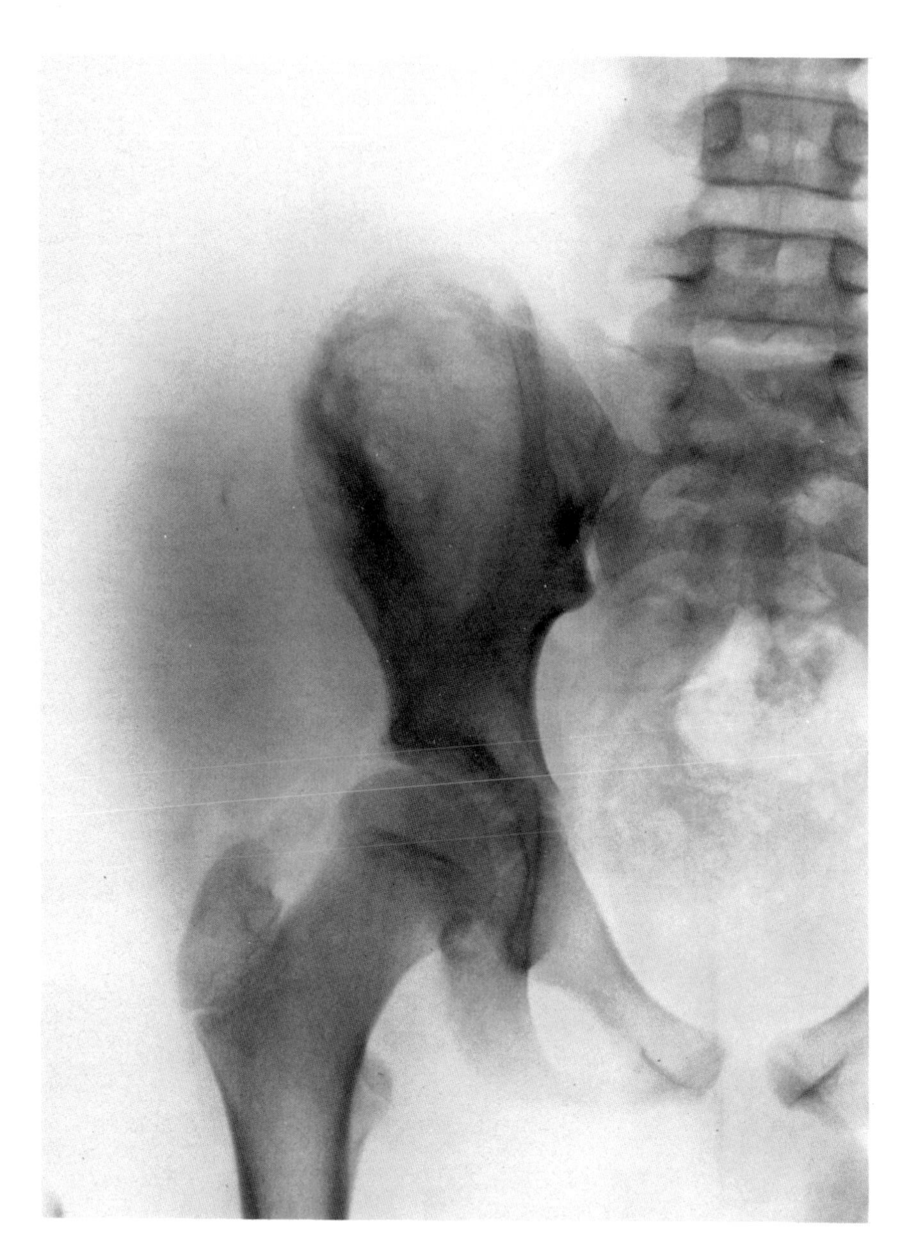

Fig. 12.2. Ewing's sarcoma of the ilium showing large soft tissue mass.

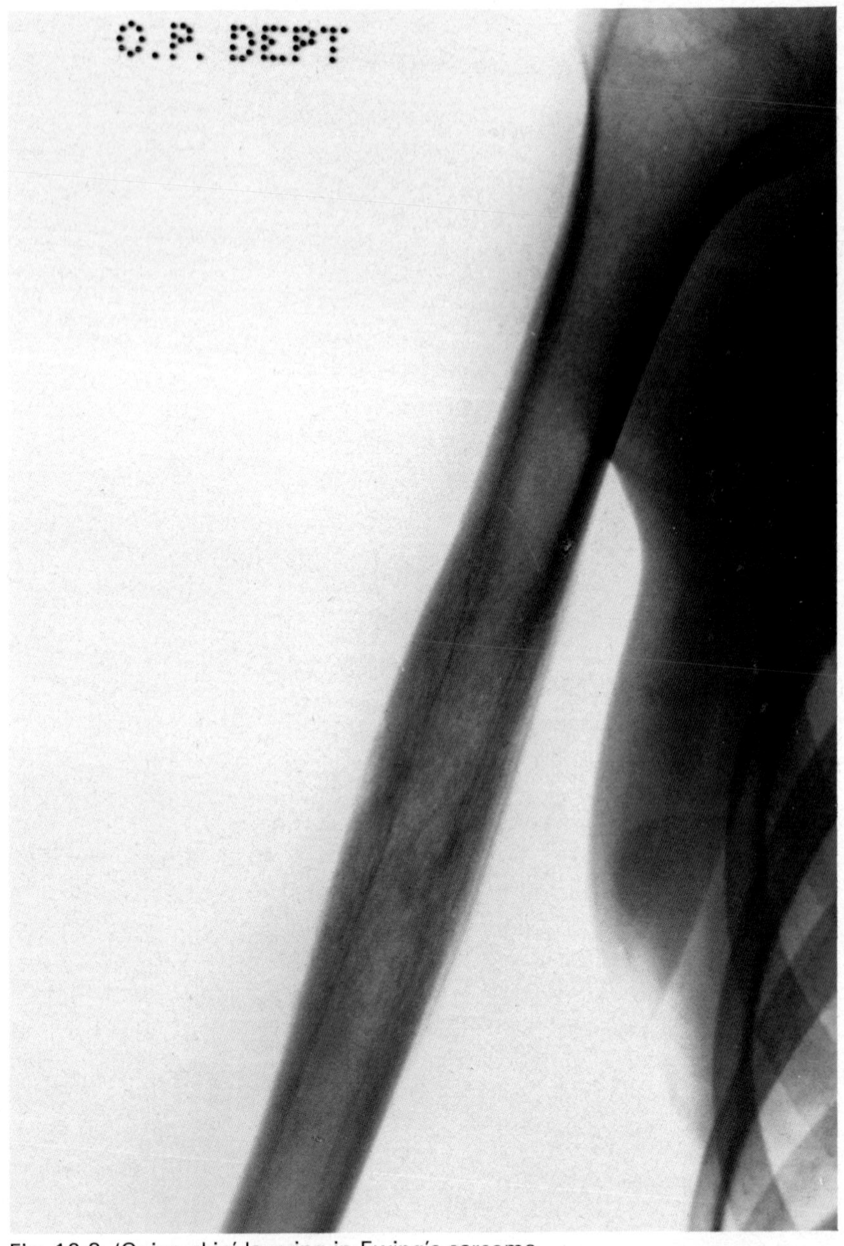

Fig. 12.3. 'Onion-skin' layering in Ewing's sarcoma.

and to other bones occurs very often, but the frequency of spread to the brain is a matter of debate. In the past, most patients have died rapidly of metastatic spread.

Ewing's sarcoma responds rapidly to radiotherapy with relief of symptoms and tumour shrinkage. This has led to the belief that local cure can be achieved easily. Recurrence at the primary site is common in cases given less than 3000 rad in 2–3 weeks. Studies of cell kinetics (Fowler, 1966) show that the probable explanation is that the stem (clonogenic) cells of Ewing's sarcoma which divide to form the main non-dividing cell mass of the tumour are no more responsive to radiation than the stem cells of many tumours considered to be relatively radio-resistant. In Ewing's sarcoma there is an unusually high rate both of cell production and of subsequent spontaneous cell death. A dose of radiation which inhibits mitosis of the stem cells will result in rapid tumour regression due to the continuing death of cells already produced by them. In a tumour with a much slower turnover of non-dividing cells, a similar dose of radiation may well inhibit mitosis of the stem cells to the same extent without producing much change in the tumour size.

The response of the stem cells in both cases is similar, however, and both tumours may need a similar high dose of irradiation to prevent regrowth. Ewing's sarcoma has been found, in fact, to require surprisingly high dosage to prevent local recurrence; the range at present being employed is between 4500 and 6500 rad in four to eight weeks, although Suit *et al.* (1972) report regrowth in three instances following doses in the neighbourhood of 7000 rad in seven weeks. All cases are treated initially by irradiating the whole of the involved bone, the field-size taking into account the estimated soft tissue spread. Treatment confined to the primary, even though locally effective, will result in about 95 per cent of all cases in death from disseminated disease within months of diagnosis, and it must be assumed that in almost all cases metastases too small to detect are widely spread by the time the condition is diagnosed.

Since a report by Hustu *et al.* (1968) that all of five children treated by a full course of radiotherapy to the involved bone, followed by prolonged cyclophosphamide and vincristine therapy, were alive and well 12–38 months after treatment, a much more optimistic attitude has developed. Other drugs which have been shown to have an effect on Ewing's sarcoma include actinomycin D, Adriamycin, BCNU and Mithramycin; other published papers have given support to Hustu's work. No final agreement is yet reached on the best combination of drugs to be used but Hustu *et al.* (1972) have since added actinomycin D to their régime giving, for each square metre of body surface area, cyclophosphamide 300 mg, vincristine 1·5 mg combined with actinomycin D 0·4 mg, by intravenous injection once weekly for six weeks, followed by a rest period of six weeks. This treatment cycle is repeated for two years. Twelve out of a total of 15 patients were alive at the time of reporting, 4–91 months after treatment, and there are now many reports of similar results from other centres. Rosen *et al.* (1974), who use Adriamycin in addition to the three drugs used by Hustu's group in a repeated 90-day cycle, feel that now the life-expectancy of this condition is beginning to look more hopeful, the long-term risks of high-dosage irradiation of young tissues must therefore be seriously taken into account and studies should be aimed at reducing the total dose of radiotherapy required.

Some radiotherapists (Jenkin, 1966; Millburn *et al.*, 1968) have tried the effect of irradiating the primary tumour to radical dosage, followed by whole body irradiation, usually giving a single treatment of the order of 300 rad at one sitting. This has been tried in a relatively small number of cases and also appears to result in longer survival, but the treatment produces quite severe bone marrow depression and small children may require skilled management to avoid lethal complications during this phase. General opinion favours the use of chemotherapy as being more effective and less dangerous even though treatment, at present, has to be prolonged.

There have been reports of surprisingly high incidence of intracranial metastases in patients with Ewing's sarcoma treated by adjuvant chemotherapy (Mehta and Hendrickson, 1974). It is suggested that more effective therapy is allowing longer survival with the development of hitherto unusual metastases, those in the brain being due to the inadequate concentration of cytotoxic agents in the central nervous system. Marsa and Johnson (1971) consider that patients given adjuvant chemotherapy should also receive irradiation of the central nervous system, combined with intrathecal methotrexate, as in the treatment of acute lymphoblastic leukaemia. Rosen *et al.* (1974), however, question the value of cerebral irradiation, and report twelve patients treated using radiotherapy alone to the primary, and energetic adjuvant chemotherapy, as alive and free of disease 10 to 37 months after diagnosis without signs of intracranial disease. The experience of Hustu *et al.* (1972) has been similar. While agreeing that CNS involvement occurs relatively frequently in lymphoma, including primary lymphoma of bone, they have not seen initial metastasis to the central nervous system in Ewing's sarcoma.

There is no doubt that effective adjuvant chemotherapy has led to increased comfort and a lengthening of the disease-free interval before recurrence in this lethal disease of young people. There is now reasonable hope that it will produce long-term remission in many and cure in some.

Primary Malignant Lymphoma (Reticulum Cell Sarcoma) of Bone

Parker and Jackson (1939) first established this condition as a separate entity, distinct from Ewing's sarcoma. Although many of these tumours contain a predominance of reticulum cells the majority contain variable numbers of lymphoblasts and lymphocytes, a few show the Reed-Sternberg cells of Hodgkin's disease and a few are purely lymphoblastic or lymphocytic. A more correct description of this rare group of tumours is therefore 'primary malignant lymphoma of bone' (Dahlin, 1967).

Since it is so much less common than secondary spread to bone of a generalised lymphoma it can be considered as primary in bone only if careful investigation reveals no evidence of disease elsewhere, although regional lymph node involvement is acceptable. As an arbitrary rule, there should be a six-month interval, at least, between the onset of symptoms referable to the primary bone focus and the appearance of any metastases. In contrast with Ewing's sarcoma there is a notable absence of general symptoms even in patients with extensive local disease. Many, but by no means all cases, run a relatively slow clinical course and have a better prognosis than most other malignant bone tumours. Quite a number give a history of symptoms present for six months or more.

There is often a considerable soft tissue mass which is usually a good

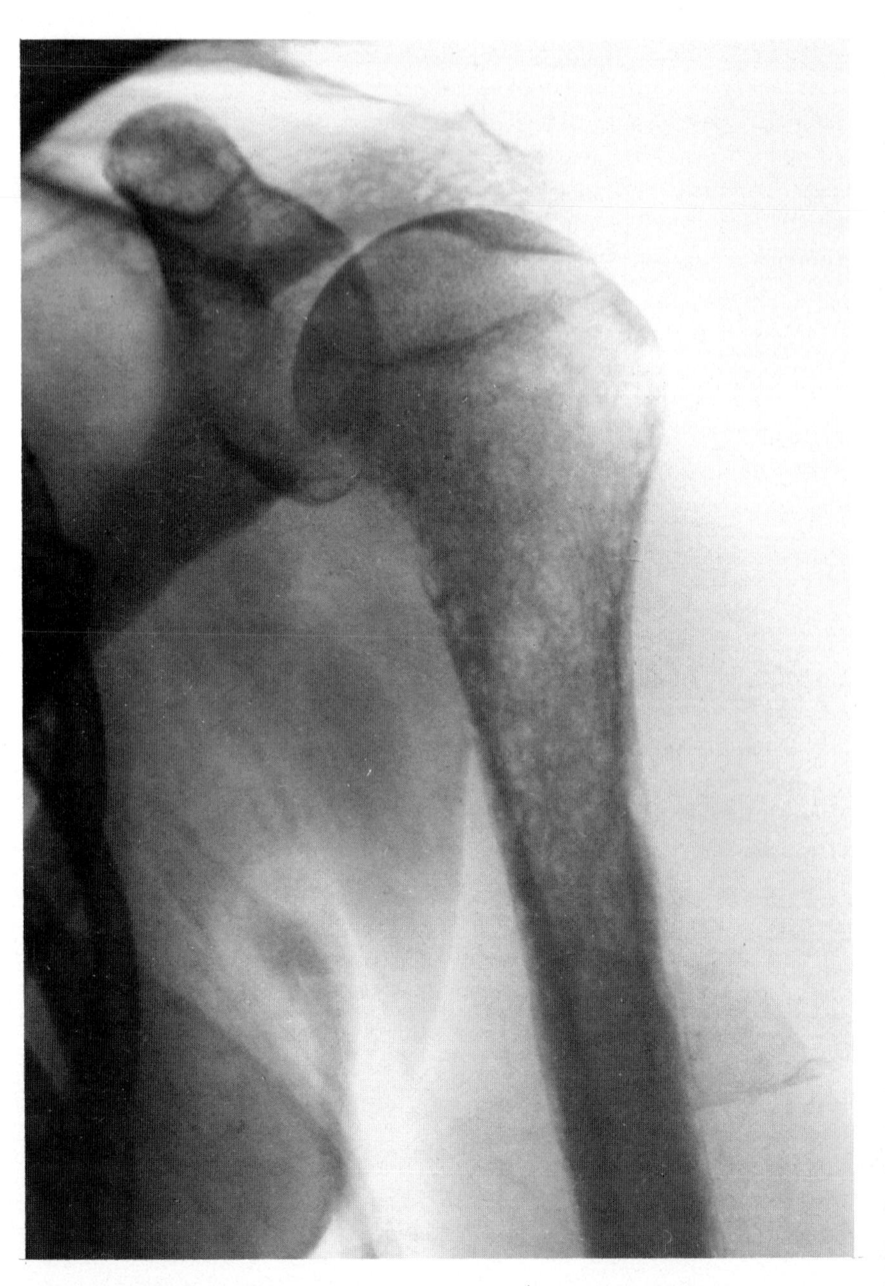

Fig. 12.4. Primary reticulosarcoma of the humerus in a woman aged 47.

deal more extensive than radiographs suggest. X-rays show a predominantly destructive and osteolytic picture (Fig. 12.4) although no characteristic appearance has been described.

Primary lymphoma of bone may occur at any age, most series showing a rather flat graph of age incidence with a peak between 30 and 50 years of age. It involves most frequently the femur, tibia, humerus and pelvic bones with spread, in some cases, to the regional lymph nodes. Deposits may occur in other bones, but involvement of other lymph node areas and viscera does not usually occur until late in the disease.

Initial investigation should include a skeletal survey, sternal marrow examination (especially in the predominantly lymphoid tumours) and, in many, lymphographic studies. It is possible that total body scanning with ^{67}Ga, or bone scanning, may also prove helpful in confirming the lesion to be a primary one.

These tumours are markedly radiosensitive and, as with extra-nodal but unifocal lymphomas at other sites, they are treated by radiotherapy using fields which include the whole of the involved bone and a generous margin to cover soft tissue extension and the regional lymph nodes. Local recurrence has been reported in some cases given less than 3000 rad in two weeks but does not occur in those given 4500–5000 rad in 4–5 weeks.

Of 87 cases reviewed by Dahlin (1967), 44 per cent lived for five years or more without evidence of disease. Shoji and Miller (1971) gave a very similar figure in 47 cases (44·2 per cent).

Chemotherapy is not used at the present time as an adjunct to initial treatment, being reserved for recurrent or disseminated disease. Nevertheless, patients who have developed metastases may sometimes be kept in good health for considerable periods with a combination of chemotherapy and palliative irradiation.

References

ALLEN, C. V. and STEVENS, K. R. (1973) *Cancer*, **31**, 1364–1366.

BRENNOVD, I. O., ROGER, Y. and HOEG, K. (1972) *24th Symposium of the Colston Research Society, Bristol*, ed. Price, C. H. G. and Ross, F. G. M. Butterworth, London, 245–249.

CADE, S. (1955) *Proceedings of the Royal College of Surgeons, Edinburgh*, **1**, 79–111.

CAMPBELL, C. J. and BONFIGLIO, M. (1972) *24th Symposium of the Colston Research Society, Bristol*, ed. Price, C. H. G. and Ross, F. G. M. Butterworth, London, 15–38.

CORTES, E. P., HOLLAND, J. F., WANG, J. J. and SINK, L. F. (1972) *Journal of The American Medical Association*, **221**, 1131–1138.

DAHLIN, D. C. (1967) *Bone Tumours*. Thomas, Springfield, Ill.

ENNEKING, W. F. (1972) *24th Symposium of the Colston Research Society, Bristol*, ed. Price, C. H. G. and Ross, F. G. M. Butterworth, London, 431–437.

FERGUSON, A. B. (1940) *Journal of Bone and Joint Surgery*, **22**, 92–96.

FOSS, O. P., BRENNOVD, I. O., MESSELT, O. T., EFSKIND, J. and LIVERUD, K. (1966) *Surgery*, **59**, 691–695.

FOWLER, J. F. (1966) *Current Topics in Radiation Research*, **2**, 305–360.

HUSTU, H. O., HOLTON, C., JAMES, D. and PINKEL, D. (1968) *Journal of Paediatrics*, **73**, 2, 249–251.

HUSTU, H. O., PINKEL, D. and PRATT, C. B. (1972) *Cancer*, **30**, 1522–1527.

JAFFE, H. L., LICHTENSTEIN, L. and PORTIS, R. B. (1940) *Archives of Pathology*, **30**, 993–998.

JAFFE, N., FARBER, S., TRAGGIS, D., GEISER, C., BYUNG SOO KIM, LAKSHMI DAS, FRAUENBERGER, G., DJERASSI, I. and CASSADY, J. R. (1973) *Cancer*, **31**, 1367–1373.

JENKIN, R. D. T. (1966) *Clinical Radiology*, **17**, 97–106.

JENKIN, R. D. T., ALLT, W. E. C. and FITZPATRICK, P. J. (1972) *Cancer*, **30**, 393–400.

LEE, E. S. and MACKENZIE, D. H. (1964) *British Journal of Surgery*, **51**, 252–274.

LE SERVE, A. W. and HELLMANN, K. (1972) *British Medical Journal*, **i**, 597–601.

LOCKSHIN, M. D. and HIGGINS, I. T. T. (1968) *Clinical Orthopaedics*, **58**, 85–101.

MARCOVE, R. C., SOUTHAM, C. M., LEVIN, A. G., HUVOS, A. G. and MIKÉ, V. (1972) *24th Symposium of the Colston Research Society, Bristol*, ed. Price, C. H. G. and Ross, F. G. M. Butterworth, London, 313–318.

MARSA, G. W. and JOHNSON, R. E. (1971) *Cancer*, **27**, 1051–1054.
MARSH, B., FLYNN, L. and ENNEKING, W. F. (1972) *Journal of Bone and Joint Surgery*, **54A**, 1367–1397.
MCDONALD, I. and BUDD, J. W. (1943) *Surgery, Gynaecology and Obstetrics*, **77**, 413–421.
MCKENNA, R. J., SCHWINN, C. P., SOONG, K. Y. and HIGINBOTHAM, N. L. (1966) *Journal of Bone and Joint Surgery*, **48A**, 1–26.
MEHTA, Y. and HENDRICKSON, F. R. (1974) *Cancer*, **33**, 859–862.
MILLBURN, L. F., O'GRADY, L. and HENDRICKSON, F. R. (1968) *Cancer*, **22**, 919–925.
NEWTON, K. A. (1972) *24th Symposium of the Colston Research Society, Bristol*, ed. Price, C. H. G. and Ross, F. G. M. Butterworth, London, 307–311.
PARKER, F. and JACKSON, H. (1939) *Surgery, Gynaecology and Obstetrics*, **68**, 45–53.
PRICE, C. H. G. (1972) *24th Symposium of the Colston Research Society, Bristol*, ed. Price, C. H. G. and Ross, F. G. M. Butterworth, London, 177–187.
REILLY, C. A., PRITCHARD, D. J., BISKIS, B. O. and FINKEL, M. P. (1972) *Cancer*, **30**, 603–609.
ROSEN, G., WOLLNER, N., TAN, C., WU, S. J., HADJU, S. I., CHAM, W., D'ANGIO, G. J. D. and MURPHY, M. L. (1974) *Cancer*, **33**, 384–393.
SHOJI, H. and MILLER, T. R. (1971) *Cancer*, **28**, 1234–1244.
SUIT, H. D., FERNANDEZ, C., SUTOW, W., SAMUELS, M. and WILBUR, J. (1972) *24th Symposium of the Colston Research Society, Bristol*, ed. Price, C. H. G. and Ross, F. G. M. Butterworth, London, 219–227.
SWEETNAM, D. R. (1972) *24th Symposium of the Colston Research Society, Bristol*, ed. Price, C. H. G. and Ross, F. G. M. Butterworth, London, 297–302.
SWEETNAM, R., KNOWELDEN, J. and SEDDON, H. (1971) *British Medical Journal*, **ii**, 363–367.
TUDWAY, R. C. (1959) *British Journal of Radiology*, **32**, 315–321.
World Health Organisation (1972) *Histological Classification of Bone Tumours*. Geneva.
WOODARD, H. Q. and COLEY, B. L. (1947) *American Journal of Roentgenology*, **57**, 464–471.

CHAPTER THIRTEEN

Computing in Radiotherapy

M. Cohen

The Scope of Computing in Radiotherapy

During the past decade a unique partnership has evolved between radiotherapy and computing. This is not to imply that digital computers are not used extensively in other branches of medicine; but radiotherapy, as a method of treatment, is able to assimilate and benefit from computer assistance more fully than other medical specialties. This ability arises from the very nature of radiotherapy.

Radiotherapy is the treatment of disease, usually malignant disease, by means of ionising radiation. Since radiation is a physical agent, the treatment may be considered to a great extent – but not, of course, entirely – in purely physical terms, and physicists are invariably closely involved in any good radiotherapy practice. When a beam of X-rays or other ionising radiation is directed into the body of a patient, the initial interactions which occur may be described in terms of the laws of radiation physics and, at least to a first approximation, the patient's tissue may be thought of as an inert tank of water. The physical interactions lead to absorption and scattering of the radiation within the body and the formation of complex patterns showing how the radiation dose, i.e. the energy absorbed by each gram of tissue, varies throughout the irradiated volume and in the adjacent tissues. The first task of the computer in radiotherapy is therefore to calculate the detailed distribution of the radiation dose in the individual patient, taking into account the anatomy of the patient and the physical characteristics of the radiation beam or beams.

The physical dose, as just defined, is an important factor, but by no means the only factor, determining the biological and clinical effects of the radiation. The actual energy deposited in the tissues by the radiation is very small (measured, for example, in terms of ability to heat the tissues) but the physical interactions trigger a complex sequence of chemical, biological and clinical events which may extend over many years. The final result, in terms of the permanent destruction of the tumour, the effects on normal tissues and the survival of the patient, cannot at present be predicted with any confidence for any individual patient, although, of course, the results for particular groups of patients subjected to particular treatment régimes are well documented.

The role of the computer in the biological and clinical aspects of radiotherapy is twofold. Firstly, the computer can assist in the testing of radiobiological *models* of the treatment, i.e. mathematical formulae which purport to quantify the killing of cells in terms of the various parameters of the irradiation and of the cells concerned. The number of relevant factors, and their possible combinations, is so large that the arithmetic of even a simple model would be extremely laborious in the absence of a computer. Secondly, the computer can play a major role in *record-keeping and statistical analysis*. In this application the computer plays a role basically similar to its function in any situation, medical or non-medical, in which a large number of factors need to be recorded and analysed. Radiotherapy records are, however, a particularly complex example of medical records because of (*a*) the great diversity of tumour types, stages and sites; (*b*) the very large number of factors which may be relevant to the outcome of any cancer treatment; (*c*) the prevalence of other types of treatment, such as surgery and chemotherapy, given in conjunction with radiotherapy; (*d*) the complex nature of the radiation treatment itself, usually involving many treatment fractions spread over a period of time; and (*e*) the necessity of following up patients for many years after treatment – effectively, for the remainder of their lives. The situation is such that, in the absence of computer assistance, it is virtually impossible to carry out an adequate analysis except on a very limited scale.

In addition to the applications already mentioned, the computer can also play a role in the preparatory work leading to the radiation treatment and in the irradiation itself. The preparatory work includes the use of specialised techniques (e.g. radiography, ultrasonics, radiation transmission and scattering, optical methods) to determine the outline and internal anatomy of the patient, and also the measurement of the fundamental characteristics of the radiation beams which are to be used. All these operations are essentially measurement procedures which may be carried out independently of a computer (as they are in many hospitals) but which can be greatly speeded up or made more reliable under computer control. The actual irradiation of the patient is also a fruitful field for computer intervention. This is a problem of setting the various parameters, such as the beam dimensions and orientation, so that their values correspond exactly to those prescribed, of delivering the correct radiation dose, and of making a permanent record of the relevant values in every treatment session. There is even the possibility – as yet only partially realised in practice – of completely automating the setting-up of the patient, under computer control. However, many people consider this development to be undesirable, even if it were feasible.

Finally, the computer can be of great value in assisting the day-to-day running of a radiotherapy department. Radiotherapy is a protracted sequence of events, starting with the initial diagnosis of the disease, continuing through a series of investigations and preparatory procedures to the formulation of a treatment plan and the calculation of the dose-distribution, and culminating in the course of treatment itself and, finally, in follow-up. The chain is such that every patient needs to make many visits to the radiotherapy department in a defined sequence. The scheduling of patients and the smooth transfer of patients along the 'chain' can present serious problems of organisation in a busy department. The computer can be of great assistance in facilitating the orderly flow of patients and, in countries where treatment has to be paid for individually, in ensuring that each patient receives the correct bill for his treatment. Indeed, some have suggested that the billing of patients has provided the main impetus for the application of computers to radiotherapy!

To summarise, computers may be used in radiotherapy for the computation of 'treatment plans', in the acquisition of radiation data and patient anatomical data, for the control of the treatment machine, in radiobiological modelling, for patient records and analysis, and in patient scheduling in a radiotherapy department. In the remainder of this chapter some of these applications will be described in more detail, with special emphasis on treatment planning. First, however, it is necessary to discuss, very briefly, the digital computer itself.

The Elements of Computing

A digital computer is a device for carrying out a large number of elementary arithmetical or logical operations in a predetermined sequence. These operations are performed very rapidly and very accurately, and they may be repeated any number of times. The 'elementary' operations comprise basic arithmetic operations plus copying and comparison of numbers. More complex operations are derived from a large number of simple operations, while the ability to compare numbers is the basis of decision-making, of the type: if A equals B, or is greater than B, do X; otherwise do Y. A set of instructions which control the sequence in which the computer carries out different operations is called a *program*. If the machine is to 'understand' the instructions directly, the program must be set out in such a way as to correspond to the machine's own method of working, i.e. the program must be written in 'machine language'. This is a very flexible language but is tedious for most people to learn and to use. Many computer programs are therefore written in a 'high level' language such as Fortran, which is more akin to ordinary English, and the computer itself 'translates' the instructions into its own language before carrying them out.

The heart of a computer comprises (Fig. 13.1) a 'memory' or 'store' and a central processing unit. The store can be regarded as a set of labelled 'boxes' or locations, each containing an item of data either permanently or temporarily. The store of a small computer may contain about 4000 locations, while a typical large machine might have

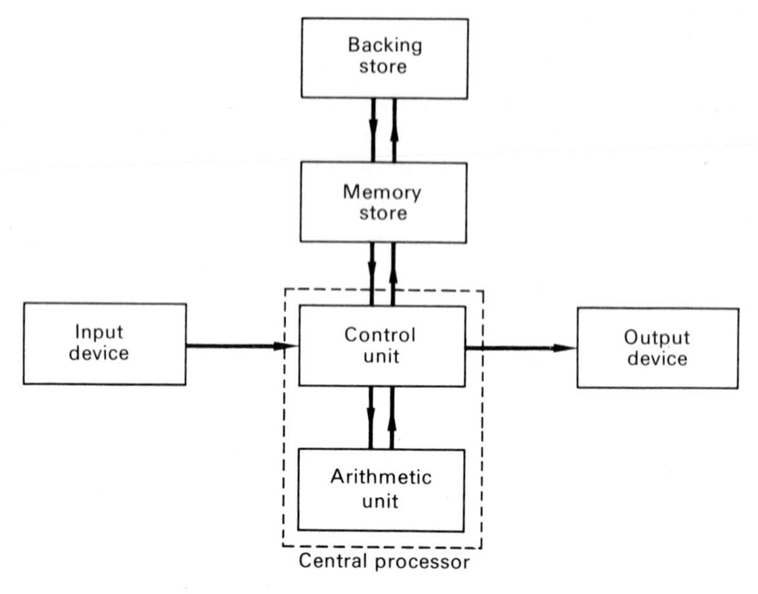

Fig. 13.1. Basic configuration of a digital computer.

256 000 storage locations. The data held permanently in the store comprise the information needed to translate any given program into machine language, while the translated program or programs in current use, and the specific input data relating to these programs, are held temporarily in store. For example, a program to compute $y = 4x^2 + c$ would comprise the set of instructions (coded in binary digits) to perform this calculation, while the input data would comprise the set of values of x and c for which the calculation is to be carried out. Storage space is also needed for data produced at an intermediate stage of a calculation, e.g. $4x^2$ in the above example. Frequently the store of a computer is insufficient and a 'backing store' (magnetic tape or disc) is also used.

The central processor comprises an arithmetic unit, which carries out the actual operations, and a control section which supervises the whole procedure. Although we speak of an 'arithmetic' unit, it must be emphasised that a computer can handle any type of data, including information in 'literary' or graphical form, provided that the data can be coded in binary arithmetic. An 'arithmetic' operation within the processor might, when decoded, have the effect of carrying out real arithmetic on real numbers, but it might equally have the effect of converting an English word into its plural or into its equivalent in French.

The memory store and central processor would be useless without some means of getting data in and out. Accordingly, every computer needs input and output devices and often several input/output stations are connected to a single processor. The input device may comprise a 'teletype' or similar typewriter-style equipment, a punched tape or card reader, a magnetic tape reader or devices which enable information in graphical form to be read-in. Whatever the initial form of the data, the input device converts the information to a series of binary digits since this is the only form the computer can accept. For example, if the input were the outline of a patient (an example of obvious importance in radiotherapy), a special position transducer would transmit the curve in the form of the (x,y) co-ordinates of a series of points lying on the curve.

Output equipment is similarly diverse. The results may be printed out, character by character or line by line, by a printer; plotted graphically on an incremental plotter; or displayed on a cathode-ray tube. Here it is necessary to point out that the program controls not only the nature of the characters displayed or printed (numbers, letters, dots, lines, etc.) but their spatial relationships. Thus the alphanumeric symbols in an output may be arranged in a tabular or any other form, including a form which simulates a two-dimensional pattern; alternatively, the output may be graphical or a combination of graphical and alphanumeric. In general, graphical output devices tend to be more expensive than alphanumeric printers, and must be supported by larger and more complex programs.

Before concluding this brief (and simplified) account of computing, it is necessary to distinguish between the various modes in which computers may be utilised. A computing centre serving many users will have at its disposal various programs, some of a general nature (e.g. for statistical analysis), others 'belonging' to individual users. A user wishing to avail himself of one of these programs (usually one of his own) will submit, via a messenger, appropriate data and other instructions in a suitable form (e.g. on punched cards or tape) and the results will be ready for collection some time, perhaps 24 hours, later. This is the *batch processing* system; it is relatively cheap and has been widely used in radiotherapy for treatment planning, but has obvious disadvantages in terms of convenience, speed and versatility.

An alternative mode is called *time-sharing*; here each user has a terminal (such as a teletype) linked by telephone line to the computer, which may be located even hundreds of miles away. When the subscriber wishes to perform some calculations or other work, he uses his teletype to 'call' the computer to indicate which program he intends to use. The computer responds, after a time-interval ranging from seconds to many minutes, depending on how busy it is, and the subscriber then uses his teletype to type in the particular data he wishes to use in the calculation. The calculation itself then proceeds, and usually occupies the processor only a matter of seconds. Finally the results are transmitted back to the subscriber and are printed out on his teletype. The whole process may occupy a considerable time, but most of this is taken up by the entering of input data and printing of the output. From the user's point of view the system can be improved and speeded up by substituting faster and more versatile input/output (I/O) devices, preferably devices permitting graphical I/O. Furthermore, the computer needs to be a large machine which is free of any priority commitment to a single main task if a reasonable service is to be given to a considerable number of terminals. An example of a large system of this kind, with up to 150 terminals, is the Dartmouth Time-sharing System at Hanover, New Hampshire (Kemeny and Kurtz, 1968), which has been successfully applied to radiotherapy (Sternick, 1971; Sternick *et al.*, 1974). In this system the response is so rapid, with the output appearing virtually immediately on a cathode-ray screen, that the user can effectively 'converse' with the computer. This is called the 'interactive' use of a computer.

Another important interactive computing mode utilises a machine, located in the user's own department, which is dedicated to a single task, or at most to a small number of tasks. The computer may be a relatively small one but is efficiently programmed (usually in 'machine language') to carry out a specialist task such as treatment planning in radiotherapy. An example of such a machine is the RAD-8 shown in

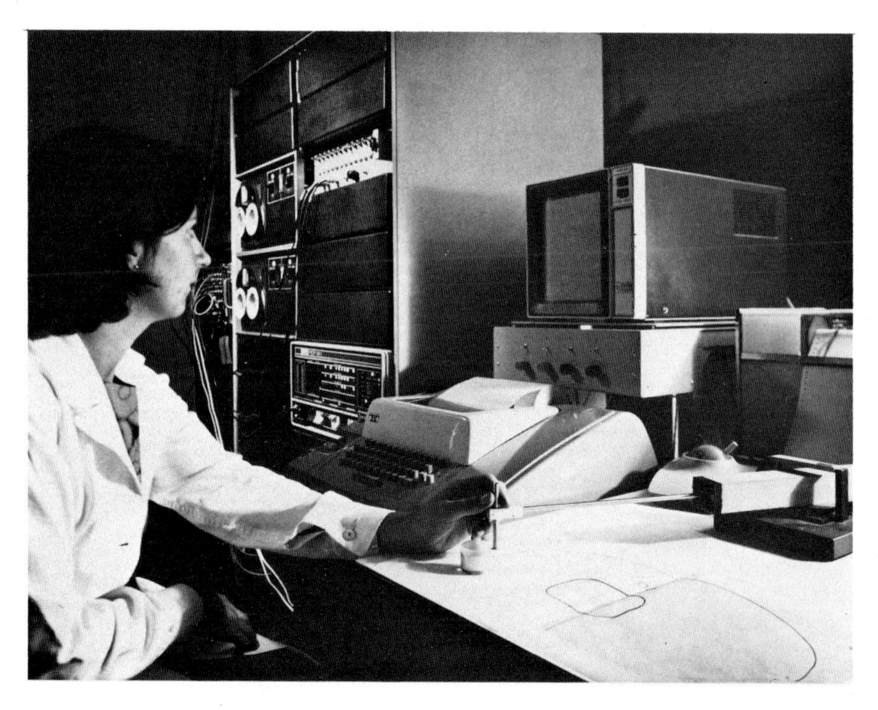

Fig. 13.2. RAD-8 interactive computing system for radiotherapy (courtesy Digital Equipment Corporation).

Fig. 13.2. This is a commerical development of the equipment devised by Bentley and Milan (1971) at the Royal Marsden Hospital in Sutton, Surrey, which was in turn based on the 'Programmed Console' developed at St Louis, Missouri (Holmes, 1970). The input and output of the RAD-8 are graphical and alphanumeric and the system is truly interactive.

The Computation of Dose-Distributions

Most radiation treatments are carried out by means of beams of radiation directed into the body from a source located outside the body and at a considerable distance, i.e. 50–100 cm, from it. This method is called *teletherapy*. A minority, but nevertheless an important sector, of treatments are performed by *brachytherapy*, i.e. small sealed sources of radiation, such as radium, ^{137}Cs or ^{192}Ir, are inserted into a body cavity, implanted in the diseased tissue itself, or placed on or close to the skin. This section will be concerned mainly with teletherapy.

Single-field Isodose Curves

When a beam of ionising radiation is directed into a homogeneous absorbing medium, such as a tank of water, the radiation dose distributes itself as shown in Fig. 13.3. This is a contour map, usually called

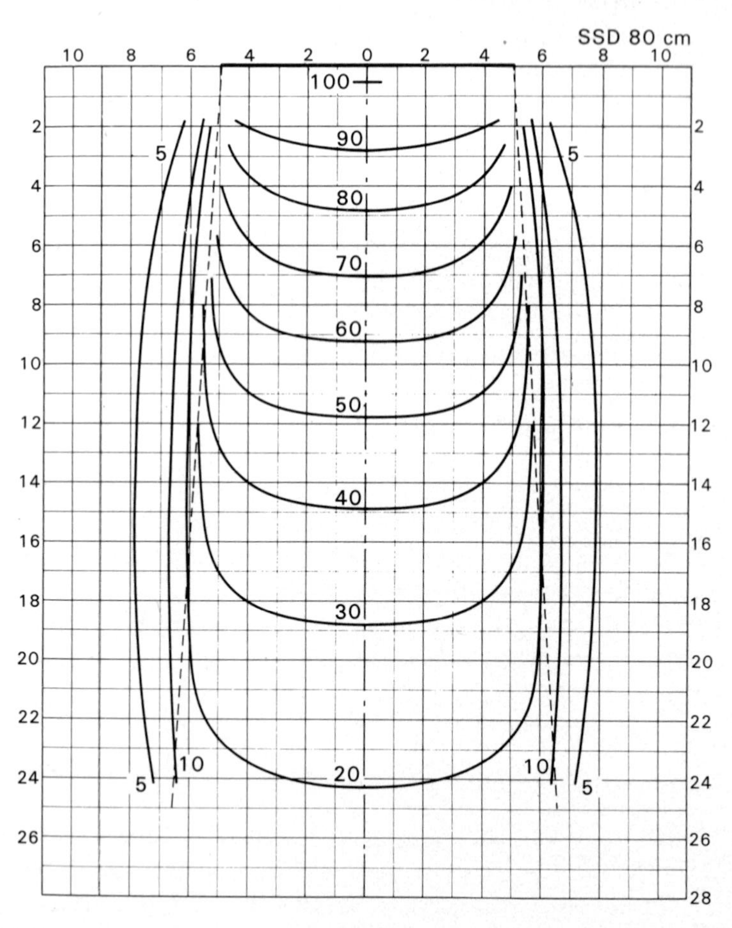

Fig. 13.3. Isodose curves of a single ^{60}Co beam, measured in a water phantom: field-size 10 × 10 cm at 80 cm source–surface distance.

an isodose chart, in which the individual isodose curves represent lines of equal relative dose. The maximum dose in such a chart, i.e. the 100 per cent point, occurs on the beam axis and either on the surface (for X-rays generated up to about 300 kV) or a little below the surface (for high-energy radiation). For example, the γ-rays from a ^{60}Co unit give rise to a maximum at 5 mm below the surface, while for X-rays generated at 8 million volts (8 MV) the corresponding point is located at 2 cm depth. This phenomenon, known as build-up, is very useful in helping to spare the skin from radiation damage, and is one of the advantages of high-energy radiation as compared with medium or low energies. Beyond the maximum point the radiation dose falls off, approximately exponentially.

The positions and shapes of the isodose curves in Fig. 13.3 depend on several factors: (*a*) the type of radiation – the curves for electron beams, for example, are different from those for X-rays shown in the figure; (*b*) the energy of the radiation – the greater the energy the greater the penetrating power of the beam and the deeper any given isodose will lie; (*c*) the field-size, larger beams being effectively more penetrating, an effect due to the increased production of scattered radiation; (*d*) the source-to-surface distance (SSD), a larger SSD giving an effectively more penetrating beam; and (*e*) the relationship between the source and the diaphragm system which defines the beam – this affects mainly the shape of the beam, particularly in the important penumbral region close to the beam edges. Note that the geometrical beam edges do not delineate the radiation completely, since some radiation is scattered outside the beam.

The isodose curves in Fig. 13.3 are symmetrical about the beam axis, but this is not always the case. Often asymmetrical beams are needed, such as that shown in Fig. 13.4, produced by inserting a wedge filter, i.e. a wedge-shaped piece of metal, in the beam. Such beams are needed for shaping the final dose-distribution, obtained by cross-firing two or more beams, in particular ways. Asymmetrical beams are also produced when irregularly shaped beams (as distinct from the usual squares, rectangles or circles) are used, or when shielding blocks are inserted within a beam to stop the radiation reaching some vital normal structure such as the eye.

As already indicated – and this will be discussed further below –

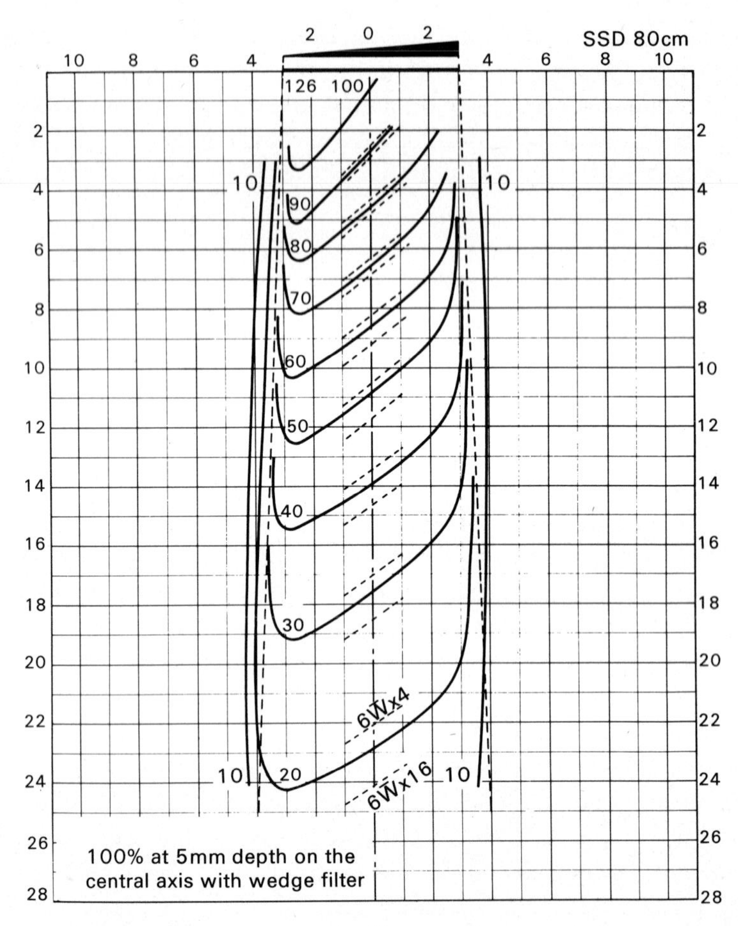

Fig. 13.4. Isodose curves of a single ^{60}Co beam, with lead wedge filter: field dimension 6 cm in the direction of the wedge, 4–16 cm in the perpendicular direction, at 80 cm source–surface distance.

most teletherapy techniques utilise two or more beams entering the patient from different directions and overlapping in the 'target volume'. The end-point of the exercise is therefore the combined dose-distribution from several beams. This can be calculated easily by hand, but it is a slow and tedious procedure; alternatively, beam addition is a comparatively trivial task for a computer – provided, of course, that the data relating to each single beam are available, and this is the difficult problem.

The data relating to single radiation beams must, in the final analysis, be obtained by direct measurement, usually by means of a small ionisation chamber moving in a tank of water ('water phantom'). In earlier computer programs, and to some extent today, the measured single beam data were digitised, i.e. the relative values of dose determined at each point on a defined grid, and the table of values held in the memory of the computer. For calculation purposes the relevant values must be transferred to the processing unit and the values for points other than those on the grid found by interpolation. This tends to be a rather slow process, and the data for many beams occupy a rather large amount of space in the store. Furthermore, it is virtually impossible to have to hand data relating to all the beam shapes, sizes and other parameters that may be needed in practice. For these reasons the calculation of dose-distributions for single beams is now often included as an integral part of a dose-distribution program.

If the radiation beam in an absorbing medium consisted only of primary radiation, i.e. rays proceeding directly from the source, calculation of the dose-distribution would present no problem. Unfortunately, much of the radiation contributing to the dose at any point comprises scattered radiation reaching the point from all directions. Calculation of this scatter has proved extremely difficult, and most of the calculation procedures now available rely to a greater or lesser extent on empirical formulae, i.e. formulae based only partly, or even not at all, on the physical processes involved, but made to 'fit' the experimental data by suitable adjustment of the values of the constants which are included in the formulae. This is not difficult if only a limited range of beam-sizes, depths, types of radiation and designs of radiation machines are concerned, but it has proved almost impossible to find a single formula which can be made to fit all the conditions encountered in modern teletherapy. Fortunately, in any given radiotherapy department, the conditions of practical interest are usually limited.

Among the many computing methods now available for single-beam dose-distribution, those of van de Geijn (1965, 1972a), Cunningham *et al.* (1972), Schoknecht (1965), Sterling *et al.* (1964) and Weinkam *et al.* (1973) are particularly worthy of note, and all are widely used. It should also be mentioned that, long before digital computers appeared on the scene, Meredith and Neary (1944) pioneered the use of empirical formulae for calculating the isodose charts of beams of medium-energy X-rays.

Whether the single-beam data are held in store or are computed mathematically, the basic dose-distribution for 'water phantom' conditions may need to be corrected in two ways. Firstly, the beam may not enter the body perpendicularly, and the surface of the body may not be flat. Secondly, the tissues through which the radiation passes may not be completely 'water-equivalent' and corrections may therefore be needed for any lung or bone tissue in the radiation path. Correction procedures for these factors are commonly incorporated in computer programs. A further procedure, usually not incorporated because of its complexity, takes account of the fact that the plane of interest for calculation purposes may not correspond to a 'principal plane' containing the axis of the beam. In other words, if more than one beam is directed towards a 'target volume', the beams are not necessarily coplanar. Although most teletherapy techniques do, in fact, employ coplanar beams, this may simply reflect the fact that dose-distributions for non-coplanar beams are very difficult to calculate; this problem undoubtedly requires further investigation.

Combination of Isodose Curves

As already indicated, most teletherapy treatments involve two or more radiation beams which cross-fire on the 'target volume', thereby increasing the dose in the tumour related to that received by normal tissues. Ideally the target volume should receive a high and uniform dose while all other tissue receives no dose at all, but this is impossible to achieve in practice. The greater the relative dose at the tumour achieved by single beams, and the more beams there are, the more closely can this ideal be reached. However, a large number of beams creates its own problems of setting-up and avoidance of sensitive structures. By rotating a beam about the tumour we effectively use an infinite number of beams, but here again there are several problems which limit the practical application of this technique.

The technical problem of adding the doses from two or more beams is simple enough. The doses at a number of points, such as the points of intersection of the single-beam isodose curves, are added arithmetically after allowing for any weighting of one beam relative to another. The combined isodose curves are determined by interpolation between the points and, if desired, the whole pattern is renormalised to the maximum dose in the target volume.

Historically, the first application of computers in radiotherapy (Tsien, 1955) was concerned with the addition of beams rather than the calculation of single-beam dose-distributions. Nowadays, however, the final addition of beams is little more than an appendix to a program

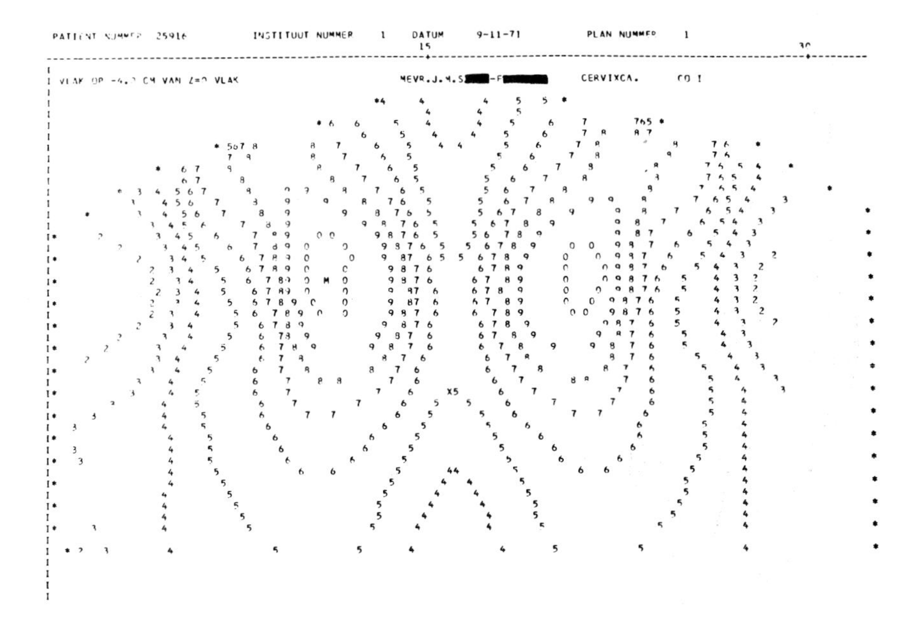

Fig. 13.5. Computer print-out of pattern composed of alphanumeric symbols (van de Geijn (1972b), reproduced by permission of the author and the Editor of *Computer Programs in Biomedicine*).

concerned mainly with single beams and the various corrections that have to be applied to them. However, there are interesting problems related to the presentation of the output. Fig. 13.5 shows a pattern derived from the printing out of a sequence of symbols, while Fig. 13.6 shows isodose curves plotted directly on an incremental plotter. The latter display represents the 'hard copy', plotted full size, of the small-scale display which appears almost instantaneously on the cathode-ray screen of a RAD-8 type of interactive computer.

Optimisation

Figures 13.5 and 13.6 show examples of radiation beams directed towards a tumour in order to deliver a high and uniform dose within the target volume while normal tissue outside this volume receives as

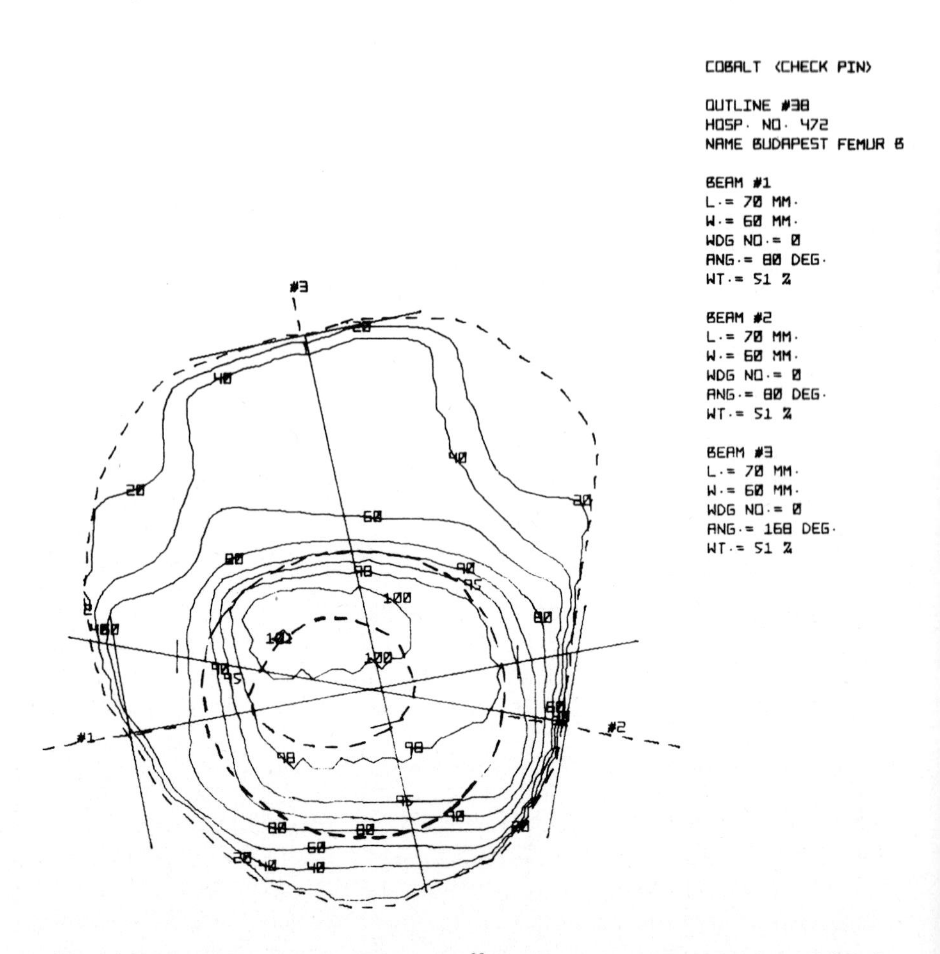

Fig. 13.6. Isodose curves of a 3-beam ^{60}Co treatment, computed by a RAD-8 type of computer and printed out on an incremental plotter.

low a dose as possible. It does not follow, however, that the particular arrangements of beams chosen are the best possible for achieving the prescribed distribution of dose. It may be that a change in beam size, angulation or relative weighting, or perhaps in the number or type of beam, will improve the uniformity of the tumour-dose or decrease the normal-tissue dose. The process of determining the optimum parameters is an important part of treatment planning.

When isodose curves are computed by hand or by a batch-processing computer system with a 24-hour 'turn-around' time, it is usually impracticable to consider more than two or three alternative plans, and frequently the first has to suffice. This is not as bad as it appears, since the planner has both general principles and previous experience to guide his choice of beams and their arrangement. He may also refer to an atlas of dose-distributions (e.g. Cohen and Martin (1966)). Nevertheless, the achievement of a truly optimum arrangement for each patient and each tumour may well require a more rigorous and lengthy iterative procedure, especially when treatment planning is carried out by inexperienced personnel.

Basically there are two approaches to this problem. If a RAD-8 or similar in-house interactive computing system is available, it is possible to alter the beam positions, orientations and other factors by a mere turn of a knob or touch of a key; recalculation of the chart and its display on the screen after such a change occupies a matter of seconds, so that a large number of possibilities can be tried in a short time. Only the solution judged to be the best need be plotted out full size in 'hard copy'.

The process just described involves judgement on the part of the planner, and this implies criteria for judgement, however subjective. If, however, the criteria could be stated objectively, agreed by all concerned, and put in mathematical form, then the process of optimisation could be carried out by the computer itself. This was the approach of Hope and his colleagues (Hope and Orr, 1965; Hope *et al.*, 1967; Orr, 1972) who introduced the concept of 'score functions'. These authors postulated a set of criteria (Fig. 13.7) for an optimum plan, embracing the dose-gradient within, and at the boundary of, the target volume; the relative dose to the target volume; the integral (whole body) dose; the relative shapes of the 'treated' and 'target' volumes; doses to specified sensitive tissues; and doses to regions of possible tumour spread. Each of these criteria was expressed mathematically so that, for any given beam arrangement, the computer could calculate a 'score' ranging from zero for an ideal situation to 1 for a situation which is just acceptable and > 1 for an unacceptable situation. The optimum plan (or plans) is that with the lowest total score. The computer is programmed to score hundreds of possible beam-arrangements but only the few with low total scores are calculated in detail and printed out.

In practice a system of this kind has to be developed over a long period by comparing the results of computer scoring with the judgement of experienced radiotherapists. Both the formulation of the criteria and their relative weighting may need to be changed as a result of such comparison.

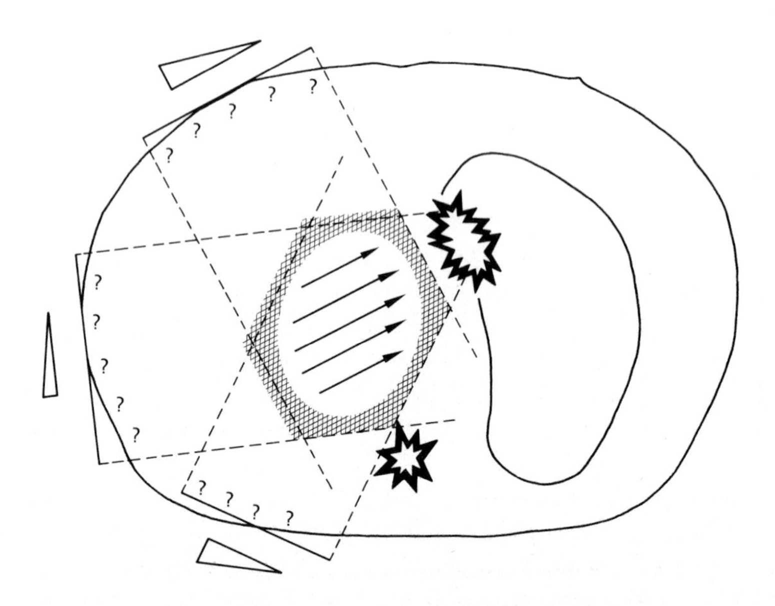

Fig. 13.7. Criteria for optimisation of treatment plans. The criteria illustrated are deviation from uniformity of tumour dose, relative shapes of 'target' and 'treated' volumes, doses to normal tissue and to sensitive organs (Orr (1972), reproduced by permission of the author and the Editor of *Computer Programs in Biomedicine*).

The work of Hope and his colleagues has led to several major attempts at computer optimisation, including the use of sophisticated mathematical techniques such as 'linear programming'. However, none of these methods has so far gained widespread acceptance and, for the time being at least, visual optimisation using an interactive computer system appears to offer the best practical solution. Finally, it must be emphasised that the optimisation discussed in this section refers only to the distribution of the dose *in space*; a further optimisation procedure, as yet much less developed, needs to be applied to the dose distribution *in time*.

Treatment Records in Radiotherapy

The number of factors which are known to influence, or may possibly influence, the results of a course of radiotherapy is very large indeed. When a vast amount of data has to be gathered, stored, tabulated, retrieved and analysed, computer assistance is virtually obligatory: otherwise the job can be done only at the cost of enormous expenditure of human labour, entailing not only time and effort but also an error-rate far in excess of that associated with a good computing system. (Computing 'errors' are, in fact, nearly always human errors in disguise.)

In view of the above, it is perhaps surprising that computing systems for radiotherapy records are not yet in widespread use. Several successful systems are, in fact, in operation (McAinsh *et al.*, 1972; Dutreix *et al.*, 1972; Snelling and Kunkler, 1970) but the number is not large in relation to the overall need. There are, indeed, several major problems in this field and it is noteworthy that, at any conference on computers in radiotherapy, the session on records is always controversial.

The first question is: how much data should be recorded? One possible answer is: everything. If a factor is not recorded, there is clearly no possibility of ever discovering a correlation between that factor and some aspect of radiotherapy. However, the more data we try to record, the greater the likelihood that physicians and others responsible for gathering the information will find the task so onerous that they will lose interest altogether. Furthermore, the larger the volume of data, the bigger the computer needed and the more complex the program.

These diffficulties point to some form of selection in the recording of information. Selection, however, implies that we know in advance the questions we will later want to ask! It also implies some major decision of the type: should radiotherapy records be limited to factors known (or thought) to be relevant to radiotherapy, or should the records be broadened so as to embrace problems of cancer epidemiology?

Many workers have addressed themselves to the above problem, and have reached conflicting conclusions (see, for example, the sections on this subject in the conference proceedings listed at the end of this chapter). The best consensus of opinion was that obtained by a Working Party set up in 1967 jointly by the British Institute of Radiology and the Faculty of Radiologists. This group produced a Minimal List of Variates which has been criticised, and ultimately accepted, by a large number of radiotherapists in the UK (see Snelling and Kunkler, 1970). The list contains over 120 variates under three major headings: personal and diagnostic data, treatment (further subdivided by mode) and follow-up. For any given patient only about 50 variates are needed because many of the treatment modes are alternatives, although frequently more than one mode may be used. On the other hand, many variates (such as anatomy site, stage, field combination) permit of a large number of possibilities, all of which have to be allowed for in any practical application of the system. Thus even a 'minimal list' quickly leads to a fairly complex overall system.

The next questions are: how shall the data be recorded, and by whom? One possibility is for the radiotherapist himself, or a trained assistant, to go through the patient's notes transferring the data, via a coding system, to punched tape or cards or other computer-compatible input forms. This method is laborious and error-prone; moreover there is a high probability that any given patient's notes will lack some items of data in the list. For this reason most workers have concentrated their efforts on the design of a pro-forma which the medical officer fills up as he examines the patient or receives the information for the first time. Such a sheet has to satisfy several criteria: for example, it should act as a check-list and be capable of rapid and easy completion, with a minimum of coding and no possibility at all of confusion or ambiguity.

The transfer of the data from the pro-forma to punched tape for computer processing may readily be carried out by punching clerks,

					2	1	2	1	2	1	2	1	2	1	2	1
Sex *M* Colour *BROWN*	MALE M	FEMALE F									WHITE	NEGRO	BROWN (COLOUR)	YELLOW	LAT. AM.	NOT KNOWN
Date of birth *12 AUG '07*	16	8	DAY 4	2	1	8	MONTH 4	2	1	64	32	YEAR 16	8	4	2	1
Duration of symptoms *13 MONTHS*	<1		DAYS 4	2	1	8	MONTHS 4	2	1	64	32	YEARS 16	8	4	2	1
Diagnosis *LEFT PARIETAL GLIOMA* System *C.N.S.*	SKIN	C.N.S.	ALIMENT'Y	RESP'Y	CARDIO VASC.	RETIC ENDOT	LOCOR	ENDOCR.	GENITAL	URINARY	SPEC SENSES	NOT KNOWN				
Site *HEAD* Position *LEFT*	HEAD	NECK	ARM	THORAX (SITE)	ABDO.	LEG	GENERAL		LEFT	RIGHT	CENTRAL	L&R (POSITION)	NOT KNOWN	NOT APPLIC.		
Detail Level A	A1	2	3	4	5	6	7	8	9	10	11	12	13	14	15	16
Level B	B1	2	3	4	5	6	7	8	9	10	11	12	13	14	15	16
Level C	C1	2	3	4	5	6	7	8	9	10	11	12	13	14	15	16
	8	DIGIT 1 4	2	1	8	DIGIT 2 4	2	1	8	DIGIT 3 4	2	1	8	DIGIT 4 4	2	1
Lymph node involvement *NONE*	CLINICAL (BEFORE RADIATION)		DISSECTION		BIOPSY		NOT KNOWN	NONE	CLINICAL (AFTER RADIATION)		DISSECTION		BIOPSY		MARROW CHANGES	NOT KNOWN
Size of lesion *5 cm*	<1	1<2	2<3	3<4	4<5	5<6	6<7	7<8	8<9	9<10	10<11	11<12	12<13	13<15	15+	NOT KNOWN
Histogenetic type *GLIOMA*	EPITH	SOFT TISSUE	BONE/CART	MUSCLE	NERVE	SEROUS MEMB.	MENINGES	VESSELS	LYMPH	MARROW	GLAND	MIXED	NOT KNOWN			

Fig. 13.8. Example of layout of form used for recording of radiotherapy data, suitable for direct reading by a lector (Ellis and Paine (1970), reproduced by courtesy of English Electric Computers).

since every item of information on the original sheet is in a separate, numbered box. Nevertheless this process, besides being laborious, is by no means error-free. The alternative method is therefore to fill up the pro-forma in ink in such a way that the marks can be read by a machine (lector) which automatically codes the data. Such a form is shown in Fig. 13.8 (Ellis and Paine, 1970), in which (for example) the date of birth of the patient is shown by marking squares 8 and 4 under 'day', 8 under 'month' and 4, 2 and 1 under 'year'. Provision is also made for erasing marks.

An important objective of computerised patient records in radiotherapy is to enable the results of treatment in small centres to be aggregated so that methods of treatment for less common cancers can be assessed. However, it should be stated that proposals of this kind, laudable as they are in principle, presuppose a reasonable measure of agreement on the interpretation (not merely the definition) of staging, histology and many other components of diagnosis and treatment, including even some physical concepts such as 'tumour-dose'. This, however, takes us well outside the scope of the present chapter.

Automation in Radiotherapy

At the present time most manufacturers of radiotherapy equipment are attempting to 'automate' their machines. This term has a range of meanings, from the simple printing-out of the treatment parameters (beam sizes, angles, etc.) after the irradiation, to the setting-up of the patient and the machine entirely under computer control. Most systems currently under development in fact aim at an intermediate solution, often called an 'open loop' system because the radiographer plays a vital role in 'closing the loop' before the irradiation can begin. An example is shown in Fig. 13.9 (von Arx and Kuphal, 1970); the machine and the couch are positioned automatically, the machine parameters are set under punched card control, and their values recorded, but the final positioning of the patient is left to the radiographer.

The impetus for automation in this field came from the United States, where trained radiographers are scarce. Even the possibility of automatic patient set-up, using marks on the skin and optical sensing

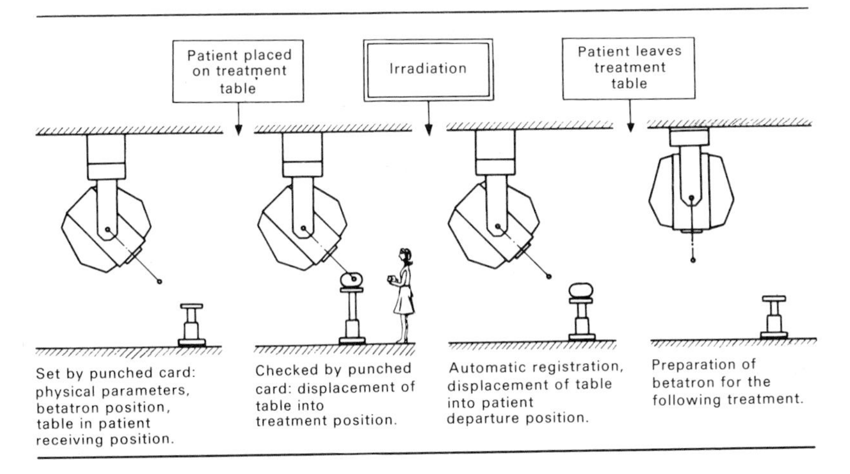

Fig. 13.9. Automation of machine set-up under computer control (von Arx and Kuphal (1970), reproduced by courtesy of the authors and S. Karger, Publishers, Basel).

devices, has been explored. The same system could be used for compensating for any patient movement during the irradiation. In Europe, however, the emphasis has been on automating only those parts of the setting-up procedure that are tedious, repetitive and liable to error, leaving the radiographer free to devote her skills to positioning, reassuring and generally 'nursing' the patient. This seems to be a good compromise, since a faster and more accurate setting of the machine, and hence greater throughput of patients, can nevertheless allow the radiographer more time to devote to the individual needs of each patient.

Conclusion

In this chapter we have sketched out some of the ways in which computing is helping to improve the practice of radiotherapy. It is often asked whether these changes are likely to be matched by an improvement in the patient survival rates. If by this is meant a sudden, dramatic jump in the survivals over a given period, the answer is no. If, however, we mean a slow but steady upward trend in the survival figures for some types of cancer (not necessarily for all), accompanied by an improvement in the quality of survival, then there is cause for optimism. We shall probably never be able to demonstrate conclusively that an upward trend in survival rates is specifically due to the use of computers, since many other improvements – in diagnosis and tumour localisation, for example – are taking place concurrently. Since, however, the computer has become closely involved in all of these aspects of radiotherapy, it is sufficient to conclude that the honorable role of the computer in this field is already beyond challenge.

References

BENTLEY, R. E. and MILAN, J. (1971) *British Journal of Radiology*, **44**, 826–833.

COHEN, M. and MARTIN, S. J. (1966) *Atlas of Radiation Dose Distributions Vol II. Multiple-field Isodose Charts.* International Atomic Energy Agency, Vienna.

CUNNINGHAM, J. R., SHRIVASTAVA, P. N. and WILKINSON, J. M. (1972) *Computer Programs in Biomedicine*, **2**, 192–199.

DUTREIX, J., DUTREIX, A. and ZUMMER, K. (1972) *Computer Programs in Biomedicine*, **2**, 232–241.

ELLIS, F. and PAINE, C. H. (1970) in *Computers in Radiology*, ed. de Haene, R. and Wambersie, A. Karger, Basel, 233–236.

HOLMES, W. F. (1970) *Radiology*, **94**, 391–400.

HOPE, C. S., LAURIE, M. J. E., ORR, J. S. and HALNAN, K. E. (1967) *Physics in Medicine and Biology*,**12**, 531–542.

HOPE, C. S. and ORR, J. S. (1965) *Physics in Medicine and Biology*, **10**, 365–373.

KEMENY, J. G. and KURTZ, T. E. (1968) *Science*, **162**, 223–228.

MCAINSH, T. F., ORR, J. S., HALNAN, K. E. and STEVENSON, J. (1972) *Bio-Medical Computing*, **2**, 137–145.

MEREDITH, W. J. and NEARY, G. J. (1944) *British Journal of Radiology*, **17**, 75–82 and 126–130.

ORR, J. S. (1972) *Computer Programs in Biomedicine*, **2**, 216–220.

SCHOKNECHT, G. (1965) *Strahlentherapie*, **127**, 217–228.

SNELLING, M. D. and KUNKLER, P. B. (1970) in *Computers in Radiology*, ed. de Haene, R. and Wambersie, A. Karger, Basel, 221–227.

STERLING, T. D., PERRY, H. and KATZ, L. (1964) *British Journal of Radiology*, **37**, 544–550.

STERNICK, E. S. (1971) in 'Computers in Radiotherapy'. Special Report No. 5, *British Journal of Radiology*, 20–22.

STERNICK, E. S., HUGHES, M., HOGAN, R. and GOODHUE, L. R. (1974) *Radiology*, **110**, 467–472.

TSIEN, K. C. (1955) *British Journal of Radiology*, **28**, 432–439.

VAN DE GEIJN, J. (1965) *British Journal of Radiology*, **38**, 369–377.

VAN DE GEIJN, J. (1972a) *Computer Programs in Biomedicine*, **2**, 169–177.

VAN DE GEIJN, J. (1972b) *Computer Programs in Biomedicine*, **2**, 153–168.

VON ARX, A. and KUPHAL, K. (1970) in *Computers in Radiology*, ed. de Haene, R. and Wambersie, A. Karger, Basel, 183–189.

WEINKAM, J. J., KOLDE, R. A. and STERLING, T. D. (1973) *British Journal of Radiology*, **46**, 983–990.

Further Reading

COHEN, M. (1970) 'Computers in Radiotherapy'. Special Report No. 4, *British Journal of Radiology*, **43**, 658–663.

Computer Programs in Biomedicine (1972) Special issue devoted to computers in radiotherapy, **2**, 125–241.

CUNNINGHAM, J. R. (1971) 'The Stampede to Compute – Computers in Radiotherapy', 1971 Gordon Richards Memorial Lecture. *Journal of the Canadian Association of Radiologists*, **22**, 242–251.

DE HAENE, R. and WAMBERSIE, A. (eds) (1970) *Computers in Radiology*, proceedings of international conference, Brussels, 1969. Karger, Basel.

DEELEY, T. J. (1972) *Computers in Radiotherapy – Clinical Aspects*. Butterworth, London.

GLICKSMAN, A. S., COHEN, M. and CUNNINGHAM, J. R. (eds) (1971) 'Computers in Radiotherapy', proceedings of international conference, Glasgow, 1970. Special Report No. 5, *British Journal of Radiology*.

GLICKSMAN, A. S., CEDERLUND, J., COHEN, M., CUNNINGHAM, J. R.,

JUNG, B., OLSEN, B. and ORR, J. S. (eds) (1973) *Computers in Radiation Therapy*, proceedings of international conference, Uppsala, 1972. Akademiska Sjukhuset, Uppsala.

WOOD, R. G. (1974) *Computers in Radiotherapy – Physical Aspects*. Butterworth, London.

INDEX